Data Analytics for Traditional Chinese Medicine Research

Josiah Poon • Simon K. Poon
Editors

Data Analytics for Traditional Chinese Medicine Research

Foreword by Kelvin Chan

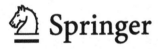

Springer

Editors
Josiah Poon
University of Sydney
Sydney, NSW, Australia

Simon K. Poon
University of Sydney
Sydney, NSW, Australia

ISBN 978-3-319-34629-8   ISBN 978-3-319-03801-8 (eBook)
DOI 10.1007/978-3-319-03801-8
Springer Cham Heidelberg New York Dordrecht London

Printed on acid-free paper

Springer is part of Springer Science+Business Media (www.springer.com)

Foreword

Facing the advances of recent science and technology developed in modern medical practice, experts of traditional Chinese medicine (TCM) have made efforts to published peer-reviewed papers to produce an enormous amount of information on the research and practice of TCM as progress towards modernization of TCM since the 1950s. These include: efficacy, safety and quality of Chinese medicines and the practice of TCM at large. To coordinate this updating information in an integrative approach is crucial to connect the multiplicity of expertise and scientific innovation and investigations that link practice of TCM to maintain good health and treatment of diseases. Several key areas can be identified in the recent 11th Annual Meeting of the Consortium for Globalization of Chinese medicine held in August 2012 in Macau Special Administrative Region, China. At this meeting a Bioinformatics Pre-meeting Workshop on *"Data Analytic Approach to Evidence-based Research for Traditional Chinese Medicine"* was organised to focus on issues mentioned above. The organiser of this Workshop was requested to collect these valuable research results and reviews for compilation of a reference book. In this way, those who were absent at the meeting, and general readers who are interested in TCM progress will benefit from the guidance and directions for future translational medicine from TCM research and practice.

Although TCM is getting popular, more evidence is required to enable it to gain official recognition in Western countries; it demands a rigorous evaluation for the effectiveness of TCM interventions. Randomized Controlled Trial (RCT) is regarded as the "gold standard" in clinical research for the efficacy and safety evaluation of a medical intervention, but its application to TCM is doubtful owing to several methodological and logistical issues. Poon and his colleagues in chapter" Searching for Evidence in Traditional Chinese Medicine Research: A Review and New Opportunities" aimed to introduce and discuss issues relating to establishing scientific evidence for TCM. It was suggested that either RCT study design is augmented to adapt to TCM principles or new methodologies such as Comparative Effectiveness Research (CER) are utilized.

Chinese Medicine Formulae are sets of herbs to address the syndromes and symptoms complained by patients. Although there are some standard formulas, practitioners often modify them according to a patient's individual condition. In chapter "Causal Complexities of TCM Prescriptions: Understanding the Underlying Mechanisms of Herbal Formulation," Poon and his team introduced a framework to explore the complex relationships amongst herbs in TCM clinical prescriptions. They applied their framework in the analysis of a large number of TCM herbal prescriptions, and it was able to show some herbs may have different pathways to affect the effectiveness; such herbs have often been overlooked in the past. Although they play a weak role in enhancing the overall effectiveness of the TCM treatment, they are however non-trivial.

To cope with challenges in data analysis on the 4 classical TCM patterns of diagnosis of syndromes and conventional symptoms of patient records collected in clinics, You and Li in chapter "Medical Diagnosis by Using Machine Learning Techniques" describe novel methods on feature selection, multi-class, and multi-label techniques in machine learning to meet the challenges. They introduce their works on discriminative symptoms selection and multi-syndrome learning, which have improved the performance of state-of-arts works.

In chapter "Network Based Deciphering of the Mechanism of TCM," the team of Yi Sun indicates that the rapid development of "-omics" platforms and systems biology has facilitated systems-level understanding of biological processes concerning the interactions of genes, proteins and environmental factors, thus affording new possibilities for uncovering the molecular mechanisms related to the therapeutic efficacy of TCM from a systematic point of view. Through integrating various high-throughput data, *in silico* models could help accelerating network-based multi-target drug discovery, especially for optimizing molecular synergy of TCM herbal formulas.

In chapter "Prescription Analysis and Mining", to unblock the massive accumulated literature in TCM prescription, Zheng and co-workers use Liuwei-Dihuang formula to show the value of network analysis by executing discrete derivative algorithm in the text mining process, prescription associated networks are mined out. These networks include prescription-pattern-disease, prescription-disease-Chinese herbal medicine, prescription-pattern-Chinese herbal medicine, prescription-Chinese herbal medicine-symptom, and prescription-pattern-symptom. They claim that such approach provides useful reference for future TCM research and clinical practices.

Applying an innovative approach of 'Latent tree analysis' methodology by Zhao and colleagues studied syndrome factors such as 'Yang Deficiency' and 'Yin Deficiency' from published data recording symptoms of 604 depressive patients in several regions of China. The authors report in chapter "Statistical Validation of TCM Syndrome Postulates in the Context of Depressive Patients" that the 'Latent tree analysis' yielded a model with 29 latent variables corresponding well to TCM syndrome factors. This type of analysis can demonstrate statistical evidence for the validity of TCM postulates in depressive patients.

Lin and Wong propose in chapter "Artificial Neural Network Based Chinese Medicine Diagnosis in Decision Support Manner and Herbal Ingredient Discoveries" describe an artificial neural network (ANN) package for fast and trusted herbal ingredient discoveries. They indicate the ANN results are trustworthy as they have been and can be ascertained in future input by TCM domain experts in real clinical environments in Hong Kong Nanning and New York. The ANN is able to learn the relationship between Chinese materia medica (CMM) ingredients and sets of information generated from TCM diagnosis and treatment principles.

In chapter "Chromatographic Fingerprinting and Chemometric Techniques for Quality Control of Herb Medicines": Zhang and co-workers recommend that the use of chromatographic fingerprint analysis of CMM can describe the maintenance of the consistent quality of samples for biological and pharmacological research. But the application as Quality Control (QC) measures for acceptable fingerprints require carefully mined fingerprint after highly scrutinised procures from smoothing, base-line correction, peak alignment and peak detection; followed by similarity analysis, exploratory data analysis, cluster analysis and classification to extract the representative pattern sample from the large dataset.

Chau and colleagues describe the approach of quantitative pattern-activity relationship (QPAR) for herbal medicines (HM) to link activity fingerprints, the chemical composition of HMs can be standardized to higher and accurate levels within the safety limits in chapter "A New Methodology for Uncovering the Bioactive Fractions in Herbal Medicine Using the Approach of Quantitative Pattern-Activity Relationship." They claim that the composition of compounds in HM formulation with more than one herbal component can be optimized to the desired level of bioactivity. They speculate personalized HM can be prepared according to the required bioactivity level to meet the needs of individual patients.

In chapter "An Innovative and Comprehensive Approach in Studying the Complex Synergistic Interactions Among Herbs in Chinese Herbal Formulae," Chau and her co-workers describe the use of an innovative and comprehensive approach using Combination Index with statistic testing to analyse multi-targeted *in vitro* data after screening an herbal formulae containing 5 CMM. They claimed that their study is one of the first applications of statistical interpretations of combination effects of herbs in complex herbal formulae. They concluded the feasibility of applying this methodology in combinatory study of herbs is a promising and low-cost means of novel drug discovery.

Zhou and colleagues introduce the application of data warehouse techniques and data mining approaches to utilise real-world TCM clinical data, which are mainly electronic medical records. In chapter "Data Mining in Real-World Traditional Chinese Medicine Clinical Data Warehouse," the main framework of clinical data mining applications in TCM field is also introduced. The sticking points and/or issues to improve the research quality are discussed and future directions are proposed. They emphases that there still needs a reliable and efficient pre-processing step to filter the useful data set from a large scale clinical data source, clean and integrate the data to provide high-quality data for further analysis.

Chan and co-workers of biomedicine, information technology and TCM practitioners express their view on evidence-based and medical informatics in TCM practice and research in chapter "An Overview on Evidence-Based Medicine and

Medical Informatics in Traditional Chinese Medicine Practice." They conclude that there is a need in using modified modalities that can focus on a holistic assessment of TCM diagnosis and treatment outcomes of individual patients. Their reported outcomes are linked with biomedical parameters for evidence of treatment efficacy. Using TCM formulae in treating female infertility they suggested that continuing feedback between practitioners in each field will help refine TCM informatics in general.

In chapter "TCM Data Mining and Quality Evaluation with SAPHRON™ System": Yang and colleagues describe the development of a proprietary SAPHON TCM data system to quantitatively evaluate the quality of TCM information, which ranks TCM prescriptions, CMM, active ingredients and lead compounds based on the reliability of available information for recommendation.

This book consists of 13 chapters arranged in no special order due to the multiplicity of experts' presentations from various disciplines. It is anticipated that more research in the Informatics for TCM will emerge in the near future as a reference point for quality data that may guide future TCM research and development. The way forward to identify evidence in TCM. Multidisciplinary collaborations among different professionals of both conventional medical and TCM practices with expertise from biomedical, bioinformatics, pharmaceutical and TCM disciplines. These approaches are particularly important for the scientific evaluation of effectiveness, safety and quality of ethnic traditional medicine. The progress in globalisation and modernisation of TCM will form the guiding example for R&D of other ethnic traditional medicine supported by the World Health Organisation.

The book serves as a gathering of the latest information from IT aspects on TCM; it also offers directions and guidance of the logical way to decipher the mystery of TCM: How an experience-based medical practice receives such an enormous attraction from the conventional scientific and medical arenas.

NSW, Australia   Kelvin Chan

Contents

About the Editors

Dr. Josiah Poon obtained his Ph.D. from the University of Sydney in 1997. He is currently a senior lecturer in the School of Information Technologies in the same university and has been a lecturer in School of Information Technology and Electrical Engineering in the University of Queensland. He held two patents in the area of adaptive multimedia display, when he worked in the Canon Information System Research Australia between 1997 and 1998. His previous projects were in the area of text mining, imbalanced data learning and evolutionary algorithms. He has published more than 60 articles in journals, conferences and book chapters.

Dr. Simon K. Poon is currently a senior lecturer and a postgraduate coursework director of the School of Information Technologies, and a postgraduate coursework coordinator for the Institute of Biomedical Engineering and Technology at the University of Sydney. He is an information systems researcher with interests in complex data analytics. He received his B.Sc. in Computer Science and Ph.D. in Information Systems from the University of Sydney. He holds a Graduate Certificate in Mathematical Sciences and a Master in Engineering Management from the University of Technology, Sydney. In 2009, he completed his Master in Public Health from the School of Public Health at the University of Sydney. He also underwent Commercial Pilot License training from British Aerospace Flying College in Scotland between 1992 and 1994. One of his current research interests is applying quantitative research methods in the health informatics domain. He was a visiting scholar at the School of Management (as well as studying Public Health at the School of Public Health) in Boston University between January and July 2008.

Back in 2009, Drs. Josiah and Simon K. Poon started to engage research in Informatics for Traditional Chinese Medicine (iTCM). They were the conveners and leaders of a multi-discipline and multi-university iTCM research team. The reputation of this team has attracted many important international collaborators, including China Academy of Chinese Medical Sciences, Longhua Hospital (teaching hospital of Shanghai University of TCM), Shanghai Innovation Research Center of Traditional Chinese Medicine, Chinese University of Hong Kong and Hong Kong Polytechnic University. As a result, the team involves in various successful international research grants, but it has also drawn the media's attention. Their achievements were reported in *Wall Street Journal*, Xinhua News and Australian TV channel.

From January to July 2011, Simon spent his sabbatical as a visiting research scientist at the Institute of Chinese Medicine in Chinese University of Hong Kong, and at the Department of Health Technology and Informatics in Hong Kong Polytechnic University. Simon has worked on a number of related iTCM research projects including analysing data from various TCM hospitals (in Beijing and Shanghai, China) in deriving analytical models for analysing complex herbal interactions from patient data records. He has been exploring ways to study formulation of Chinese Medicine within the data analytics perspective by integrating methodologies from diverse research fields to assist TCM drug formulation. His research interest includes studying effects from various forms of the synergistic effects. Models and techniques developed from his research have been shown in diverse research publications, including information systems, data mining, health informatics and pharmacology.

Josiah aims to make TCM an evidence-based treatment. He approaches iTCM from two avenues. The first one is to apply data mining techniques to analyse patient records to identify the core herbs for a certain treatment and study the interaction of herbs leading to positive outcome. The second avenue is to use text-mining techniques on textual documents, such as ancient literature, research papers and clinical notes, so that valuable information (especially causal relationship) can be captured from the text. By integrating the relational graph from clinical data analysis and causal graph from textual analysis, the integrated graph can help re-confirm existing knowledge and/or discover new knowledge. Josiah has been fully funded as invited speaker on iTCM research in many international meetings and summer schools.

Drs. Poon have served in several organising committees including International Workshop on "Information Technology for Chinese Medicine" at the IEEE International Conference on Bioinformatics and Biomedicine (BIBM), Shanghai in 2013 and Hong Kong in 2011; Workshop on "Evidence-Based Research for TCM Data Mining", at the 11th Meeting of Consortium for Globalization of Chinese Medicine (CGCM), Macau in 2012; Workshop on "Advances and Issues in Traditional Chinese Medicine Clinical Data Mining", at the Pacific-Asia Conference on Knowledge Discovery and Data Mining (PAKDD), Shenzhen in 2011; Workshop for "Advances and Issues in Biomedical Data Mining" at the Pacific-Asia Conference on Knowledge Discovery and Data Mining (PAKDD), Bangkok, Thailand, in 2009; and track co-chair for "ICT and Health" at the Pacific Asia Conference on Information Systems (PACIS), Suzhou, China, in 2008.

University of Sydney, Sydney, NSW, Australia   Josiah Poon
                                                                               Simon K. Poon

Searching for Evidence in Traditional Chinese Medicine Research: A Review and New Opportunities

Simon K. Poon, Shagun Goyal, Albert Cheng, and Josiah Poon

Abstract Traditional Chinese medicine (TCM) is growing in popularity worldwide. In order for this complementary medicine system to gain official recognition in the health-care policies of Western countries, the evidence for the effectiveness of TCM interventions will need to be rigorously established. It is generally agreed that many research techniques used for evaluating western medicine (such as the randomized controlled trial study design) are not methodologically suited to appraise the efficacy and safety of TCM interventions. In this chapter, we aim to introduce and discuss issues relating to establishing scientific evidence for TCM.

1 Introduction

Traditional Chinese Medicine (TCM) has been practiced over thousands of years. The underlying principles of TCM are found to be quite different from the current popular western medical approaches. The underpinning philosophies like theory of Yin-Yang and Five Elements subscribe to a holistic approach that pays attention to interrelations between different parts of the body. It is different to the reductionist approach in Western Medicine (WM) in the way that TCM treatments are personalized rather than standardized.

Each TCM prescription is personalized for a particular diagnostic assessment, i.e. the herbs in a prescription and their dosages not only vary among patients, but they may be different for the same patient at different times according to the current circumstances of that patient. Hence, the TCM prescriptions taken by a patient have usually not undergone clinical trial assessment as compared to biomedicines prescribed by WM doctors. Standard formulae exist but they often serve as a template

S.K. Poon (✉) • S. Goyal • A. Cheng • J. Poon
School of Information Technologies, University of Sydney, Sydney, NSW 2006, Australia
e-mail: simon.poon@sydney.edu.au; sgoy3681@uni.sydney.edu.au; albertc@doctor.com; josiah.poon@sydney.edu.au

J. Poon and S.K. Poon (eds.), *Data Analytics for Traditional Chinese Medicine Research*,
DOI 10.1007/978-3-319-03801-8_1, © Springer International Publishing Switzerland 2014

Table 1 Key differences between TCM and Western Medicine

	TCM	Western Medicine
	(Syndrome-differentiation approach)	(Disease-based approach)
Diagnosis	TCM tongue diagnosis, TCM pulse diagnosis, looking, listening, smelling, asking	Standardised and straightforward procedure for each patient
Treatment recipient	A particular patient can receive distinct TCM remedies from different TCM practitioners based on the syndrome-patterns detected by each practitioner	A particular patient will receive the same biomedical treatment from all WM doctors
Treatment provision	'Personalized' – a TCM practitioner will provide personalized treatment to each patient depending upon the patient's unique syndrome-patterns	'One-size-fits-all'– the WM doctor will offer similar biomedical treatment to all patients with a particular disease
Treatment focus	Restoring the flow of 'Qi' through the meridians in the entire body	Treating the specific disease, reducing the known symptoms
Treatment procedure	Multiple modalities – such as combination of different herbs, acupuncture, dietary therapy etc	Single medication or combination of medications and surgery

for modification and adaption during the personalization process. These standard formulae have been passed down from history without the rigorous biomedical examinations or clinical trials found in WM. They were essentially created from the clinical experience of the master TCM doctors.

There are several pragmatic differences between the underlying mechanisms of TCM and WM. While TCM operates on a 'syndrome-differentiation' approach, a 'disease based' methodology is followed in WM. The distinctions between these approaches are summarized in the table above (Table 1).

It is not uncommon to find around 10 to 20 different kind of herbs in a typical TCM formula. A herb in a formula carries a particular role in the treatment process; however the same herb may have a different role in another formula. This is unlike WM that aims to focus on the efficacy of a singleton drug, i.e. interactions between the drugs are to be minimized. It is known that the efficacy of a TCM formula comes from the synergistic interaction of herbs. Although these formulae are considered useful and effective, they have not been necessarily validated or supported by scientific or statistical evidence.

Randomized controlled trials (RCT) are widely accepted in medical research for evaluating the efficacy and safety of a medical intervention. This study type is commonly accepted as the gold standard for conducting evidence-based medicine (EBM) research. However, the RCT study design has distinct limitations when used to evaluate TCM due to several methodological and logistical issues. Thus, many TCM interventions have wrongly been shown to be ineffective or even harmful by applying conventional RCT procedures (Tang and Wong 1998). Accurate clinical evaluation for TCM can only be sought if the RCT study design is augmented to make it adaptable with the TCM principles or if new methodologies such as Comparative Effectiveness Research (CER) are utilized.

In order to advance this traditional practice in the modern world, rigorous scientific methods are sought to search for evidence. Owing to the long history of TCM, there are many sources of literature and clinical records available for analysis. The methods and techniques to study TCM can be large and diversified; it stretches from system biology all the way up to systematic reviews. In the next sections, we seek to explore the augmentation of Randomized Controlled Trials (RCT) and Comparative Effectiveness Research (CER) in establishing scientific evidence for TCM.

2   Augmentations to the RCT 'Gold Standard'

In this section, we systematically examine novel augmentations presented in the literature for adapting the 'design', 'conduct' and 'evaluation' phases of a RCT study. The aim of these modifications is to augment the RCT methodology in a manner that will make the clinical trial procedures appropriate for examining TCM interventions.

The conventional RCT procedure has many limitations when it is applied to evaluate the efficacy and safety of TCM. This is because the interventions in TCM follows the *'patient-centered research'* paradigm which involves varying the medical approach based on the unique characteristics associated with each individual patient. This approach is inconsistent with the *'evidence-based research'* paradigm which involves assessing the average effects of a homogeneous treatment provided to a group of participants (Verhoef et al. 2002). Hence, without proper adaptation, the RCT study design is not suitable for evaluating TCM and it could lead to inconsistent results (Lee and Shen 2008).

There are three main reasons for the proposition that the notions of TCM and conventional RCT are contradictory with one-another. *Firstly*, patients in a RCT study are given a particular intervention based on the treatment arm that they were randomly assigned at the commencement of the clinical trial. Such methodological basis is inconsistent with the fundamental TCM notions of personalized medicine. *Secondly*, conducting a placebo-controlled clinical trial becomes complex when physical TCM treatments such as acupuncture and acupressure are involved. This is because according to the EBM guidelines, a true placebo should have no therapeutic impact on the patient. However, when sham acupuncture or acupressure massages are provided, it acts as a stimulus to generate a 'limbic touch response' that can result in psychosomatic benefits for the patient (Lund et al. 2009). *Lastly*, it is known that the RCT methodology usually tries to limit the impact of the patient-provider relationship on the outcomes measured in the study. However, the therapeutic effects of the patient-provider relationships are a crucial component of TCM practice (Verhoef et al. 2002).

The adaptations described below are based on three perspectives of the RCT study, namely the 'design', 'conduct' and 'evaluation' phases. The aim is to make the clinical trial methodology suitable for evaluating the efficacy and safety of TCM interventions.

2.1   RCT Adaptations from the 'Design' Perspective

Adaptations from the 'design' perspective of a RCT study include variations made to the manner in which patients are selected into the study. The two solutions discussed below are two-stage stratified protocol and n-of-1 trials.

2.1.1   The Two-Stage Stratified Protocol

A two-stage stratified protocol has been put forth by Zhang et al. (2011) in order to incorporate information about TCM syndrome-patterns in the RCT study design. The stage-1 is an open-label trial which aims to explore which types of symptoms (i.e. TCM syndrome-patterns) correlate with better efficacy of the herbal formulations. It begins by administering the TCM herbs for a particular ailment to all the patients in the clinical trial. This is followed by performing correlation analysis between the TCM herbs and the symptoms of the patient sub-groups that made the most recovery i.e. the participants who had the optimal outcomes at the end of the study period. The stage-2 of the clinical trial is a typical double blind, placebo-controlled RCT comparing TCM herbs to WM. However, the key differentiating aspect in comparison to regular trials is that the group of symptoms identified in stage-1 of the trial (which formulate the TCM syndrome-patterns) will become part of the inclusion criteria for all the participants entering stage-2 of the trial. Hence, the stage-2 trial evaluates the comparative effectiveness of TCM and WM among only those participants who display the specific TCM syndrome-patterns correlating to the given TCM herbs.

A growing number of researchers are using similar concepts of stratified trials in the design of RCT studies. For instance, Tong et al. (2010) only included participants with '*damp-heat accumulation*' syndrome in a clinical trial conducted for examining the efficacy of Composite Sophora Colon-Soluble Capsule (CSCC) in the treatment of ulcerative colitis. Similarly, Wang et al. (2013) are conducting a RCT to verify the efficacy of Shenyan Kangfu tablet (SYKFT) for diabetic nephropathy in only those patients that display the '*qi-yin deficiency*' syndrome. About a decade back, Qi et al. (2004) conducted a stratified trial to evaluate the efficacy and safety of Shugan Yiyang Capsule for treating erectile dysfunction in male patients with '*Gan stagnation and Shen-deficiency*' syndrome.

In summary, the two-stage stratified protocol utilizes the TCM syndrome-pattern differentiation concept. Stage-1 of the trial uncovers the group of TCM symptoms that correlate with the given TCM herbal formulations and these symptoms become part of the inclusion criteria for participants entering stage-2 of the RCT.

2.1.2   The N-of-1 Trials

The adoption of n-of-1 trial design has been advocated by Lillie et al. (2011) as an optimal way of establishing the evidence-base for personalized medicine. The authors have argued that conventional patient care does not take into account the specific genetic composition and environmental circumstances of a patient. As such, the physicians work on a "hit-and-miss" basis when choosing an intervention for a particular patient from a given set of comparable treatments; as this is done mostly without any systematic evidence or decision-making process behind their choice. This problem can be solved by conducting 'n-of-1' trials in which only a single patient is the subject for the study. That patient is given the alternative treatments (for instance 'treatment A' and 'treatment B') in a random sequential order (AABB/ABAB/ABBA), and health outcomes are measured extensively throughout the study period. However, it is important to note that confounding can be induced into this study if there are carryover effects of the intervention or if the washout period is not appropriate. In addition, while n-of-1 trials have the potential of contributing significantly to personalized patient care, the generalizability of the results from these trials to benefit the population at large is limited. This raises questions about the cost effectiveness of the RCT and resource utilization by the researchers, physicians and the study subject during the research study. The authors have suggested that through conducting the meta-analysis of several n-of-1 trials, it will be feasible to derive meaningful results that can be used in the treatment plan for wider sets of patients. In addition, the advancements in wearable medical monitoring devices will make the data-collection process efficient, thereby facilitating the conduct of the single-subject trials.

One of the earlier examples of the application of n-of-1 trial design has been by Satoh et al. (2005). The researchers applied this framework when conducting a clinical trial at the Toyama Medical and Pharmaceutical University in Japan to verify the efficacy of Hochuekkito medicine in elderly patients suffering from general weakness. Moreover, Chen (2008) highlights that *"Chinese medicine stresses on single case study and treats each individual on a case-by-case basis"*. This signifies the crucial role that n-of-1 trials will play in establishing the evidence for TCM in the coming years. Finally, Li et al. (2013) have proposed three recommendations that will enable greater use of this trial methodology, namely a call for increased government funding of n-of-1 trials, systematic training of researchers and clinicians who are involved in the conduct of these trials, and increasing awareness about the significance of single-subject studies in meeting the medical needs of patients.

In summary, n-of-1 trials technique seems to have promising potential in researching efficacy of TCM treatments in the near future. This RCT methodology enables the co-existence of personalized medicine as well as the rigorousness required by the EBM guidelines.

2.2 RCT Adaptations from the 'Conduct' Perspective

Adaptations from the 'conduct' perspective of a RCT study include variations made to the manner in which treatment is administered to the patients. The two solutions discussed below are Creation of Treatment Manuals an conducting Pragmatic Trials.

2.2.1 Creation of Treatment Manuals

The method of creating 'treatment manuals' was proposed by Schnyer and Allen (2002) to enable the co-existence of standardization as well as flexibility during treatment provision in the clinical trials of TCM interventions. The authors explain that the guidelines for the treatment provision in a RCT study should be carefully constructed using a two-part process and needs to be documented in a reference manual. In Part I, the conceptual framework for the TCM intervention is established by conducting meticulous literature reviews and by surveying a number of TCM practitioners. In Part II, the contents of the manual are created which includes sections on the biomedical perspective of the intervention, theoretical framework, clinical developments, applications of theoretical framework during diagnosis and treatment, assessment of treatment provision, case studies and clinical issues. As a result, the final treatment manual will consist of guidelines for the uniform procedure to be followed when TCM interventions are given to the patients during the clinical trial, as well as description of the scenarios where modifications to the standardized procedures could be made at the discretion of the TCM provider.

This proposed solution of creating treatment manuals has been applied in many acupuncture trials. This technique was referred by Napadow et al. (2004) as a current development to improve the RCT methodology whereby "*a fixed set of acupoints are augmented depending on individualized signs and symptoms (TCM patterns)*". Indeed, the process of creating treatment manuals was followed in the German Acupuncture Trials (GERAC) study which sought to evaluate the efficacy of acupuncture in restoring the health of patients who had migraine or 'tension-type headaches' (Molsberger et al. 2006). The researchers in that study established a semi-structured treatment protocol through carrying out a broad literature review of acupuncture treatment procedure, along with conducting face-to-face, email and phone interviews with acupuncture specialists. Similarly, in a RCT conducted to evaluate the effectiveness of Japanese acupuncture as an intervention for endometriosis-related pelvic pain, the research team created treatment manuals as well as carried-out focus group sessions for establishing the diagnostic criteria (Schnyer et al. 2008).

In summary, it is recommended that treatment manuals should be created prior to administering the TCM interventions in a RCT study. This will enable a balance between the conflicting requirements of 'standardization' as mandated by the EBM guidelines with the need for providing 'personalized' treatment which is a core aspect of TCM.

2.2.2 Pragmatic Trials

MacPherson (2004) proposed the use of pragmatic trials for evaluating complementary medicine systems such as TCM. Pragmatic trials allow for the comparison of two active treatments in the backdrop of every-day community settings. The author's proposal is based on the rationale that TCM offers a 'package' of care comprising multiple modalities unlike western medicine which provides standardized treatment to patients. Moreover, the therapeutic impact of the patient-provider relationships and the patient's expectations of the treatment effect are a key component of this 'package' provided by TCM. These aspects can only be incorporated reasonably in a RCT study through conducting a pragmatic trial. Finally, pragmatic trials involves the comparison of two active treatments, and hence do not involve a placebo intervention. This has twofold advantages in terms of evaluating TCM: firstly, it is not always possible to provide a suitable placebo for physical TCM interventions like acupuncture or acupressure. Secondly, the results from the pragmatic trials will be more useful as patients normally have to make choices between active treatments in real-life, and therefore the findings regarding the effectiveness of a treatment in comparison with a placebo are irrelevant to them.

During pragmatic trials, very few exclusion criteria are set for participants so that patients with diverse characteristics can enter the study. This increases the generalizability of the results for all members of the population. In addition, MacPherson (2004) has suggested that pragmatic trials should be conducted for conditions such as 'lower back pain' where the WM treatments are not satisfactory. This will allow the outpatient clinics to easily gauge the interest of their patients for taking part in the RCT and subsequently becoming a participant in the TCM treatment arm of the clinical study. The author is also a supporter of using treatment manuals during the trials to ensure that the practitioners operate using a defined framework, whilst having the flexibility to provide personalized treatment within the realms of the guidelines. Finally, the outcomes measured in a pragmatic trial are of a holistic nature, i.e. measures such as 'quality of life' indicators are evaluated rather than just assessing the physical improvements (for instance, variation of pain level in a particular joint etc). This is because TCM interventions have an effect over a longer period of time and this affect is not limited to a particular organ, but instead it has broad implications on the physical, mental and social health of the patient.

It is interesting to note that many researchers in western countries have used pragmatic trials for evaluating the effectiveness of TCM. MacPherson et al. (2010) conducted a pragmatic trial in the United Kingdom to examine the efficacy of acupuncture in treating irritable bowel syndrome. Patients were recruited from 10 GP databases and they were provided with acupuncture plus usual GP care or only the usual GP care. In Germany, a pragmatic trial was conducted by Molsberger et al. (2010) to assess the effectiveness of Chinese acupuncture in comparison with conventional orthopedic treatment for patients with chronic shoulder pain who attended one of the 31 outpatient centers taking part in the RCT. In Australia, an acupuncture RCT based on pragmatic trial notions was commenced in 2012 involving patients with chronic knee pain (Hinman et al. 2012).

In summary, it is suggested that conducting a pragmatic trial is an efficient and more realistic way of evaluating TCM interventions in a RCT study. This is because pragmatic trials involve examining the therapeutic benefit of TCM for a heterogeneous group of patients in routine clinical settings, rather than evaluating the impact of the intervention on a group of homogeneous participants in an experimental setting.

2.3   RCT Adaptations from the 'Evaluation' Perspective

Adaptations from the 'evaluation' phase of a RCT study includes variations made to the manner in which the outcomes of the clinical trial are interpreted and communicated. The two solutions discussed below are qualitative assessment of outcomes and 'CONSORT for TCM' publication guidelines.

2.3.1   Qualitative Assessment of Outcomes

It has been argued that many RCT studies have disproved the effectiveness of TCM because the clinical trials failed to assess the impact of the intervention on holistic health outcomes (Verhoef et al. 2002). The statistical measures of frequency and association do not always capture the overall therapeutic impact of 'whole-body' treatments such as TCM. The authors have recommended that in order to accurately evaluate the effectiveness of TCM remedies in a clinical trial, qualitative research methods such as interviews, focus groups and patient observations should be used in conjunction with quantitative tools like standardized questionnaires and laboratory tests.

Alraek and Malterud (2009) utilized a qualitative assessment technique to understand the impact of acupuncture on women with menopausal hot flashes. The participants in the clinical trial were asked to record their experiences and write about any perceived impact of acupuncture on their health. The written records were assessed using systematic text condensation, which allowed the researchers to comprehend the therapeutic impact of acupuncture in a more enhanced manner compared with solely relying on the quantitative results. It is important to note that qualitative assessment becomes even more crucial in assessment of interventions directed at having a psychosomatic impact. In a RCT conducted to assess the impact of *TuiNa* (or remedial massage) on children with autism, Silva et al. (2011) did not limit themselves to only conducting objective assessment of sensory and self-regulation outcomes. The research team collected additional data from the school teachers and the parents of the participating children to comprehensively understand the impact of the *Tui Na* intervention on the severity of autism and parental stress respectively. In another example of qualitative assessment, Thompson et al. (2012) conducted interviews with the TCM practitioners who took part in a RCT that evaluated the impact of acupuncture on women with ovarian dysfunction. After the conclusion of treatment administration, the acupuncturists were asked to describe their views about the clinical trial through written questionnaires, open-ended interviews and focus group sessions. It was concluded that by striving to understand the clinician's perspective about the treatment provision, the results from the RCT can be evaluated in the right context.

In summary, the meaning and impact of TCM interventions can be understood more thoroughly from the perspective of the patients, patient's family, and the practitioners if qualitative assessments are conducted in conjunction with quantitative measurements. This is vital for gaining insight into the real-life impact of TCM outside of 'controlled' clinical settings.

2.3.2 'CONSORT for TCM' Publication Guidelines

It has been argued repeatedly that evidence created through clinical trials adds little value to enhance adoption of TCM because of inadequately written RCT publications. A study of 70 Cochrane Database System Review (CDSR) of TCM found that evidences are inconclusive due to poor methodology and heterogeneity of the studies reviewed (Manheimer et al. 2009). The reporting of TCM clinical trials has been generally of poor quality because the researchers do not provide sufficient information about the trial methodology in the publications. The meaning and quality of the results cannot be fully understood and validated by the users of the publications. Hence, it has been proposed that the 'CONSORT for TCM' publication guidelines should be adopted to increase the accuracy of the research reports published about clinical trials of TCM interventions (Bian et al. 2011). It is not only to standardize the reporting of trial results, and also to enable TCM evaluations to be conceptualized and improved, but also as a way to help TCM research studies into the "mainstream" literature. The CONSORT (Consolidated Standards of Reporting Trials) is an internationally accepted guide for reporting of RCT studies. It includes a checklist of 25 items which the author must discuss in the journal paper. The customized 'CONSORT for TCM' guidelines ensure that discussion about specific Chinese medicine principles are also included in the publication report (such as the impact of TCM 'zheng' classification on the inclusion criteria for participants in the RCT, diagnosis of baseline characteristics, and interpretation of results).

It has been stated that encouraging the reporting of trials based on CONSORT guidelines will be highly beneficial and it will help in assessing the scientific rigour and the ethical implications of the clinical trial (Zhong et al. 2010). The significance of this solution can be understood further by putting it in the context of the report by Wang et al. (2007). After conducting a systematic search of RCT studies in TCM journals from mainland China, the researchers found that the quality of reporting was generally poor. This is because on average only 39.4 % of the items from the modified CONSORT statement were published in the reports which disseminated the results of the clinical trial. Similar findings were stated in a study by Wei et al. (2009) who found that though the quality of reporting for TCM trials is improving, it remains relatively poor in comparison with clinical studies conducted for western medicine. The researchers called for leading journals to endorse the CONSORT statement so as to guarantee high-quality reporting.

In summary, the quality of reporting can be improved if all researchers who conduct clinical trials for TCM are required to publish results using the 'CONSORT for TCM' guidelines. The policy-makers, physicians, and patients will then be able to objectively evaluate and understand the results of those RCT studies, and the results will be more acceptable by various stakeholders in the medical field.

3 Using Comparative Effectiveness Research for TCM

A critical component of Comparative Effectiveness Research (CER) is to generate evidence about the effectiveness, benefits and harms of a particular intervention in comparison with the alternative therapies available for treating the given ailment (AHRQ 2013) In 2010, the Unites States government legislated the Patient Protection and Affordable Care Act (PPACA), and with it a new organization called Patient-Centered Outcomes Research Institute (PCORI) was established to promote the development and adoption of CER in health-care research. D'Arcy and Rich (2012) have stated that better information on the clinical effectiveness of alternative treatments and other complementary interventions is needed to improve the quality of medical care and restrain growth in health-care expenditures.

The establishment of PCORI is a positive step for EBM in terms of shifting research funding solely from RCT-based evidence to now incorporating other sources such as data from observational studies and decision analysis (Pedulli 2013). One of key agenda promoted by PCORI is to reframe the focus of research studies by placing less emphasis on 'internal validity' and more emphasis on 'external validity' (i.e. the typical patients). This view recognizes that data for evaluating the effectiveness of an intervention is not just generated by the experimental clinical trials, but rather the data can come from multiple real-world sources such as electronic health records (EHR) and health insurance claims forms.

The Multi-Payer Claims Database (MPCD) was developed by PCORI in 2011 to become a repository of Medicare data and private health insurance claims, thereby facilitating the researchers to implement observational studies (Mohr 2012). In addition, funding has been allocated to create a National Clinical Research Network that has the potential to revolutionize the manner in which data for health-care research is generated. The significance of it can be best summed up in a quote by NIH Director Francis Collins *"if each patient were an active and informed participant in clinical research as part of their regular health care, a visit to a doctor's office would have the potential to transform the health of millions of individuals"* (Rukovets 2013). As part of this initiative, the clinical data research networks (CDRNs) and patient-powered research networks (PPRNs) will be developed (Winkler 2012).

3.1 Progress of CER

Historically, the research community has placed great emphasis on using evidence from RCT studies based on the rationale that if a drug/medical device is effective for a group of participants in the clinical trial, then it can be reasonably inferred that it will be effective in an individual patient as well. But this notion is beginning to come under scrutiny, as many clinical trials are now conducted to find out the risk and benefit of an intervention at not only the population level, but also with a sharp focus to identify the individuals who could benefit the most from the therapy. This trend is synonymous with the syndrome-differentiation approach of TCM. Shi et al. (2012)

marked the beginning of linking the CER methodology with TCM research and proposed various ways to harness the retrospective study and compare effectiveness based on historical data to provide insights and partial evidence prospective studies.

Many statistical methods have been developed to overcome the main drawback regarding the absence of randomization in observational studies (Velentgas et al. 2013). Propensity Score Method (PSM) is a technique that has gained popularity and is known to be able to mimic the advantage of randomization in terms of limiting the influence of confounding factors. The ability to develop computational techniques that can harness a diversity of data sources and subsequently process data with statistical rigor will be an important factor in establishing evidence for TCM by using CER.

With CER, the focus has shifted from group medicine to personalized medicine, and this brings new hope for TCM which is rooted in a patient's individual syndrome diagnosis. Even in WM, there is growing acceptance of individualization of treatment based on a patient's unique characteristics, particularly at the genetic level. In the past, the use of n-of-1 or single subject clinical trial has been sparingly used in medical research, possibly because of the difficulty in monitoring the patient's health outcomes throughout the RCT. As discussed previously, the concept of n-of-1 trial is synonymous with TCM philosophy since it assumes there is variability from individual to individual, so treatment should be personalized based on an individual's particular characteristics. Furthermore, it has been showed that results from individual treatment can be combined to give comparative treatment effect estimates at the population level by using Bayesian mixed method (Zucker et al. 1997).

3.2 PICOTS Typology and Its Potential for TCM Research

As the basis for developing a protocol for CER, the Agency for Healthcare Research and Quality (AHRQ) outlined the six elements of the PICOTS typology that enables the development of research questions for CER (Velentgas et al. 2013). The six elements shown in Table 2 highlight the various factors to consider when conducting a CER study.

PICOTS, as recommended by PCORI, could be a valuable protocol for evaluating comparative effectiveness of TCM as the model has similarities with the classical Chinese medicine philosophy. These six components should form the basis for designing any observational studies for CER that evaluates the effectiveness of TCM interventions:

1. Population – As treatment assignment in TCM is based on syndrome differentiation, it is expected that patient characteristics will be matched within each syndrome subgroup. By making comparison across different subgroups, it can be uncovered which syndrome would most benefit from the treatment, or alternatively which patient subgroup would suffer the greatest harm. This additional homogeneity will enable analysis of treatment effect within each subgroup to be more meaningfully performed.

Table 2 PICOTS typology for developing research questions

Component	Relevant questions
Population	What is the patient population of interest? Are intervention effects expected to be homogeneous or heterogeneous between different subgroups of the population? What subgroups will be considered in terms of age, gender, ethnicity, etc....?
Intervention	What is the intervention of interest (e.g. a drug, device, procedure, or test)?
Comparator	What are the alternatives?
Outcomes	What are the outcomes and endpoints of interest?
Timing	What is the time frame of interest for assessing outcomes? Are stakeholders interested in short-term or long-term outcomes?
Setting	What is the clinical setting of interest (e.g. hospital, private practice, community health center, etc.)?

Source: Velentgas et al. (2013)

2. *I*ntervention – Various modalities of interest in TCM under different contexts can be explored or compared such as interventions for etiology, prevention, diagnosis, prognosis or treatment.
3. *C*omparators – There are many possible scenarios of comparison: TCM vs. TCM, TCM vs. Western Medicine (WM), or TCM vs. Integrative Medicine (TCM + WM). One of the challenges of comparing Chinese herbal treatments is that they are multi-agent and multi-target, i.e. a concoction usually consists of multiple herbs, with each of them having its own effects and targets. Hence, one single herbal formulation may need to be considered as many simultaneous treatments when performing statistical analysis.
4. *O*utcomes – Use of Patient Reported Outcome (PRO) is gaining popularity in CER, and it is also an integral part of many TCM treatments. Quality of Life (QoL) measures such as ability to walk (mobility) or eat (appetite) are commonly used in addition to biomedical diagnostic tests like X-Rays. TCM remedies has the further benefit of having relatively few side effects, and this argument is often used to justify TCM as an adjunct treatment. CER studies involving integrative medicine can provide evidence about the impact of TCM in countering the side-effects of WM interventions like chemotherapy or radiotherapy used in treatment of cancer. When comparing TCM with WM, it is also important to select common endpoints or surrogate endpoints as evidence of analyzing the treatment effects.
5. *T*iming – The timeframe for measuring treatment outcome should be carefully considered as TCM often has a longer time to response (TTR).
6. *S*ettings – The clinical settings for the delivery of TCM treatments is a key factor as different clinics can offer varying quality of TCM treatments. Analyzing the research data by using the clinical settings as a data parameter is important for reducing selection bias. For instance, patients going to hospital versus patients visiting a TCM community clinic could have very different health status or severity of disease. Moreover, it is generally considered that patients often choose to visit the local TCM clinic if they have a chronic condition rather than a terminal illness.

3.3 Future of CER: Big Data Analytics

Recent literature suggests that the future of conducting CER will not solely rely on RCTs or its derivatives, but rather a big data approach will be followed that leverages on semantic web technology, linked data and data mining. Patient information and treatment prescriptions will need to be captured at the point of care in the community rather than only being generated by research institutions during the conduct of clinical trials. Electronic health records can be mined to identify research patient objects which would have satisfied the inclusion and exclusion criteria for a clinical trial. By linking data across diverse healthcare organizations (such as primary GP care, private and public hospitals) together with insurance claims data from multiple insurance providers, the CER researchers can have a more longitudinal view of the patient's treatment progress and uncover novel insights about the comparative effectiveness of alternative interventions.

Big data could essentially save millions of dollars by enabling more efficient planning, selection and analysis of patient data. Big data also has the potential to efficiently implement n-of-1 trials in which remote monitoring medical devices used by millions of individual patients can be networked together to provide real-time treatment results for analytical research. Undoubtedly, the advent of big-data will revolutionize the manner of evaluating the effectiveness of medical interventions, but how fast this can be realized will depend on whether a mutually agreeable CER standard or protocol can be established for generating credible evidence from comparative effectiveness analysis.

4 Conclusion

A rigorous evidence-base of Chinese medicine remedies will lead to far-reaching acceptance of TCM amongst the general population, greater use of TCM techniques by the medical community, and incorporation of TCM in the health-care policies by governments world-wide. In the previous sections, the benefits of augmenting the design, conduct and evaluation phases of the RCT methodology were articulated to partially account for the perspectives of personalized medicine prescribed in TCM philosophy. The principles and concepts of Comparative Effectiveness Research (CER) were explored so that a procedure can be developed by using the PICOTS typology that will enable researchers to aggregate evidence for TCM interventions in comparison with biomedicine. Observational research using electronic-health records and insurance-claims data with such considerations will be highly useful as the studies will take into account the distinct TCM notions of syndrome-based personalized prescriptions and the focus on restoring the holistic health of the patients. Nevertheless, both RCT and CER have restricted scope when attention is drawn towards the extensive monetary cost, time-consumption and resource utilization by these studies. This makes it vital that going forwards, new methods using advanced computational and pharmacological techniques are devised with the aim of establishing evidence for TCM.

Many data-driven techniques (also called knowledge discovery approaches) have been developed to uncover the implicit patterns in patient data. The main goal of using machine learning and data mining to discover implicit patterns from prescription records is to establish evidence for the effectiveness of TCM in treating a given medical condition. These techniques have the potential to tap into the clinician's experience and thereby, facilitate the transition of novel insights into new drug discovery and improved patient care. For example, Poon et al. (2011) proposed a new statistical technique to facilitate the extraction of all high dimensional statistically significant synergistic interactions amongst herbs in TCM prescriptions. Zhou et al. (2010) and Yan et al. (2013) utilized association rules in conjunction with networks analyses to find subsets in TCM prescriptions that are effective in treating a condition. As well, Poon et al. (2012) incorporated the evolution approach to search for relationships amongst symptoms and herbs in prescriptions. Zhang et al. (2008) and Ouyang et al. (2011) used the Bayesian methods to model the concept of 'syndrome' which is uniquely found in TCM philosophy.

At the current state of research, electronic health records are still not fully uniform and data systems across institutions are not compatible to each other, particularly between TCM and Western Medicine databases. Greater effort is needed in the coming years to build an electronic information infrastructure that can be used for big data analytics. This chapter aimed to familiarize the readers with the advancements in the RCT methodology and the emergence of CER protocol. But given the restrictions of these research studies, this rest of the book aims to introduce the reader to the prime computational and pharmacological techniques used for evaluating TCM interventions. We aim to enable readers to appreciate the kind of diverse solutions that can be applied by researchers to establish evidence for TCM and, hence we explore issues surrounding computations of data and analytics of evidence. The foci are particularly placed on study of clinical data and the analysis of herbal data.

References

AHRQ, What is comparative effectiveness research. Agency for Healthcare Research and Quality (AHRQ) (2013), http://effectivehealthcare.ahrq.gov/index.cfm/what-is-comparative-effectiveness-research1/. Accessed 11 Aug 2013

T. Alraek, K. Malterud, Acupuncture for menopausal hot flashes: a qualitative study about patient experiences. J. Altern. Complement. Med. 15(2), 153–158 (2009). doi:10.1089/acm.2008.0310

Z. Bian, B. Liu, D. Moher, T. Wu, Y. Li, H. Shang, C. Cheng, Consolidated standards of reporting trials (CONSORT) for traditional Chinese medicine: current situation and future development. Front. Med. 5(2), 171–177 (2011)

K.-j. Chen, Clinical service of Chinese medicine. Chin. J. Integr. Med. 14(3), 163–164 (2008)

L.P. D'Arcy, E.C. Rich, From comparative effectiveness research to patient-centered outcomes research: policy history and future directions. Neurosurg. Focus 33(1), E7 (2012)

R. Hinman, P. McCrory, M. Pirotta, I. Relf, K. Crossley, P. Reddy, A. Forbes, A. Harris, B. Metcalf, M. Kyriakides, Efficacy of acupuncture for chronic knee pain: protocol for a randomised controlled trial using a Zelen design. BMC Complement. Altern. Med. 12(1), 161 (2012)

M.M. Lee, J.M. Shen, Dietary patterns using traditional Chinese medicine principles in epidemiological studies. Asia Pac. J. Clin. Nutr. **17**(supplement 1), 79–81 (2008)

J. Li, J. Tian, B. Ma, K. Yang, N-of-1 trials in China. Complement. Ther. Med. **21**, 190–194 (2013)

E.O. Lillie, B. Patay, J. Diamant, B. Issell, E.J. Topol, N.J. Schork, The n-of-1 clinical trial: the ultimate strategy for individualizing medicine? Personalized. Med. **8**(2), 161–173 (2011). doi:10.2217/pme.11.7

I. Lund, J. Näslund, T. Lundeberg, Minimal acupuncture is not a valid placebo control in randomised controlled trials of acupuncture: a physiologist's perspective. Chin. Med. **4**(1), 1 (2009)

H MacPherson, Pragmatic clinical trials. Complement. Ther. Med. **12**(2–3), 136–140 (2004). doi:http://dx.doi.org/10.1016/j.ctim.2004.07.043

H. MacPherson, M. Bland, K. Bloor, H. Cox, D. Geddes, A. Kang'ombe, J. Reynolds, E. Stamuli, T. Stuardi, H. Tilbrook, Acupuncture for irritable bowel syndrome: a protocol for a pragmatic randomised controlled trial. BMC Gastroenterol. **10**(1), 63 (2010)

E. Manheimer, S. Wieland, E. Kimbrough, K. Cheng, B.M. Berman, Evidence from the cochrane collaboration for traditional Chinese medicine therapies. J. Altern. Complement. Med. **15**(9), 1001–1014 (2009). doi:10.1089/acm.2008.0414

P. Mohr, Looking at CER from medicare's perspective. J. Manag. Care Pharm. **18**(4), S5 (2012)

A.F. Molsberger, G. Boewing, H.C. Diener, H.G. Endres, N. Kraehmer, K. Kronfeld, M. Zenz, Designing an acupuncture study: the nationwide, randomized, controlled, German acupuncture trials on migraine and tension-type headache. J. Altern. Complement. Med. **12**(3), 237–245 (2006)

A.F. Molsberger, T. Schneider, H. Gotthardt, A. Drabik, German randomized acupuncture trial for chronic shoulder pain (GRASP)–a pragmatic, controlled, patient-blinded, multi-centre trial in an outpatient care environment. Pain **151**(1), 146–154 (2010)

V. Napadow, J. Liu, T.J. Kaptchuk, A systematic study of acupuncture practice: acupoint usage in an outpatient setting in Beijing, China. Complement. Ther. Med. **12**(4), 209–216 (2004)

W.-w. Ouyang, X.-z. Lin, Y. Ren, Y. Luo, Y.-t. Liu, J.-m. Yuan, A.-h. Ou, G.-z. Li, TCM syndromes diagnostic model of hypertension: study based on Tree Augmented Naive Bayes, in *Bioinformatics and Biomedicine Workshops (BIBMW), 2011 IEEE International Conference on*, 2011. IEEE, pp. 834–837

L. Pedulli, PCORI announces $68 M in grants for national clinical research network (2013). http://www.clinical-innovation.com/topics/interoperability/pcori-announces-68m-grants-national-clinical-research-network. Accessed 12 Aug 2013

S.K. Poon, J. Poon, M. McGrane, X. Zhou, P. Kwan, R. Zhang, B. Liu, J. Gao, C. Loy, K. Chan, A novel approach in discovering significant interactions from TCM patient prescription data. Int. J. Data. Mining. Bioinform. **5**(4), 353–368 (2011)

J. Poon, D. Yin, S. Poon, R. Zhang, B. Liu, D. Sze, Co-evolution of symptom-herb relationship. In: Evolutionary computation (CEC), 2012 IEEE Congress on, 2012. IEEE, pp. 1–6

W. Qi, Y. Ji-xiang, L. Guo-xin, X. Zhong-yuan, W. Bin, L. Xian-chu, H. Hai-xiang, B. Huan-zhou, X. Fu-song, H. Ying, Treatment of patients with erectile dysfunction by Shugan Yiyang capsule: a multi-centered randomized controlled trial. Chin. J. Integr. Med. **10**(2), 96–101 (2004)

O. Rukovets, New national research network to unite patients, researchers, and health care delivery organizations. Neurology Today (2013)

N. Satoh, S. Sakai, T. Kogure, E. Tahara, H. Origasa, Y. Shimada, K. Kohoda, T. Okubo, K. Terasawa, A randomized double blind placebo-controlled clinical trial of Hochuekkito, a traditional herbal medicine, in the treatment of elderly patients with weakness <i>N</i> of one and responder restricted design. Phytomedicine **12**(8), 549–554 (2005)

R.N. Schnyer, J.J. Allen, Bridging the gap in complementary and alternative medicine research: manualization as a means of promoting standardization and flexibility of treatment in clinical trials of acupuncture. J. Altern. Complement. Med. **8**(5), 623–634 (2002). doi:10.1089/107555302320825147

R.N. Schnyer, D. Iuliano, J. Kay, M. Shields, P. Wayne, Development of protocols for randomized sham-controlled trials of complex treatment interventions: Japanese acupuncture for endometriosis-related pelvic pain. J. Altern. Complement. Med. **14**(5), 515–522 (2008)

H. Shi, Q. Xie, X. Li, B. Liu, Z. Wen, Thinking of comparative effectiveness research of the combination in the real traditional Chinese medicine world, In *e-Health Networking, Applications and Services (Healthcom), 2012 IEEE 14th International Conference on, 2012*. IEEE, pp. 7–9, Beijing, China, October 10-13

L.M. Silva, M. Schalock, R. Ayres, A model and treatment for autism at the convergence of Chinese medicine and western science: first 130 cases. Chin. J. Integr. Med. **17**(6), 421–429 (2011). doi:10.1007/s11655-011-0635-0

J. Tang, T.W. Wong, The need to evaluate the clinical effectiveness of traditional Chinese medicine. Hong Kong Med. J. **4**, 208–210 (1998)

M.E. Thompson, J. Jenkins, A. Smucker, S. Smithwick, D. Groopman, L.M. Pastore, Acupuncturist perceptions of serving as a clinical trial practitioner. Complement. Ther. Med. **20**(4), 183–189 (2012). doi:10.1016/j.ctim.2012.01.002

Z.-q. Tong, B. Yang, B.-y. Chen, M.-l. Zhao, A multi-center, randomized, single-blind, controlled clinical study on the efficacy of composite sophora colon-soluble capsules in treating ulcerative colitis. Chin. J. Integr. Med. **16**, 486–492 (2010)

P. Velentgas, N.A. Dreyer, P. Nourjah, et al., editors, Developing a Protocol for Observational Comparative Effectiveness Research: A User's Guide. Rockville (MD): Agency for Healthcare Research and Quality (US); 2013 Jan. Available from: http://www.ncbi.nlm.nih.gov/books/NBK126190/

M.J. Verhoef, A.L. Casebeer, R.J. Hilsden, Assessing efficacy of complementary medicine: adding qualitative research methods to the" gold standard". J. Altern. Complement. Med. **8**(3), 275–281 (2002)

G. Wang, B. Mao, Z.Y. Xiong, T. Fan, X.D. Chen, L. Wang, G.J. Liu, J. Liu, J. Guo, J. Chang, T.X. Wu, T.Q. Li, The quality of reporting of randomized controlled trials of traditional Chinese medicine: a survey of 13 randomly selected journals from mainland China. Clin. Ther. **29**(7), 1456–1467 (2007). doi:10.1016/j.clinthera.2007.07.023

H. Wang, W. Mu, J. Zhai, D. Xing, S. Miao, J. Wang, Y. Deng, N. Wang, H. Chen, H. Yang, The key role of Shenyan Kangfu tablets, a Chinese patent medicine for diabetic nephropathy: study protocol for a randomized, double-blind and placebo-controlled clinical trial. Trials **14**(1), 165 (2013)

X. Wei, L. Tiejun, W. Cheng, Current situation on the reporting quality of randomized controlled trials in 5 leading Chinese medical journals. J. Med. Coll. PLA. **24**(2), 105–111 (2009)

J. Winkler, Multi-payer claims database (MPCD) (2012), http://www.academyhealth.org/Programs/ProgramsDetail.cfm?itemnumber=7554. Accessed 11 Aug 2013

S. Yan, R. Zhang, X. Zhou, P. Li, L. He, B. Liu, Exploring effective core drug patterns in primary insomnia treatment with Chinese herbal medicine: study protocol for a randomized controlled trial. Trials **14**(1), 61 (2013). doi:10.1186/1745-6215-14-61

N.L. Zhang, S. Yuan, T. Chen, Y. Wang, Latent tree models and diagnosis in traditional Chinese medicine. Artif. Intell. Med. **42**(3), 229–245 (2008)

C. Zhang, M. Jiang, A. Lu, A traditional Chinese medicine versus western combination therapy in the treatment of rheumatoid arthritis: two-stage study protocol for a randomized controlled trial. Trials **12**(1), 137 (2011)

Y.-Q. Zhong, J.-J. Fu, X.-M. Liu, X. Diao, B. Mao, T. Fan, H.-M. Yang, G.-J. Liu, W.-B. Zhang, The reporting quality, scientific rigor, and ethics of randomized placebo-controlled trials of traditional Chinese medicine compound formulations and the differences between Chinese and non-Chinese trials. Curr. Ther. Res. **71**(1), 30–49 (2010)

X. Zhou, J. Poon, P. Kwan, R. Zhang, Y. Wang, S. Poon, B. Liu, D. Sze, Novel two-stage analytic approach in extraction of strong herb-herb interactions in TCM clinical treatment of insomnia. In: medical biometrics (Springer, 2010), pp. 258–267, Lecture Notes in Computer Science 6165, Springer Press, Germany

D. Zucker, C. Schmid, M. McIntosh, R. D'Agostino, H. Selker, J. Lau, Combining single patient (N-of-1) trials to estimate population treatment effects and to evaluate individual patient responses to treatment. J. Clin. Epidemiol. **50**(4), 401–410 (1997)

Causal Complexities of TCM Prescriptions: Understanding the Underlying Mechanisms of Herbal Formulation

Simon K. Poon, Alan Su, Lily Chau, and Josiah Poon

Abstract Traditional Chinese Medicine (TCM) is a holistic approach to medicine which has been in use in China for thousands of years. The main treatment, Chinese Medicine Formulae is prescribed by combining sets of herbs to address the patient's syndromes and symptoms based on clinical diagnosis. Although herbs are often combined based on various classical formulas, TCM practitioners personalize prescriptions by making adjustments to the formula. However, the underlying principles for the choice of herbs are not well understood. In this chapter, we introduce a framework to explore the complex relationships amongst herbs in TCM clinical prescriptions using Boolean logic. By logically analyzing variations of a large number of TCM herbal prescriptions, we have found that our framework was able to show some herbs may have different pathways to affect effectiveness and such herbs have often been overlooked but can play a weak yet non-trivial role in enhancing the overall effectiveness of the TCM treatment. To achieve this goal, two computational solutions are proposed. An efficient set-theoretic approach is first proposed to study the effectiveness of herbal formulations, and followed by complex network analysis to study the role each herb plays in affecting the outcome.

1 Introduction

TCM prescriptions depend on not just the herbs that make up a prescription, but the inter-relatedness between herbs. The interactions may strengthen the positive effects of a herb, reduce harmful effects, or produce a new effect not seen with only one of the components. Each prescription may contain as many as 20 components selected from a wide range of potential herbs. Quantitative assessment of the effect of

S.K. Poon (✉) • A. Su • L. Chau • J. Poon
School of Information Technologies, University of Sydney, Sydney, NSW 2006, Australia
e-mail: simon.poon@sydney.edu.au; kasu4088@uni.sydney.edu.au; lily@it.usyd.edu.au;
josiah.poon@sydney.edu.au

J. Poon and S.K. Poon (eds.), *Data Analytics for Traditional Chinese Medicine Research*,
DOI 10.1007/978-3-319-03801-8_2, © Springer International Publishing Switzerland 2014

prescriptions depends on models that are capable of measuring the complex interactions that are part of the final treatment outcome (Poon et al. 2011a).

Traditionally, analysis of causality has relied on a correlational approach such as multivariate regression, however, it has been demonstrated by several researchers that such an approach cannot account for the phenomena of *conjunctural causation*, *equifinality* and *causal asymmetry* (Ragin 2000; Fiss 2007) which are critically relevant to study causal complexities of TCM.

Conjunctural causation is derived by the fact that an outcome can be achieved from the interaction between multiple causal variables whereas interactions of more than two variables are difficult to interpret using correlational methods such as regression (Fiss 2007). The phenomenon of equifinality suggests that outcomes can be achieved by utilizing different combinations of variables (Katz and Kahn 1978), however, correlational methods such as multivariate regression analysis is unable to account for equifinality as the model produces only a single solution (Fiss 2007). Finally, causal asymmetry addresses the fact that causal relations are asymmetrical in nature (Ehring 1982) which cannot be addressed through correlational analysis as the correlational connections established are symmetrical in nature (Ragin 2008).

Motivated by the inefficiencies with the correlational approach, a new methodology called *Qualitative Comparative Analysis* (QCA) was outlined in (Ragin 1987). QCA is described by Ragin as "an analytic technique designed specifically for the study of cases as configurations of aspects, conceived as combinations of set memberships". Unlike in correlational methods whereby variables are considered "analytically separable", the set-theoretic approach combines variables into sets thus enabling its asymmetric nature (Ragin 2008). This is to address the fact that some factors may have asymmetrical effects on outcome. The set of factors that affect positively to effectiveness can be different from the set of factors hindering the effect, i.e. factors that positively affect project success do not necessarily have a reverse effect when they are reduced or removed. In view of the above, we apply an efficient method to analyze data such as prescription records for effective configurations of herbs. The output of our framework is both a measure of the effectiveness of herbal configurations and the consistencies of the analysis.

2   Background of QCA

The implementation of the original QCA that we will discuss here is called *Crisp-Set QCA*, (or cs/QCA), which deals with cases that have membership scores that are binary in nature (Ragin 1987). For example, in our application to TCM prescriptions, the membership score for a herb is either zero (0) if it is not used in the prescription, or one (1) if there is a presence of the herb in that particular prescription. Note that the dosage information of herbs is ignored in this study to keep our focus on the logical selection of suitable herbs based on inclusion (or exclusion) of a herb in the TCM prescription. The underpinning procedure in cs/QCA is a process of logically eliminating the herbs in the prescription dataset until only the most important herbs remain – this process is termed Boolean minimization.

In cs/QCA, the algorithm used to implement Boolean minimization is called the Quine-McCluskey algorithm first introduced in (Quine 1952, 1955) and later extended in (McCluskey 1956). The algorithm uses a two-level approach similar to solving a *Karnaugh map*.

The first stage of the Quine-McCluskey algorithm generates a set of *prime implicants* from a given truth table. An implicant is defined as a covering of one or more minterms[1] of a Boolean function, and a prime implicant is an implicant that cannot be covered by a more general implicant. The process of generating prime implicants is as follows:

1. Rows in the dataset truth table are grouped based on the number columns with a 1-membership score.
2. Rows in the truth table are combined if they differ by a single variable and this produces an implicant. (e.g. 1,0,1,1,0,1 and 1,1,1,1,0,1 is combined to form the implicant 1,–,1,1,0,1).
3. Repeat step 2 until no more merges are possible in the truth table.
4. Terms which cannot be combined are termed the *prime implicants*.

Once the prime implicants are determined, a prime implicant chart is generated from the output of the first step of the algorithm and the final solution is generated by the second stage of the algorithm. The solution is achieved by removing essential prime implicants, and implicants with row and column dominance and repeating the process until no further reduction can be achieved (Jain et al. 2008).

While the Quine-McCluskey algorithm produces the exact minimal solution for the problem, there is a tradeoff for runtime. It is the problem that is NP-Complete with exponential runtime complexity proportional to the number of causal conditions (Hong et al. 1974; Jain et al. 2008), which presents a major overhead for large-scale analysis. Since the QCA framework was first applied to social and political sciences research, the number of causal conditions that QCA has been used to analyze have been relatively small in quantity and this limitation has gone largely unnoticed. However, in our research, the scale of data analysis that is required is immense as the dataset contains hundreds or even of remedies – for datasets of this magnitude, the Quine-McCluskey algorithm is unable to perform analysis within an adequate timeframe due to the vast number of logical comparisons that will have to be performed.

In order to overcome this issue, we use an alternative algorithm as substitute for the Quine-McCluskey algorithm called BOOM developed by (Fiser and Hlavicka 2003). This algorithm originated from a field of research known as computer aided design and was motivated by the same inefficiencies discussed previously in existing Boolean minimization algorithms. The intended application for the BOOM algorithm was for programmable logic arrays (PLAs), which, similar to our application in TCM prescription data, have vast numbers of variables. Unlike the Quine-McCluskey algorithm which produces an exact solution using a two-level logic

---

[1] A minterm is a product term of n-variables whereby each variable appears only once. For example, given an input function with variables *a*, *b* and *c*, there are $2^3 = 8$ minterms, *abc, abc', ab'c, ab'c', a'bc, a'bc', a'b'c*, and *a'b'c'* respectively.

minimization process, the BOOM algorithm produces a near minimal solution using a three-level heuristic approach, which we found to be much more efficient in our testing than previous methodologies.

3 Methodological Implementations

In this work we apply a two-step framework to analyze causal complexities from TCM patient data record for insomnia treatment. This approach integrates two techniques to provide a holistic analysis of the complex structures of resource interdependencies. It also helps to abstract complexities through the notions of synergistic bundle. The first step of this framework is to identify core herbal components from data using Network Analysis (NA). The second step is to analyze herbal prescriptions using a more efficient QCA algorithm. The aim is to identify herbal combinations that are likely to appear on configuration leading to effective herbal treatment, as hidden relationships amongst herbs in prescriptions.

3.1 Network Analysis

A descriptive summary of a binary herb usage data can be visualised with a frequency network. A frequency network can be constructed by drawing an undirected edge for every pair of herbs that is used in one prescription record. The thickness of the edge connecting two herbs increases proportionally to the fraction of the prescription records that contain the herbs together. Where an undirected edge appears in the next set of a prescription record, the edge will increase in weight and thickness. When all edges and weights have been established, the number of edges for each node is computed as a means to adjust the node size. This measure is known as degree centrality in Network Analysis. In a core herb network, a high degree centrality indicates the importance of a herb to working effectively with many other herbs in achieving a treatment. The calculation of the degree centrality is essential in the purpose of breaking ties in next stage of the methodology, the BOOM algorithm.

Strong usage and correlated herbs can be summarised and visualised in a core herb framework. Introduced in the computation of centrality values, a core-herb network based on the frequency of herbs summarises the common herbal combination usage by TCM practitioners. This network is constructed by computing from the raw data, the number of records where Herb A and Herb B are used together. This is the support of the association rule, indicating the proportion of transactions which contain an edge itemset. An undirected edge is therefore constructed between Herb A and Herb B with edge weights determined by the support. For each edge, confidence calculations are also useful in order to determine if the edge itemset has a large percentage of transactions leading to a positive outcome. Confidence in association rule determines the strength and reliability of the edge itemset. Herb A and Herb B are represented by nodes and the existence of non-zero support and confidence calculations between the two nodes is indicated by an undirected edge. A correlation-based network can similarly be constructed with strength and reliability estimators of herbal combinations.

A core-herb network based on pairwise correlation summarises the association between two herbs as an effective pair. As the raw data is binary, the correlation between herbs is computed using the phi correlation coefficient defined in Eq. 1. The phi coefficient has a maximum value determined by the distribution of the two herb variables A and B. Assuming the data has an equal distribution of positive and negative combinations, the ϕ coefficient will range from -1 to $+1$. ϕ closer to ± 1 indicates strong association while a phi closer to zero indicates weak association.

$$\phi = \frac{n_{11}n_{00} - n_{10}n_{01}}{\sqrt{n_{1\cdot}n_{0\cdot} - n_{\cdot0}n_{\cdot1}}} \tag{1}$$

where

$n_{11}, n_{00}, n_{10}, n_{01}$ are record counts of two herb usage; 1 indicates the presence of the herb and 0 indicates the absence of the herb

n is the total number of observations

Similar to the frequency-based core herb network, Herb A and Herb B is represented by nodes and the correlation between the two nodes is represented by an undirected edge. To estimate the reliability of each correlation coefficient, confidence values are also calculated for each edge. Foundational frequency and correlation networks can therefore be constructed with strength and reliability estimators on each herbal combination edge.

3.2 BOOM Algorithm

The three stages of the BOOM algorithm are *Coverage-Directed Search, Implicant Expansion* and *Covering Problem Solution*, respectively. These will now be discussed in detail.

3.2.1 Coverage-Directed Search

The coverage directed search (CD-Search), is named by (Fiser and Hlavicka 2003) as the most innovative part of the algorithm. The algorithm searches for suitable literals (or variables), which are added iteratively to construct an implicant. The strategy for the selection of the initial literal is to use the most frequent literal as it covers the $(n-1)$-dimensional hypercube. If the $(n-1)$-dimensional hypercube found does not intersect with the off-set, it becomes an implicant, otherwise, another literal is added in the same manner described above (Fiser and Hlavicka 2003). One other advantage of the CD-Search is the use of immediate implicant checks when adding literals to a hypercube – when two or more literals have the same frequency, the only ones that will be combined to form a new hypercube is if the new hypercube does not intersect with the off-set. This improves the runtime comparing to the Quine-McCluskey algorithm and generates a higher quality result.

Algorithm 1 CD_Search(F,R) (Fiser and Hlavicka 2003).

Input: F – the set of prescriptions with positive outcomes; R – the set of prescriptions with negative outcomes.

Output: A set of implicants covering F.

```
CD_Search(F, R) {
  H=∅
  do
  F' =F
  t  =∅
    do
      v=most_frequent_literal(F')
      t=t·v
      F' =F'  - cubes_not_including(t)
    while (t ∩ R !=∅)
  H=H ∪ t
  F=F - F'
  until (F == ∅)
  return H
}
```

In the Algorithm (1), F is the on-set, R is the off-set, and H is the set of implicants.

One modification that we have made to the original CD-Search algorithm is that we incorporate the use of domain knowledge in the form of *centrality values* obtained by analyzing the data using network analysis in part A of the methodology. The degree centrality values measure the amount of interaction that a particular herb may have with other herbs in the network. Essentially the centrality values are a measure to influence the selection algorithm when there exists a tie for the most frequent literal – instead of a randomized selection for the most frequent literal, we propose the use of the centrality value ranking as a tie breaker in order to produce a more meaningful result. This approach would favor herbs that have less direct effect on the outcome, but have strong interactions with other herbs, to higher probably to be selected.

Example

Given the data set in Fig. 1, we will follow the BOOM outlined algorithm to find an implicant.

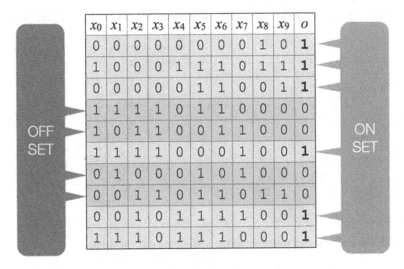

x_0	x_1	x_2	x_3	x_4	x_5	x_6	x_7	x_8	x_9	o
0	0	0	0	0	0	0	0	1	0	1
1	0	0	0	1	1	1	0	1	1	1
0	0	0	0	0	1	1	0	0	1	1
1	1	1	1	0	1	1	0	0	0	0
1	0	1	1	0	0	1	1	0	0	0
1	1	1	1	0	0	0	1	0	0	1
0	1	0	0	0	1	0	1	0	0	0
0	0	1	1	0	1	1	0	1	1	0
0	0	1	0	1	1	1	1	0	0	1
1	1	1	0	1	1	1	0	0	0	1

Fig. 1 Example dataset used to demonstrate the BOOM algorithm

In the first iteration, the most common literal in the on-set is x_3', but as this term intersects with the off-set, it cannot be an implicant, and as a result, another literal will have to be appended (Fig. 2).

x_0	x_1	x_2	x_3	x_4	x_5	x_6	x_7	x_8	x_9	o
0	0	0	0	0	0	0	0	1	0	1
1	0	0	0	1	1	1	0	1	1	1
0	0	0	0	0	1	1	0	0	1	1
1	1	1	1	0	0	0	1	0	0	1
0	0	1	0	1	1	1	1	0	0	1
1	1	1	0	1	1	1	0	0	0	1

	x_0	x_1	x_2	x_3	x_4	x_5	x_6	x_7	x_8	x_9
0	3	4	3	5	3	2	2	4	4	4
1	3	2	3	2	4	3	3	2	2	2

x_0	x_1	x_2	x_3	x_4	x_5	x_6	x_7	x_8	x_9	o
0	0	0	0	0	0	0	0	1	0	1
1	0	0	0	1	1	1	0	1	1	1
0	0	0	0	0	1	1	0	0	1	1
1	1	1	1	0	1	1	0	0	0	0
1	0	1	1	0	0	1	1	0	0	0
1	1	1	1	0	0	0	1	0	0	1
0	1	0	0	0	1	0	1	0	0	0
0	0	1	1	0	1	1	0	1	1	0
0	0	1	0	1	1	1	1	0	0	1
1	1	1	0	1	1	1	0	0	0	1

Fig. 2 Coverage-directed search algorithm demonstrating the intersection of x_3 with the off-set

Ignoring the previously discovered term x_3' and the row in the on-set which is not covered by the term, we continue to find the next literal. In this next step, there are four literals that have the same frequency, in this case, all four combinations with x_3' are tried, with the combinations that intersect with the off-set removed and the literal with the greatest centrality value is then chosen from the remaining literals (Fig. 3).

The only combination which intersects with the off-set is x_3'x_5 and thus

	x_0	x_1	x_2	x_3	x_4	x_5	x_6	x_7	x_8	x_9	o
	0	0	0		0	0	0	0	1	0	1
	1	0	0		1	1	1	0	1	1	1
	0	0	0		0	1	1	0	0	1	1
	1	1	1	1	0	0	0	1	0	0	1
	0	0	1	0	1	1	1	1	0	0	1
	1	1	1	0	1	1	1	0	0	0	1
0	3	4	3	-	2	1	1	4	3	3	
1	2	1	2	-	3	4	4	1	2	2	

x_0	x_1	x_2	x_3	x_4	x_5	x_6	x_7	x_8	x_9	o
0	0	0	0	0	0	0	0	1	0	1
1	0	0	0	1	1	1	0	1	1	1
0	0	0	0	0	1	1	0	0	1	1
1	1	1	1	0	1	1	0	0	0	0
1	0	1	1	0	0	1	1	0	0	0
1	1	1	1	0	0	0	1	0	0	1
0	1	0	0	0	1	0	1	0	0	0
0	0	1	1	0	1	1	0	1	1	0
0	0	1	0	1	1	1	1	0	0	1
1	1	1	0	1	1	1	0	0	0	1

Fig. 3 Coverage-directed search algorithm demonstrating ties in literals

x_3'x_1', x_3'x_6, and x_3'x_7 form the three possible implicant candidates as these sum of products do not intersect with the off-set.

Suppose x_6 has the highest centrality value rank out of the three remaining literals, we choose x_3'x_6 as an implicant, and then the next step would be to find another implicant which covers the remainder rows, shown in green in the diagram below (Fig. 4):

	x_0	x_1	x_2	x_3	x_4	x_5	x_6	x_7	x_8	x_9	o
	0	0	0	0	0	0	0	0	1	0	1
	1	0	0	0	1	1	1	0	1	1	1
	0	0	0	0	0	1	1	0	0	1	1
	1	1	1	1	0	0	0	1	0	0	1
	0	0	1	0	1	1	1	1	0	0	1
	1	1	1	0	1	1	1	0	0	0	1
0	1	1	1	1	2	2	2	1	1	2	
1	1	1	1	1	0	0	0	1	1	0	

Fig. 4 Coverage-directed search algorithm demonstrating the next stage of finding implicants that cover the remaining rows

The previous steps are repeated until all rows of the on-set are covered and the resultant sum of products (or implicants) is the solution to the coverage-directed search, in this case, a possible solution to the CD-search is $x_3'x_6+x_5'x_6'$.

The original CD-search algorithm was non-deterministic in nature due to the randomized selection in the presence of multiple literals that are equally frequent. Our modification to the algorithm, which introduces the use of centrality values, aims to eliminate the uncertainty by using a centrality value rank as the tie-break selection criteria.

3.2.2 Implicant Expansion

With the set of implicants generated from the CD-search, the next stage of BOOM called implicant expansion is run in order to produce the prime implicants. The term expansion can be somewhat misleading, as the number of literals in the implicants is actually reduced. However, by removing literals from implicants, their coverage is expanded and thus the name.

Individual literals in each implicant are tried for removal and if the new expression does not intersect with the off-set, then the literal removal is made permanent (Fiser and Hlavicka 2003). There are three strategies for implicant expansion, which are *exhaustive expansion, sequential expansion* and *multiple sequential expansion,* respectively. In our testing it was found that the sequential expansion strategy's performance was the most acceptable and the results produced were adequate.

The sequential expansion method simply tries to remove all literals from the implicants one by one and once no further removals are possible, then the newly reduced implicant becomes a prime implicant (Fiser and Hlavicka 2003). One minor downside of this expansion strategy is that it is a greedy algorithm, that is, for each original implicant; only one prime implicant is produced because it does not consider the benefits and costs of removing one implicant as opposed to another. Nonetheless, as noted by the authors, the "simplest sequential expansion is better for very sparse functions" which is the case for our research due to the limited diversity present in the dataset (Fiser and Hlavicka 2003).

3.2.3 Covering Problem Solution

Once the prime implicants are obtained from the implicant expansion process, ideally we would like to reduce the number of prime implicants so that a minimal number of them still cover the given dataset. This is an instance of an NP-hard problem called the *Unate Covering Problem*, i.e. the best known algorithms have exponential complexity. As noted in (Fiser and Hlavicka 2003), an exact solution to the covering problem is time consuming and that a heuristic approach is the only viable method.

The heuristic proposed in BOOM is called *Least Covered, Most Covering* (LCMC) whereby prime implicants covering minterms which are covered by the least number of other prime implicants are preferred and if there are more than one such prime implicant, then the one which covers the most number of minterms which are not yet covered is chosen (Fiser and Hlavicka 2003).

While the performance of this heuristic is efficient, we felt like the quality of the results could be improved. As a result, we introduce an alternative heuristic as a slight modification to BOOM called *Literal Weights and Output Weights* (WLWO) proposed in (Kagliwal and Balachandran 2012). The Unate Covering Problem can be transformed into a well-known *Set Cover Problem*. This heuristic, unlike the LCMC heuristic, is designed for the sole purpose of logic minimization and takes into account the relationship between implicants and minterms.

This heuristic defines several weights:

1. Literal Weights (LW) – this is defined to be the number of prime implicants which contain such a literal
2. Output Weights (IC) – this is defined to be the number of implicants in the on-set or don't-care-set for each output. In our case with only a single output function, this is simply the cardinality of the on-set and don't-care-set.

Along with the weights, the sub-section then goes on to define several weight functions:

1. Weighted Literal Count (WL): $WL_i = \sum_{x \in X_i} LW_x$
2. Weighted Output Count (WO): $WO_i = \sum_{y \in Y_i} IC_y$

Using these weight functions, the sub-section introduces a three-stage heuristic. Firstly, select prime implicants for inclusion into the final solution if they cover the most number of yet uncovered minterms. If there is a tie, then select the 'shortest' implicant, that is, the one with the lowest literal count. Finally, if there is another tie, then the prime implicant with the highest WLWO heuristic value is used whereby $WLWO_i = WL_i \times WO_i$. (Kagliwal and Balachandran 2012)

The final set of prime implicants produced by the solution to the covering problem forms our final causal configurations with each prime implicant forming a single configuration that leads to the outcome.

3.3 Integration of Results

The set of prime implicants can subsequently be super-imposed on the Herbal Network to verify and determine strong herb-herb interactions and other interesting patterns. Note that as analysing the prime implicant's negative or NOT(herb) result is confounded by the ambiguous definitions of negative, therefore these negative herbs will be ignored in visualisation. Two comparative core herb networks can therefore be generated and compared to observe interesting patterns; a herb frequency of usage network; and a pairwise herbal correlation network.

Atop either of the two foundational base networks, prime implicants can be super-imposed to visualise interesting results. For each prime implicant set, an undirected edge is created between every pair of herbs in the set. This undirected edge will have a thick line if this edge exists in the base network and a dashed line otherwise. When all edges and weights have been established, the number of edges for each node is computed based on the degrees centrality measures. Interesting factors can thus be inferred by super-imposing positive outcome prime implicants.

4 Data

The described methodology was performed on the insomnia dataset described in (Zhou et al. 2010a). A clinical data warehouse was developed (Zhou et al. 2010b) to integrate and to manage large-scale real-world TCM clinical data. This data warehouse consists of structured electronic medical record from all TCM clinical encounters, including both inpatient and outpatient encounters. There are about 20,000 outpatient encounters of the TCM expert physicians. These encounters included clinical prescriptions for the treatment of various diseases, in which insomnia is a frequently treated disorder.

Total of 460 insomnia outpatient encounters were extracted. The outcome of each encounter was annotated by TCM clinical experts who went through the changes of the insomnia-related variables over consecutive consultation; these include the sleep time per day, sleep quality and difficulty in falling asleep. The outcomes are then classified into two categories: good and bad. When a treatment was effective, which means that if the patient recovered completely or partly from insomnia in the next encounter, then the prescription of the current encounter would be categorized as 'good'; otherwise, the herb prescription would be categorized as 'bad'. After labelling these 460 outpatient encounters, there are 68 encounters with bad outcomes in this dataset; in other words, it is an imbalanced dataset to the advantage of the target class. The average good outcome rate (GOR) of the whole data set is 392/460 = 85.21 %. There are 261 distinct herbs in the dataset and there are on average 14 herbs in a formula.

5 Results

5.1 Analytical Results from Set-Theoretic

Another important modification to the BOOM algorithm was made such that when two prescriptions are present in the dataset but contributes to both a positive outcome and a negative outcome. Instead of marking these as don't-care terms (whereby the outcome is marked by '-' instead of 0 or 1), we calculate the ratio of the desirable outcome and the occurrence of this prescription. This is similar to calculating the odds ratios in a case-control study where effectiveness is compared between a set of herbs in a prescription and another prescription with one of more herbs removed. If this ratio were higher than a threshold value, the outcome for this prescription would be set to the desired outcome, otherwise, the undesired outcome. In our case, the threshold used was the overall ratio of desirable outcomes to the total number of prescriptions (Su et al. 2013).

5.1.1 Results from Analysis of Positive Outcomes

We first analyze the causal configurations that lead to a positive outcome, in this case, the on-set of the dataset is set to where the outcome equals to 1. The results produced along with the frequency of these configurations in the prescriptions are shown in Table 1:

5.1.2 Results from Analysis of Negative Results

Next we analyze the causal configurations that attribute to a negative outcome, in this case, the on-set of the dataset is where the outcome is equal to 0. The results produced along with the frequency of these configurations in the prescriptions are as follows (Table 2):

5.2 Results from Network Analysis

Prior to analysis, it is possible to observe descriptive statistics summaries from the described core herbal network. A larger node size indicates a herb is core to a desired outcome. The edge weights between two nodes indicate a dependent association between two nodes. To visualise core herb summaries, both frequency and correlation networks can be generated from the insomnia dataset. The insomnia frequency-based network is shown in Fig. 5 with frequency and confidence of pairwise herb usage indicated on the edges. As the full graph is too dense to quickly extract any important information visually, a threshold of 46 frequency counts was used for visualisation purposes only. This 46 threshold is equivalent to a 10 % support threshold in association rules. The centrality values are derived from the frequency network, as used in the BOOM algorithm. The centrality values are tabulated in Table 3.

After converting the frequencies for each prime implicant (shown in Fig. 5) into pair-wise edge weights, the results generated by this approach are shown to be consistent to the earlier work described in (Zhou et al. 2010b). In regards to the

Table 1 Positive prime implicant results from insomnia dataset

Configuration	Freq.
~VAR117•~VAR202•**VAR235•VAR237**	79
~(陈皮)•~(炒白术)•(制远志)•(炒酸枣仁)	
VAR34•~VAR43•**VAR200**	76
(黄连)•~(淡豆豉)•(生甘草)	
~VAR43•~VAR120•**VAR196**•~VAR235	53
~(淡豆豉)•~(五味子)•(大枣)•~(制远志)	
~VAR1•~VAR5•~VAR34•~VAR35•~VAR39•~VAR113•~VAR200•~VAR236•~VAR241•~VAR242	46
~(太子参)•~(百合)•~(黄连)•~(黄芩)•~(莲子心)•~(生地黄)•~(生甘草)•~(知母)•~(牡蛎)•~(川芎)	
VAR175•VAR237	45
(山药)•(炒酸枣仁)	
VAR40•~VAR112•~VAR210•~VAR238	44
(石菖蒲)•~(浮小麦)•~(法半夏)•~(柴胡)	
~VAR76•**VAR117**	37
~(竹茹)•(陈皮)	
~VAR151•~VAR178•~VAR235•**VAR236•VAR237**•~VAR242	36
~(煅紫贝齿)•~(炒枳壳)•~(制远志)•(知母)•(炒酸枣仁)•~(川芎)	
VAR79•VAR203	36
(肉桂)•(白芍)	
VAR33•VAR34•~VAR113•~VAR196•**VAR237**	34
(茯苓)•(黄连)•~(生地黄)•~(大枣)•(炒酸枣仁)	
~VAR34•**VAR113•VAR235**	34
~(黄连)•(生地黄)•(制远志)	
~VAR8•~VAR48•~**VAR79**•~VAR202•~VAR236•**VAR237**	29
~(党参)•~(夜交藤)•~(肉桂)•~(炒白术)•~(知母)•(炒酸枣仁)	
VAR40•~VAR235	29
(石菖蒲)•~(制远志)	
VAR35•VAR237•VAR238	28
(黄芩)•(炒酸枣仁)•(柴胡)	
~VAR33•~VAR35•~VAR46•~VAR112•~VAR113•~VAR175•~VAR198•~VAR202•~VAR238	26
~(茯苓)•~(黄芩)•~(炒枳实)•~(浮小麦)•~(生地黄)•~(山药)•~(山萸肉)•~(炒白术)•~(柴胡)	
~VAR8•~VAR112•~VAR113•~VAR175•~VAR196•**VAR202**•~VAR241	22
~(党参)•~(浮小麦)•~(生地黄)•~(山药)•~(大枣)•(炒白术)•~(牡蛎)	
VAR117•~VAR202•~VAR210	18
(陈皮)•~(炒白术)•~(法半夏)	
VAR33•~VAR36•**VAR174•VAR236**	17
(茯苓)•~(麦冬)•(当归)•(知母)	
VAR43•~VAR196•~VAR238	14
(淡豆豉)•~(大枣)•~(柴胡)	
VAR46•**VAR203**•~VAR241	13
(炒枳实)•(白芍)•~(牡蛎)	
~VAR5•**VAR35•VAR113**•~VAR236	13
~(百合)•(黄芩)•(生地黄)•~(知母)	
~VAR34•**VAR178•VAR210•VAR238**	
~(黄连)•(炒枳壳)•(法半夏)•(柴胡)	

Table 2 Negative prime implicant results from insomnia dataset

Configuration	Freq.
VAR33•~VAR113•~VAR117•~VAR178•~VAR201•~VAR202•~VAR235•~VAR237	14
(茯苓)•~(生地黄)•~(陈皮)•~(炒枳壳)•~(生姜)•~(炒白术)•~(制远志)•~(炒酸枣仁)	
~VAR40•~VAR113•~VAR117•~VAR130•VAR175•~VAR237	11
~(石菖蒲)•~(生地黄)•~(陈皮)•~(龙齿)•(山药)•~(炒酸枣仁)	
VAR33•~VAR34•~VAR36•~VAR196•~VAR198•~VAR202•~VAR235•~VAR238•~VAR241	10
(茯苓)•~(黄连)•~(麦冬)•~(大枣)•~(山萸肉)•~(炒白术)•~(制远志)•~(柴胡)•~(牡蛎)	
~VAR34•~VAR40•~VAR84•~VAR113•~VAR117•~VAR196•VAR200•~VAR202•~VAR235	7
~(黄连)•~(石菖蒲)•~(薄荷)•~(生地黄)•~(陈皮)•~(大枣)•(生甘草)•~(炒白术)•~(制远志)	
~VAR79•~VAR113•~VAR117•~VAR175•VAR203•~VAR236•VAR241	7
~(肉桂)•~(生地黄)•~(陈皮)•~(山药)•(白芍)•~(知母)•(牡蛎)	
VAR34•~VAR40•~VAR79•~VAR117•~VAR198•~VAR202•~VAR203•~VAR241	7
(黄连)•~(石菖蒲)•~(肉桂)•~(陈皮)•~(山萸肉)•~(炒白术)•~(白芍)•~(牡蛎)	
VAR39•~VAR43•~VAR113•~VAR120•~VAR200•~VAR203•~VAR241•~VAR242	7
(莲子心)•~(淡豆豉)•~(生地黄)•~(五味子)•~(生甘草)•~(白芍)•~(牡蛎)•~(川芎)	
VAR76•~VAR130•~VAR178•VAR200•VAR210•~VAR241	6
(竹茹)•~(龙齿)•~(炒枳壳)•(生甘草)•(法半夏)•~(牡蛎)	
~VAR46•~VAR120•~VAR130•~VAR175•~VAR196•~VAR200•~VAR202•~VAR235•VAR236	6
~(炒枳实)•~(五味子)•~(龙齿)•~(山药)•~(大枣)•~(生甘草)•~(炒白术)•~(制远志)•(知母)	
VAR35•~VAR40•~VAR46•~VAR79•~VAR113•~VAR210•~VAR237	5
(黄芩)•~(石菖蒲)•~(炒枳实)•~(肉桂)•~(生地黄)•~(法半夏)•~(炒酸枣仁)	
VAR8•~VAR35•~VAR79•~VAR174•~VAR200•~VAR201•~VAR242	4
(党参)•~(黄芩)•~(肉桂)•~(当归)•~(生甘草)•~(生姜)•~(川芎)	
~VAR35•VAR113•~VAR174•~VAR202•~VAR237•~VAR242	3
~(黄芩)•(生地黄)•~(当归)•~(炒白术)•~(炒酸枣仁)•~(川芎)	
~VAR34•~VAR35•~VAR39•~VAR48•~VAR200•~VAR201•VAR203•~VAR210•~VAR241•~VAR242	3
~(黄连)•~(黄芩)•~(莲子心)•~(夜交藤)•~(生甘草)•(白芍)•~(法半夏)•~(牡蛎)•~(川芎)	
VAR1•VAR235•~VAR238	2
(太子参)•(制远志)•~(柴胡)	
VAR34•VAR113•VAR202•VAR238	1
(黄连)•(生地黄)•(炒白术)•(柴胡)	

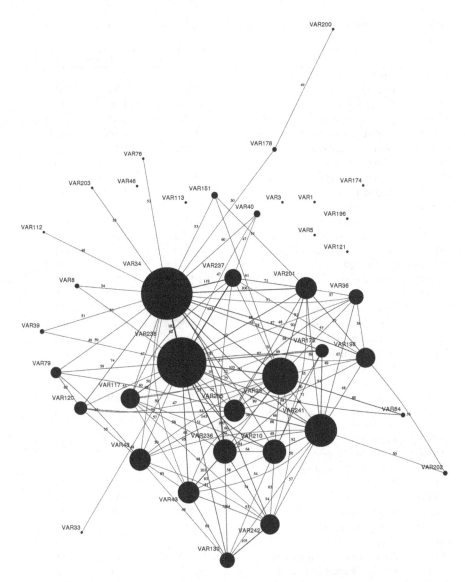

Fig. 5 Energy layout of insomnia frequency-based core herb network with 46 frequency threshold (10 % support threshold). The node size represents frequency of interaction and the edge label highlights the pairwise interaction frequency. (Figure 5 in high resolution with colour can be accessed at http://www.sydney.edu.au/it/~itcm/book/images/figure2-5.jpg). The full color version of this image may be viewed in the eBook edition

correlation network, in order to identify reasonably strong pairwise correlations, correlations greater than 0.2 threshold and less than −0.2 threshold of the insomnia dataset is shown in Fig. 6. The ±0.2 threshold is arbitrarily chosen to avoid a heavily dense network and thus to ensure a quick visual summary of core herbal combinations. Negatively correlated combinations are indicated with a dashed line and

Table 3 Degree centrality values and frequency calculated for each herb, using the full insomnia frequency network

Herb	Herb name	Chinese name	Centrality	Frequency
VAR237	Stir-frying spine date seed	炒酸枣仁	2,419	257
VAR33	Indian bread	茯苓	2,249	253
VAR34	Golden thread	黄连	1,580	165
VAR238	Chinese thorowax root	柴胡	1,576	174
VAR235	Prepared thinleaf milkwort root	制远志	1,554	166
VAR200	Fresh liquorice root	生甘草	1,456	165
VAR203	White peony root	白芍	1,377	153
VAR236	Common anemarrhena rhizome	知母	1,362	151
VAR210	Prepared pinellia tuber	法半夏	1,358	148
VAR196	Chinese date	大枣	1,248	132
VAR174	Chinese angelica	当归	1,200	139
VAR40	Grassleaf sweetflag rhizome	石菖蒲	1,167	130
VAR113	Dried/fresh rehmannia [root]	生地黄	1,127	131
VAR241	Oyster shell	牡蛎	1,111	120
VAR121	Dragon bone	龙骨	1,028	105
VAR79	Cassia bark	肉桂	995	98
VAR117	Dried tangerine peel	陈皮	972	106
VAR46	Stir-frying immature orange fruit	炒枳实	969	106
VAR242	Szechwan lovage rhizome	川芎	958	112
VAR35	Baical skullcap root	黄芩	940	109
VAR76	Bamboo shavings	竹茹	858	87
VAR39	Lotus plumule	莲子心	754	79
VAR130	Dragon teeth	龙齿	750	77
VAR202	Stir-frying largehead atractylodes rhizome	炒白术	673	86
VAR5	Lily bulb	百合	640	72
VAR36	Dwarf lilyturf tuber	麦冬	617	84
VAR48	Tuber fleeceflower stem	夜交藤	594	74
VAR8	Tangshen	党参	565	64
VAR112	Light wheat	浮小麦	565	58
VAR201	Fresh ginger	生姜	557	58
VAR175	Common yam rhizome	山药	536	70
VAR84	Peppermint	薄荷	510	54
VAR198	Asiatic cornelian cherry fruit	山黄肉	455	58
VAR120	Chinese magnoliavine fruit	五味子	372	46
VAR178	Stir-frying orange fruit	炒枳壳	357	50
VAR3	Phyllanthus ussuriensis	蜜甘草	317	40
VAR43	Fermented soybean	淡豆豉	278	33
VAR151	Arabic cowry shell	煅紫贝齿	275	26
VAR1	Heterophylly falsestarwort root	太子参	121	14

positively correlated combinations with a solid line where phi correlation values are indicated on the edges. Foundational frequency and correlation networks can therefore be constructed with strength and reliability estimators on each herbal combination edge.

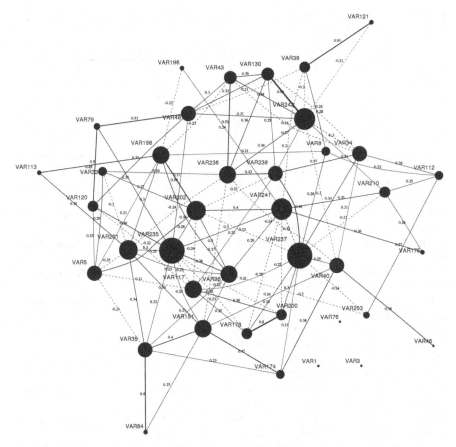

Fig. 6 Energy layout of insomnia correlation-based core herb network with ±0.2 threshold and correlation weighted edge weights, *dotted edges* indicate negative correlation, and node size indicate frequency of interaction for the given node. (Figure 6 in high resolution with colour can be accessed at http://www.sydney.edu.au/it/~itcm/book/images/figure2-6.jpg)

5.3 Results from Interaction Analysis

Frequency and correlation networks can suggest possible interactions between herbs that are interesting to test for. As the reduced frequency network displayed the majority of threshold prime implicant sets, only the cycles will be analysed as possible pair-wise interactions. Mathematically, this is expressed in Eq. 2 and can be similarly expanded for higher dimensions (e.g. Poon et al. 2011b).

$$(n_{11} + n_{00}) > (n_{01} + n_{10}) \tag{2}$$

where n_{ij} is the frequency of Herb i and Herb j where 1 indicates the presence of a herb and 0, absence.

Table 4 Interaction analysis of pairwise combinations derived from prime implicant connections in frequency and correlation networks

	Combination	Frequency	Good outcomes	Good outcome rate	Additiveness
VAR241	11+00	35+122	31+102	84.71	Sub-additive
VAR33	01+10	218+85	190+69	85.48	
VAR210	11+00	81+140	70+112	82.35	Sub-additive
VAR33	01+10	172+67	151+59	87.87	
VAR210	11+00	46+238	41+204	86.27	Super-additive
VAR241	01+10	74+102	59+88	83.52	
VAR175	11+00	46+179	46+142	83.56	Sub-additive
VAR237	01+10	211+24	191+13	86.81	
VAR113	11+00	56+219	53+174	82.55	Super-additive
VAR235	01+10	110+75	99+66	89.19	
VAR113	11+00	51+227	47+186	83.81	Super-additive
VAR203	01+10	102+80	87+72	87.36	
VAR113	11+00	24+244	21+200	82.46	Super-additive
VAR35	01+10	85+107	73+98	89.06	
VAR203	11+00	34+232	31+195	84.96	Super-additive
VAR35	01+10	75+119	63+103	85.57	
VAR200	11+00	90+220	89+180	86.77	Super-additive
VAR34	01+10	75+75	60+63	82.00	
VAR237	11+00	48+142	47+108	81.58	Sub-additive
VAR35	01+10	61+209	47+190	87.78	
VAR235	11+00	143+180	132+135	82.66	Super-additive
VAR237	01+10	114+23	105+20	91.24	
VAR203	11+00	46+247	43+214	87.71	Super-additive
VAR46	01+10	60+107	44+91	80.84	
VAR113	11+00	34+293	34+248	86.24	Super-additive
VAR175	01+10	36+97	25+85	82.71	
VAR203	11+00	100+150	93+114	82.80	Super-additive
VAR237	01+10	157+53	144+41	88.10	
VAR238	11+00	37+211	34+169	81.85	Super-additive
VAR242	01+10	75+137	68+121	89.15	
VAR33	11+00	32+175	32+144	85.02	Sub-additive
VAR8	01+10	32+221	27+189	85.38	

Table 4 summarises results of pairwise interaction analysis. Interpretation of the interaction analysis results will not be described here as the purpose of this chapter is to introduce a cause and effect methodology between herbs. Common node and cycle analysis can therefore identify effective higher order combinations by taking advantage of low correlated or low frequently ignored herbs.

5.4 Overall Results and Visualization

In order to visualise causal herb combinations, prime implicants are superimposed on the base frequency and correlation networks. The resulting frequency and

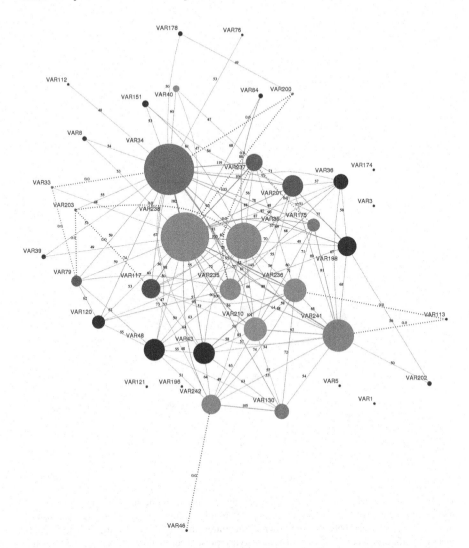

Fig. 7 Insomnia frequency network with superimposed prime implicants; *green edges* represent base frequency network; *red edges* represent prime implicant edges whereby the node pair results in a sub-additive effect; *blue edges* represent prime implicant edges whereby the node pair results in a super-additive effect. The node size represents degree of interaction in the base graph. *Blue nodes* represent nodes in the base network whereas the *red nodes* are prime implicant nodes. The degree of redness indicates frequency of presence in prime implicants (Figure 7 in high resolution with colour can be accessed at http://www.sydney.edu.au/it/~itcm/book/images/figure2-7.jpg)

correlation graphs are shown in Figs. 7 and 8. An energy layout is similar to the Kamada-Kawai algorithm was used for both core herb networks in Pajek (Batagelj and Mrvar 2003). This layout positions the graph such that the edge weights represent the edge length between two nodes. Higher frequency and correlated edges are therefore positioned closer together, and outlier frequency and correlation are further away from the primary network.

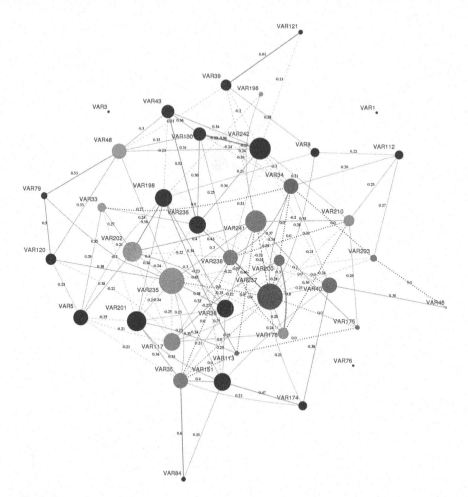

Fig. 8 Insomnia correlation network with super-imposed prime implicants; *green edges* represent base frequency network; *red edges* represent prime implicant edges whereby the node pair results in a sub-additive effect; *blue edges* represent prime implicant edges whereby the node pair results in a super-additive effect. Edges with a dashed style represent correlation <−0.2, edges with a solid style represent correlation >0.2 and edges with a dotted style represent correlation between −0.2 and 0.2. The node size represents degree of interaction in the base graph. *Blue nodes* represent nodes in the base network whereas the *red nodes* are prime implicant nodes. The degree of redness indicates frequency of presence in prime implicants (Figure 8 in high resolution with colour can be accessed at http://www.sydney.edu.au/it/~itcm/book/images/figure2-8.jpg) (The full color version of this image may be viewed in the eBook edition)

6   Discussion

The previous section describes the methodology and demonstrates its application on the insomnia dataset. Thus, general observations can be made from visualization of the results, though further analysis is necessary to conclude its validity.

Although two base visualisation and analysis methodologies, frequency and correlation, have been introduced the complexity of herb-herb interactions may affect the validity of these inferences. In the illustrated network construction, negative NOT(herb) results were ignored. These confounding factors remain to be addressed in future work. Confounding in statistics is where a factor that may exert an effect is not measured in the experiment; thus biasing any analysis performed. Herbal combinations that appear in both positive and negative frequency and correlation networks indicate there may be possible confounding herbal or background factors that are affecting accurate analysis of core herbs. Confounding may arise through herb to herb interactions and extend to different and higher order herbal configurations, particularly when herbs are interacting amongst other herbs. Auxiliary herbs may also give rise to confounding due to their dependencies on other core herbs. While auxiliary herbs may not contribute to core therapeutic effects, their high frequency of usage may cumulate to significant effects. In complex disease patterns, the use of auxiliary herbs may exceed those of principal herbs. Further, though confounding herbs may be observed, this does not necessitate the removal of those herbs, which may further bias and confound the analysis. Addressing confounding and the absence of an herb can therefore be useful to illuminating more significant core herbs and less useful herbs.

7 Conclusion

Successful TCM prescriptions depend on not just the presence of chosen herbs that make up a prescription, but the absence of other herbs may be equally important, especially for those herbs that are tightly connected to other herbs, as the later may impact negatively on the outcome. In this chapter, we have described and demonstrated an approach to discover the intertwining patterns of herbs in TCM prescriptions. Applying techniques in set-theoretic may distil the configuration where necessary herbs are required for the successful treatment. In addition, a network tool based on frequency of usage and correlation aided the understanding of domain knowledge choice of herbs as well as interesting factors that are worthwhile testing for. By further super-imposing positive outcome prime implicant results, a map of strong herb combinations with large positive outcome coverage can be inferred. This framework not only has validated results in consistence with earlier work performed by Zhou et al. (2011b), and also introduced a more efficient approach to reach configuration solutions form the causal complexity perspective.

Although this chapter introduces a computational approach for finding the useful herb combinations in the context of clinical outcomes. Several key issues still exist to be addressed in the future work. Firstly, two important information components, namely herb dosage and clinical manifestation (e.g. symptoms, co-morbid conditions), of the clinical data should be considered. Because it is widely recognized in the medical field that the herb dosage has an important effect for treatment and also performs a significant role for complex interactions amongst herbs. Secondly, by incorporating dosage information, the computing cost of moving crisp-set QCA to fuzzy-set QCA to find the optimal complex herbal formulations should be further studied.

References

V. Batagelj, A. Mrvar, *Pajek – Analysis and Visualization of Large Networks*. Graph Drawing Software, 3ed edn. (Springer, Berlin, 2003)

D. Ehring, Causal asymmetry. J. Philos. **79**(12), 761–774 (1982)

P. Fiser, J. Hlavicka, BOOM – a heuristic Boolean minimizer. Comput. Inform. **22**, 1001–1033 (2003)

P.C. Fiss, A set-theoretic approach to organisational configurations. Acad. Manage. Rev. **32**(4), 1180–1198 (2007). doi:10.5465/amr.2007.26586092

S.J. Hong, R.G. Cain, D.L. Ostapko, MINI: a heuristic approach for logic minimization. IBM. J. Res. Dev. **18**(5), 443–458 (1974). doi:10.1147/rd.185.0443

T.K. Jain, D.S. Kushwaha, A.K. Misra, Optimization of the Quine-McCluskey method for the minimization of the Boolean expressions, in *Autonomic and Autonomous Systems, 2008. ICAS 2008. Fourth International Conference on*, 16–21 Mar 2008, pp. 165–168. doi:10.1109/icas.2008.11

A. Kagliwal, S. Balachandran, Set-cover heuristics for two-level logic minimization, in *VLSI Design (VLSID), 2012 25th International Conference on*, 7–11 Jan 2012, pp. 197–202. doi:10.1109/vlsid.2012.70

D. Katz, R.L. Kahn, *The Social Psychology of Organizations*, 2nd edn. (Wiley, New York, 1978)

E.J. McCluskey, Minimization of Boolean functions. Bell. Syst. Tech. J. **35**(5), 1417–1444 (1956)

S.K. Poon, K. Fan, J. Poon, C. Loy, K. Chan, X. Zhou, R. Zhang, Y. Wang, J. Xie, B. Liu, P. Kwan, J. Gao, D. Sze, Analysis of herbal formulation in TCM: infertility as a case study, in *Proceedings of the International Workshop on Information Technology for Chinese Medicine, In Conjunction with the IEEE International Conference on Bioinformatics & Biomedicine (BIBM 2011)*, Atlanta, 12–15 Nov 2011a.

S.K. Poon, J. Poon, M. McGrane, X. Zhou, P. Kwan, R. Zhang, B. Liu, J. Gao, C. Loy, K. Chan, D. Sze, A novel approach in discovering significant interactions from TCM patient prescription data. Int. J. Data. Mining. Bioinform. **5**(4), 353–367 (2011b)

W.V.O. Quine, The problem of simplifying truth functions. Am. Math. Mon. **59**(8), 521–531 (1952)

W.V.O. Quine, A way to simplify truth functions. Am. Math. Mon. **62**, 627–631 (1955)

C.C. Ragin, *The Comparative Method: Moving Beyond Qualitative and Quantitative Strategies* (University of California Press, Berkeley, 1987)

C.C. Ragin, *Fuzzy Set Social Science* (Unuversity of Chicago Press, Chicago, 2000)

C.C. Ragin, *Redesigning Social Inquiry: Fuzzy Sets and Beyond* (University of Chicago Press, Chicago, 2008)

A. Su, S.K. Poon, J. Poon, Discovering causal patterns in TCM clinical prescription data using set-theoretic approach, in *Proceedings of the International Workshop on Information Technology for Chinese Medicine, In Conjunction with the IEEE International Conference on Bioinformatics & Biomedicine (BIBM 2013)*, Shanghai, 18–21 Dec 2013

X. Zhou, S. Chen, B. Liu, R. Zhang, Y. Wang, P. Li, H. Zhang, Z. Gao, X. Yan, Development of traditional Chinese medicine clinical data warehouse for medical knowledge discovery and decision support. Artif. Intell. Med. **48**(2-3), 139–152 (2010a)

X. Zhou, J. Poon, P. Kwan, R. Zhang, Y. Wang, S.K. Poon, B. Liu, D. Sze, Novel two-stage analytic approach in extraction of strong herb-herb interactions in TCM clinical treatment of insomnia, in *Medical Biometrics*, ed. by D. Zhang, M. Sonka, vol. 6165 (Springer, Berlin/Heidelberg, 2010b)

Medical Diagnosis by Using Machine Learning Techniques

Mingyu You and Guo-Zheng Li

Abstract There are many challenges in data analytic research for TCM (Traditional Chinese Medicine), like various clinical record sources, different symptom descriptions, lots of collected clinical symptoms, more than one syndrome attached to one clinical record and etc. Novel methods on feature selection, multi-class, and multi-label techniques in machine learning field are proposed to meet the challenges. Here in this chapter, we will introduce our works on discriminative symptoms selection and multi-syndrome learning, which have improved the performance of state-of-arts works.

1 Introduction

With the increasing digitized data collection, TCM clinical data analysis has attracted more interests from TCM researchers and machine learning scientists. Various established machine learning techniques help to achieve remarkable improvements in TCM data analysis. Considering its own characteristics, TCM data analytic research still brings great challenges to machine learning techniques.

- Numerous symptoms can be recorded in clinical process. But high dimensional features will hurt the modeling performance of machine learning methods. How to select appropriate symptom subset for a certain disease in the data analytic process is a critical problem for data modeling and understanding.
- Usually, a patient is diagnosed as having more than one syndrome in TCM. Clinical data modeling can be abstracted as multi-class or even multi-label problem. Existing machine learning techniques are excellent on binary classification. Multi-class and multi-label modeling is still a challenge to machine learning researches.

M. You · G.-Z. Li (✉)
Department of Control Science and Engineering, Tongji University, Shanghai, China
e-mail: gzli@tongji.edu.cn

J. Poon and S.K. Poon (eds.), *Data Analytics for Traditional Chinese Medicine Research*,
DOI 10.1007/978-3-319-03801-8_3, © Springer International Publishing Switzerland 2014

To face the above challenges in clinical data analysis, this chapter describes the novel techniques on discriminative symptoms selection and multi-syndrome learning. Applications include feature selection for lip diagnosis, symptom selection for inquiry diagnosis of coronary heart disease, multiple syndrome classification for medical diagnosis and syndrome classification of hypertension with feature fusion.

Most TCM machine learning works does not consider the medical meaning and links among features. However, TCM data contain a large quantity of symptoms or syndromes which have specific medical meaning. Therefore, seeking the links between features including symptoms and syndromes in TCM data analysis is also important.

Among a large number of symptoms in TCM diagnosis data sets for a certain disease, some symptoms may be redundant. Therefore, selecting major or relevant symptoms is crucial to the performance of machine learning. Wang et al. (2009a) used SVM (Support Vector Machine) to generalize symptom weights in CHD (Coronary Heart Disease) predictions. Liu et al. (2010)used symptom frequency analysis to enhance modeling results in learning. Zhou et al. (2010) developed a clinical RIM (Reference Information Model) and a physical data model to manage various entities and relationships in TCM clinical data. PCA (Principal component analysis) (Jolliffe 1986), PLS (Partial Least Squares) (Helland 1990), MRMR (Maximum Relevance and Minimum Redundancy) (Peng et al. 2005) have been used to perform symptom selection to improve prediction accuracy.

The results from conventional primary symptom selection or reduction methods are difficult to be interpreted in TCM. For instance, PCA reduces symptom dimensionality at the expense of losing medical meaning (Lu et al. 2011). Although MRMR can predict fairly using only a few major symptoms (Hu and Wu 2007), the results are often inconsistent with basic TCM theory (Deng 1984; Wang 2004). This study aims to use RAD (Relative Associated Density) to perform symptom selection, and evaluate whether the results can be better explained by TCM theory (Deng 1984; Wang 2004).

Multi-label learning is usually referred to high-dimensional data, but there are very few dimension reduction methods and feature selection methods available for multi-label data due to the complexity of multi-label learning. As to feature dimensionality reduction, the recently published MDDM (Multi-label Dimensionality reduction via Dependence Maximization) (Zhang et al. 2010) is a feature extraction method which uses the HSIC as the performance criteria and attempts to project the original data into a lower-dimensional feature space to maximize the dependence of the original feature description on the associated class labels. Experiments show MDDM is slightly superior to PCA and nonlinear dimensionality reduction method LPP, and is significantly superior to the multi-label dimensionality reduction method MLSI (Yu et al. 2005). Linear Dimensionality Reduction (Ji et al. 2009) shows improved performance when the least squares and other loss functions, including the hinge loss and the squared hinge loss, are used in multi-label classification. One problem of MDDM and Linear Dimensionality Reduction is that the original low-dimensional features cannot be obtained, which poses an obstacle to scientific understanding of scientific problems.

Feature selection attempts to remove irrelevant and redundant features and entails choosing the smallest number of features to adequately represent the data and maximizing the prediction or classification accuracy. Feature selection distinctly improves the comprehensibility of the classification model and builds a model which can better predict the unknown samples. It has practical significance. For example, extensive experiences are needed to grasp the main symptom in TCM differential treatment. The current feature selection methods are divided into three broad categories: wrappers, filters, and embedded methods (Guyon and Elisseeff 2003). Wrappers depend on the learning machine and utilize the learning machine of interest as a black box to score feature subsets according to their predictive power. Although the wrapper methods are comparative time-consuming, they are widely used in scientific data analysis because the selected feature subset is optimal to the specific learning machine due to its mechanism that the selection result is based on the learning algorithms. In multi-label feature selection, MEFS (Embedded Feature Selection for Multi-Label Learning) (Ge et al. 2009) was proposed last year, in which sequential backward search algorithm is adopted to search the feature subset, and the prediction risk criterion (Moody and Utans 1992) is used to evaluate the performance of the feature subset. In wrappers, a comparatively good result was achieved when the genetic algorithm was introduced (Zhang et al. 2009).

Multiple possible syndromes in TCM clinical diagnosis result raise a multi-class problem, which is more popular in real-world applications. Meanwhile, a few works have been devoted to the study of multi-class data sets with skew distribution (Zhou and Liu 2006). In designing data mining algorithms, it is often easier first to devise algorithms for distinguishing between only two classes. Some data mining algorithms, such as K-Nearest-Neighbour, Neural Network and C4.5 (Quinlan 1993) can then be naturally extended to handle the multi-class case. For other algorithms, such as AdaBoost (Schapire and Singer 1999) and the SVM algorithm (Cortes and Vapnik 1995), a direct extension to the multi-class case may be problematic. Typically, in such cases, the multi-class problem is reduced to multiple binary classification problems that can be solved separately. SVM is a classifier widely researched and applied. There are many ways designed to use a combination of several binary SVM classifiers to solve a given multi-class problem. In one-versus-rest SVM, the ith SVM will be trained with the examples in the ith class with positive labels, and all other examples with negative labels. In one-versus-one SVM, each classifier will be trained on only two out of N classes. DAG (Directed Acyclic Graph) SVM is a decision tree structured graph, with each node distinguishing two classes (Platt et al. 2000). Hastie and Tibshirani (1998) proposed a strategy called pairwise coupling for combining posterior probabilities provided by individual binary classifiers for multi-class classification. As SVMs do not naturally output posterior probabilities, they suggested a particular way of generating these probabilities from the binary SVM outputs. Based on their idea, Platt (1999) suggested a properly designed sigmoid applied to the SVM (shortly, sig_SVM) output to form these probabilities. All these methods are sophistically designed and propose superior performance. However, the imbalanced data distributions among classes are not taken into consideration.

The imbalanced problem is concerned by many researchers (He and Garcia 2009). Sampling methods, cost-sensitive methods and kernel-based methods are all devoted to imbalanced classification. Most of them concentrate on two-class imbalanced mining problem. In the previous works, an APLSC (Asymmetric PLS Classifier) is proposed to balance the sensitivity of minority class and the specificity of majority class (Qu et al. 2010). It inherits the advantage of PLSC, which is prone to protect the minority class and to boost the performance on the majority class. However, APLSC is still confined to binary problems. In this paper, we focus on the multi-class problem, which is a remarkable characteristic of TCM clinical data. In addition, the severe distribution imbalance among classes is elaborated researched. As APLSC is devised for binary classification, this paper ensembles multiple APLSCs to establish MAPLSC (Multiple Asymmetric PLS Classifier) for the multi-class problem. Each APLSC classifier in MAPLSC distinguishes a pair of classes and the posterior probability calculated from the classifier's output is used for finally combination. A new coming example is labeled as the class with maximal posterior probability sum.

Syndrome in TCM means a characteristic profile of all clinical manifestations that can be identified by a TCM practitioner. In the field of data mining, differentiation of syndrome is modeled as a classification problem. For traditional classification methods, every instance should have one and only one label. However, TCM diagnostic result usually consists of several syndromes. In other words, one patient could have more than one syndrome. Professionally, it is called multi-label data, the learning of which is a rather hot topic recently in the fields of data mining and machine learning. International workshops about multi-label learning are held in recent 3 years respectively to promote the development of this topic (Zhang 2010; Tsoumakas et al. 2009). Multi-label learning has been applied to TCM (Guo-Ping et al. 2010), which compared the performance of ML-kNN and kNN on a coronary heart disease dataset. You et al. and Shao et al. proposed embedded multi-label feature selection method MEFS (Ge et al. 2009) and wrapper multi-label feature selection method HOML (Shao et al. 2011) respectively to improve multi-label classification's performance on a coronary heart disease dataset.

One characteristic of TCM syndrome differentiation is "Fusion use of four classical diagnostic methods". Inspection, auscultation and olfaction, inquiry and palpation are the four classical diagnostic methods in TCM. How to use information from these four diagnostic methods to make better syndrome differentiation is an important research area in TCM field. Some theories of traditional Chinese medicine diagnosis even claim that only by using information from all the four classical diagnostic methods can we differentiate correctly the syndrome (Deng 2004). And "Fusion use of the four classical diagnostic methods" is treated as an important direction in computerization of TCM diagnosis (Wang 2010). In fact, it is called information fusion in the field of data mining. Therefore, fusion of information from different sources should be considered seriously in building syndrome classification with multi-label learning techniques. Nowadays, no researchers have tried to bring techniques of information fusion into the field of multi-label learning. Wang et al. have done some work in TCM information fusion using traditional single-label methods, which mainly focus on the data acquisition and medical analysis on experiment results (Wang 2010; Wang et al. 2009a, b). But as described above, multi-label learning should be more appropriate for syndrome classification. So more attentions should be paid on the research of information fusion for multi-label learning.

In this chapter we will introduce our works on medical diagnosis processing by using novel machine learning techniques, we focus on how to select appropriate symptom features, and improve the medical diagnosis performance. RAD (relative associated density) and HOML (Hybrid Optimization based Multi-Label) feature selection methods, MAPLSC (Multiple Asymmetric Partial Least Squares Classifier) and Fusion-MLKNN (Fusion-Multilabel K Nearest Neighbor) analytic models will be described and demonstrated on CHD, lip color, and hypertension data sets. The rest of this chapter is arranged as follows: Sect. 1 presents computational methods including RAD, HOML, MAPLSC and Fusion-MLKNN; Sect. 2 describes the TCM applications of all the methods proposed; Then Sect. 3 gives the description of data sets. The chapter ends in the summery of Sect. 4.

2 Computational Methods

2.1 The RAD Method

Conventional methods usually use only one numerical value to describe the relationship of two symptoms. In this study, we use a pair of characteristic values to describe a relative link between the symptoms as a relative associated density (RAD). By analyzing the characteristic value pairs, we searched significant one-way links between symptoms and confirmed the links according to CM theory (Deng 1984; Wang 2004). The RAD method was also used to find one-way links among multiple syndromes in the clinical data.

Probability and statistics in the medical diagnosis of CHD, frequency of symptom occurrence may be different. For instance, the chest tightness symptom and the dizziness symptom are frequent symptoms, while the sleepiness symptom and the diarrhea with undigested food symptom are rare symptoms. In the data analysis, the first step is to distinguish between the frequent and the rare symptoms.

In probability of symptoms, Pf_i stands for the appearance probability of the ith symptom across all cases, which is defined as

$$Pf_i = \frac{\sum_{m=1}^{N} F_{im}}{N} \tag{1}$$

where $F_{im} = 1$ if the ith symptom appears in the mth case, or else $F_{im} = 0$. N denotes the number of the cases.

Similarly, Pl_i stands for the appearance probability of the ith syndrome across all cases, which is defined as

$$Pl_i = \frac{\sum_{m=1}^{N} L_{im}}{N} \tag{2}$$

where the ith syndrome appears in the mth sample, $L_{im}=1$, or else $L_{im}=0$.

2.1.1 Building the Symptom-Symptom Interaction Network

Equations 1 and 2 calculate the appearance probability of all symptoms and syndromes. But these values cannot reveal their potential connections. Symptom symptom interaction (SSI) network in the same manner as used for human social networks was used to find the connections (Hu and Wu 2007; Kerstin and Wolfgang 2009).

When two different symptoms occur simultaneously in the same case, sign $G_{ijm}=1$ indicating that symptom F_i and symptom F_j appear at the same time in the mth case, or else $G_{ijm}=0$. F_iF_j stands for the number of simultaneous occurrences of F_i and F_j. Then for N cases,

$$F_iF_j = \sum_{m=1}^{N} G_{ijm} \tag{3}$$

which contains two types of information: the frequency of features and the relevancy of two features.

2.1.2 Relative Associated Density

Equation 3 is largely concerned with the frequency of symptoms. In other words, frequent relationships between symptoms are obvious, while less frequent relationships are hard to be detected. The difference is even more than 300 folds. Therefore, this study used RAD, which uses conditional probability to measure the relationships of symptoms and syndromes.

The term $C(F_i, F_j)$ represents the RAD values of symptom F_i associated with F_j and use $C(F_i, F_j)$ represents the RAD values of symptom F_i associated with F_j. According,

$$C\left(F_i, F_j\right) = \frac{F_iF_j}{\sum_{m=1}^{N} F_{im}} \tag{4a}$$

$$C\left(F_j, F_i\right) = \frac{F_iF_j}{\sum_{m=1}^{N} F_{jm}} \tag{4b}$$

2.1.3 Symptom Selection with RAD

In the mth case, if symptom F_i appears with syndrome L_j, $H_{ijm}=1$; otherwise, $H_{ijm}=0$. Then for all N cases,

$$F_i L_j = \sum_{m=1}^{N} H_{ijm} \tag{5}$$

RAD estimates the influence of the appearance probability on the interaction between a symptom and a syndrome. Equation 6 calculates the RAD value between symptoms and syndromes,

$$C(F_i, L_j) = \frac{F_i L_j}{\sum_{m=1}^{N} L_{jm}} \tag{6}$$

This kind of association could be recognized as the contribution of one symptom to the syndrome.

Each syndrome was considered a single label; thus we selected corresponding symptoms regardless of their RAD values. For each single label prediction, the symptoms with low RAD values were removed one by one, and the predictions were calculated with SVM and KNN. The symptoms that lead to the highest prediction were recorded as the result of symptom selection.

2.2   The HOML Algorithm

Genetic algorithm has been used to analyze feature selection for multi-label data (Ge et al. 2009), but the algorithms only combine the MLNB algorithm, and the genetic algorithm has its limitation in optimization. The performance of feature selection may be further improved if advantages of different optimization techniques are combined together to search for an optimal subset of features. We propose to combine three search algorithms in this chapter: mutation-based simulated annealing, genetic algorithm and the greedy algorithm hill-climbing. HOML combines the ability to avoid being trapped in a local minimum of simulated annealing algorithm with a very high rate of convergence of the crossover operator of genetic algorithm and the strong local search ability of the greedy algorithm to obtain the optimal feature subset. Some work has shown that a hybrid technique generated better feature subsets than separate search algorithms (Gheyas and Smith 2010).

Selection is an important aspect of evolutionary computation. It dictates what members of the current population affect the next generation. More fit individuals are generally given a higher chance to participate in the recombination process. The primary concern of all selection schemes is what's known as the loss of diversity. As

HC (FN)
Input : FN: Feature subset
Output : BF: The optimized feature subset

while (Th>0)
   HC(BF) {
     if (Th > 0) then
       [NF] = CreateNeighbours(BF) ;   %Change one feature each time and get N neighbors of BF
       [EM] = EvaluateFitness(NF);   %Evaluate the new feature subset
       [ACC] = Replace(FS, NF);   %If EM(i)>E(i), replace FS[i] with NF[i]. ACC represents set
                                       % which contains improved feature subset.
       for i=1:Num(ACC)   %Make hill-climbing on each improved feature subset
         BF = HC(ACC(i));
       end for;
       UpdateTime (Th);   %Update time available for HC.
     end if;
   end for;}

Fig. 1 Procedure of hill climbing

a result, information encoded in the current population is not transferred into the next generation in its entirety. Loss of diversity has been measured and analyzed for a number of popular selection algorithms (Blickle and Thiele 1996; Motoki 2002). For the problem of loss of diversity, unbiased tournament selection (Sokolov and Whitley 2005) yields better results, and it is used in HOML.

In the feature selection process of HOML, experiment shows better result when using Average Precision than using (hammingloss + rankingloss). And Average Precision is used as the fitness of feature subset. That is to say, in the training process, we adopt the test result Average_Precision, which is obtained by modeling the validation set using multi-label learning techniques such as ML-KNN (Zhang and Zhou 2007), BP-MLL (Zhang and Zhou 2006), Rank-SVM (Elisseeff and Weston 2002) and MLNB-BASIC (Zhang et al. 2009), as the fitness function to evaluate the performance of feature subset.

Hill climbing is a recursive process, as shown in Fig. 1. Figure 2 shows the algorithm flow of HOML, which organizes a search in three stages.

Stage 1: HOML employs a SA (simulated annealing) to guide the global search in a solution space. As long as the temperature is very high, SA accepts every solution, thus yielding a near random search through the search space. On the other

HOML (X , Y, Tk, Tg, Th)

Input :

X: $N \times D$ feature matrix
Y: $N \times Q$ label matrix
Tk: Run time for Simulated Annealing (SA)
Tg: Run time for Genetic Algorithm (GA)
Th: Run time for Hill Climbing (HC)

Output :

BF   :Optimal feature subset

Procedure :

FS = InitIndividual();   %Initialize FS with 100 feature subsets
%Simulated annealing
E = EvaluateFitness(FS);   % E(i)=Average_Precision(FS(i))
Tc = UpdateTime(Tk);   %Update the time available time for SA
while (Tc > 0)
    FM = Mutate(FS, Pm);   %Mutate FS with probability Pm, Pm =
0.5-0.5exp(Tc/ λ) , λ=Tk/log2(0.5)
      for i=1:100
        if (Fitness(FM(i)) >= E(i))
            FS(i) = FM(i);   %Replace FS(i) with FM(i)
        else if (exp(-(E(i)-Fitness(FM(i)) < rand)   %Selectively accept the new feature subset
            FS(i) = FM(i);
        end if;
        UpdateTime(Tc);   %Update time available for SA.
      end for;
end while;
%Genetic algorithm
while (Tg>0)
    [FS,E] = Select(FS);   %Select with unbiased tournament selection
    [FS,E] = Crossover(FS, 0.65);   % Cross with probability 0.65
    [FS,E] = Mutation(FS,0.01);   % Mutate with probability 0.01
    [E] = EvaluateFitness(FS);   % Evaluate the new solutions
    UpdateTime(Tg);   % Update time available for GA
%Hill climbing
while (Th > 0){
    Order(FS);   %Sort FS by fitness value descending.
    for   i=1:100
      BF = FS(i);
      BF = HC(BF);
    End for;
End while.

Fig. 2 Procedure of HOML

hand, as the temperature becomes close to zero, only improvements are accepted. The SA is run for approximately 50 % of the total time available.

Stage 2: HOML employs a GA (genetic algorithm) to perform optimization. The GA population is set at 100. The initial population consists of the best solutions detected by SA. The crossover operator enables the good solutions to exchange information, and the mutation operator in GA introduces new genes into the population and retains genetic diversity. The GA runs for about 30 % of total time spent by HOML to find the optimal feature subset solution.

Stage 3: HOML applies a hill-climbing feature selection algorithm. The greedy algorithm performs a local search on the k-best solutions on the k-best (k represents the dimensionality of feature) solutions given by two global optimization algorithms (SA and GA) and selects the best neighbors. The hill-climbing algorithm is run in the remaining execution time.

The HOML algorithm is implemented on the platform of MATLAB, which is downloaded at http://levis.tongji.edu.cn/gzli/code/homl-code.zip.

2.3 The MAPLSC Algorithm

APLSC is an asymmetric PLS classifier, which sophisticatedly researches into the imbalanced distribution between classes. MAPLSC is an extension of classifier APLSC to the multi-class problem. Before demonstrating the algorithm of MAPLSC, we review the main steps of APLSC (Qu et al. 2010). The APLSC algorithm can be summarized as the following two steps. Firstly, normalized feature vectors are conducted feature extraction by PLS method. Secondly, compressed vectors are classified by translated hyper plane, which is influenced by the variance of low dimensional data.

PLS is a supervised feature extraction method (Li et al. 2008; Zeng et al. 2009). Consider a set of M-dimensional features and its class label vector denoted as $X \in R^{N \times M}$ and $y \in R^N$, where N is the number of examples. PLS is used to model the relations between the two blocks. Its classical form is based on the Nonlinear Iterative Partial Least Squares (NIPALS) algorithm (Wold 1975). NIPALS finds appropriate weight vectors w and c such that:

$$\max \left[\text{cov}(\mathbf{t}, \mathbf{u}) \right]^2 = \max \left[\text{cov}(\mathbf{Xw}, \mathbf{yc}) \right]^2 \qquad (7)$$

where $\mathbf{t}$ and $\mathbf{u}$ are score vectors of X and yy, respectively. $\text{cov}(\mathbf{t}, \mathbf{u}) = \mathbf{t}^T \mathbf{u}/N$ denotes the sample covariance between score vectors. The iteration process of PLS is summarized as Fig. 3.

Introduce a two-dimensional binary toy data set for illustration in Fig. 4. The majority class is signed by 'cross', whereas the minority class by 'circle'. Class distribution obeys Gaussian distribution. As observed from Fig. 4, feature vectors after PLS have prominent separable property. The first projection direction of PLS (the dot dash line in Fig. 4) contains most of the feature information and a dashed

Input: Feature set $\mathbf{X}$
           Label $\mathbf{y}$

           Number of components k
Output: Projection matrix $\mathbf{W}$, score vectors $\mathbf{T}$ and $\mathbf{U}$, parameter $\mathbf{V}$ and loading $\mathbf{Q}$

1: $\mathbf{E}_0 = \mathbf{X}$, $\mathbf{F}_0 = \mathbf{y}$, $\mathbf{w} = []$; $\mathbf{T} = []$; $\mathbf{U} = []$; $\mathbf{V} = []$; $\mathbf{Q} = []$; $\mathbf{u}_0 = \mathbf{y}$

2: **for** $i = 1$ to k **do**

3:      $\mathbf{w}_i = \mathbf{E}_{i-1}^T \mathbf{u}_{i-1} / (\mathbf{u}_{i-1}^T \mathbf{u}_{i-1})$;

4:      $\mathbf{w}_i = \mathbf{w}_i / \|\mathbf{w}_i\|$;

5:      $\mathbf{t}_i = \mathbf{E}_{i-1} \mathbf{w}_i$;

6:      $\mathbf{c}_i = \mathbf{F}_{i-1}^T \mathbf{t}_i / (\mathbf{t}_i^T \mathbf{t}_i)$;

7:      $\mathbf{c}_i = \mathbf{c}_i / \|\mathbf{c}_i\|$;

8:      $\mathbf{u}_i = \mathbf{F}_{i-1} \mathbf{c}_i$;

9:      $v_i = \mathbf{u}_i^T \mathbf{t}_i / (\mathbf{t}_i^T \mathbf{t}_i)$;

10:     $q_i = \mathbf{F}_{i-1}^T \mathbf{u}_i / (\mathbf{u}_i^T \mathbf{u}_i)$;

11:     $\mathbf{E}_i = \mathbf{E}_{i-1} - \mathbf{t}_i \mathbf{t}_i^T \mathbf{E}_{i-1} / (\mathbf{t}_i^T \mathbf{t}_i)$;

12:     $\mathbf{F}_i = \mathbf{F}_{i-1} - v_i \mathbf{t}_i q_i$;

13:     $\mathbf{w} = [\mathbf{w}, \mathbf{w}_i]$; $\mathbf{T} = [\mathbf{T}, \mathbf{t}_i]$; $\mathbf{U} = [\mathbf{U}, \mathbf{u}_i]$; $\mathbf{V} = [\mathbf{V}, v_i]$; $\mathbf{Q} = [\mathbf{Q}, q_i]$;

14: **end   for**

Fig. 3 Partial Least Squares (PLS)

line going through the data centre point and perpendicular to the first projection direction can act as a distinguish line between the two classes. The PLS classification model is represented as:

$$\tilde{Y} = sign\left(\sum_{i=1}^{k} m_i \mathbf{t}_i\right) = sign(\mathbf{t} \cdot \mathbf{m}) \tag{8}$$

Fig. 4 A toy dataset for APLSC demonstration (see online version for colours)

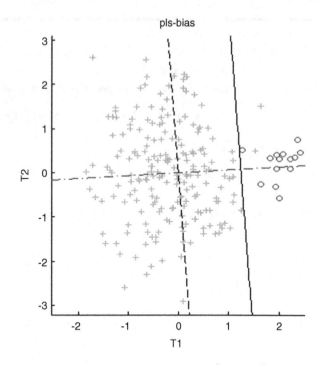

where $\mathbf{t}_i$ is the ith score vector of $\mathbf{X}$, and $m_i = v_i q_i$.

Because of the imbalanced distribution, the data center point is closer to the examples of majority class. As the distinguish line passes across the majority class and away from the minority class (shown in Fig. 4), the PLS Classifier (PLSC) misclassifies some majority class examples to minority class. The previous work (Qu et al. 2010) solves the problem of PLSC by moving the distinguishing line, which is demonstrated in Fig. 4. Classification model is revised as (namely APLSC):

$$\tilde{Y} = sign\left(\mathbf{t} \cdot \mathbf{m} - b\right) \tag{9}$$

where $b = m_1 \times (M_o - r_o \times c)$, $c = (M_o - M_c)/(r_o + r_c)$. M_o and M_c are the centers of score vectors belonging to the positive and negative classes on the first dimension, r_o and r_c indicates radius of two circles. For more information about APLSC, please refer to Qu et al. (2010).

APLSC is designed for binary problems. Multiple APLSC classifiers are combined to form MAPLSC for multi-class classification. Hastie and Tibshirani (1998) suggested a pairwise coupling strategy for combining the probabilistic outputs of all the one-versus-one binary classifiers to obtain estimates of the posterior probabilities $p_1, p_2, \cdots, p_n$ for all candidate classes. The p_is are computed using the following iterative procedure in Algorithm 2.

In Fig. 5, $\mu_{ij} = p_i/(p_i + p_j)$, n_{ij} is the number of examples in class C_i and class C_j. r_{ij} is the posterior probability of the positive class in the binary classifier. Output

Algorithm 2. The Pairwise coupling Algorithm
1). Start from an initial guess of p_i s and corresponding μ_{ij} s
2). Repeat $(i = 1, 2, \cdots, K, 1, \cdots)$ until convergence:
$-p_i \leftarrow p_i \cdot \dfrac{\sum_{j \neq i} n_{ij} r_{ij}}{\sum_{j \neq i} n_{ij} \mu_{ij}}$
– renormalize the p_i s
– recompute μ_{ij} s

Fig. 5 The pairwise coupling algorithm

function of APLSC is $f = \mathbf{t} \cdot \mathbf{m} - b$, and it cannot be interpreted as probability. Platt (1999) proposes approximating the posterior by a sigmoid function for SVM, which can be easily transferred to APLSC:

$$\Pr ob\left(C_i \mid x\right) = \frac{1}{1 + \exp\left(Af + B\right)} \tag{10}$$

where f is the output of the APLSC associated with example x. Platt (1999) uses a Levenberg-Marquardt (LM) algorithm to calculate the parameters A and B in Eq. 4. Li et al. (2008) and Lin et al. (2007) criticise the disadvantage of LM algorithm when solving Eq. 4, and propose Newton's method. In MAPLSC, we adopt Newton's method to decide the parameters A and B.

For combining the posterior probabilities from multiple binary APLSC, pairwise coupling described in Fig. 5 is adopted in MAPLSC. Actually,

$$\tilde{p}_i = 2 \sum_j r_{ij} / k\left(k - 1\right) \tag{11}$$

is an easier way for binary combination. In which, k is the number of classes. As proved by the theorem 1 in (Hastie and Tibshirani 1998), $\tilde{p}_i > \tilde{p}_j$ if and only if $p_i > p_j$, which is also revealed in our experimental results stated in section 3.3. In MAPLSC, we actually want to get the sequencing of the p_is of all classes, instead of the exact value of each p_i. So, for simplicity, $\tilde{p}_i$ instead of p_i is mostly employed in MAPLSC implementation.

The algorithm of MAPLSC is summarized in Fig. 6.

Algorithm 3. The MAPLSC Algorithm

Training section

Input: training dataset D, the number of classes k

Output: MAPLSC classifier

1) Set up $k(k-1)/2$ subsets from the dataset D, each subset S_{ij} is composed of the

   examples from class C_i and class C_j.

2) Train classifier $APLSC_{ij}$ with the examples in S_{ij}, and obtain output f_m from

   $APLSC_{ij}$ for each example x_m in S_{ij}.

3) Calculate parameters A_{ij} and B_{ij} in Equation (4), with output f_ms of examples x_ms

   in S_{ij}.

4) Output classifier MAPLSC with $k(k-1)/2$ $APLSC_{ij}$ and the corresponding posterior

   probability parameters A_{ij} and B_{ij}.

Test section:

Input: MAPLSC classifier and the corresponding posterior probability parameters, test example
x_t

Output: predicted label $\tilde{y}_t$ for test example x_t

1) Calculate the output f_t^{ij} from $APLSC_{ij}$ for test example x_t, $k(k-1)/2$ outputs

totally.

2) Calculate the posterior probability output $r_{ij} = \text{Prob}(C_i or C_j | x_t)$ by Equation (4), with

parameters A_{ij} and B_{ij} and the output f_t^{ij}.

3) Combine the $k(k-1)/2$ output f_t^{ij}s, by Equation (5), get the probabilities on k

classes $(\tilde{p}_1, \tilde{p}_2, \cdots, \tilde{p}_k)$.

4) Predict label for x_t by $y_t = \arg\max_i p_i$

Fig. 6 The MAPLSC algorithm

2.4 The Fusion-MLKNN Algorithm

In this work, we only discuss information fusion on the level of feature (Ross and Govindarajan 2005; Ross and Jain 2003). Let A, B, C, D, E denote respectively the five feature vectors with different dimensions illustrated in Tables 13, 14, 15, 16 and 17. The target is to combine these five feature sets in order to yield a new feature vector, Z, which would better represent the individual or help build better classification model (Ross and Govindarajan 2005). Specifically, information fusion is accomplished by simply augmenting the information (feature) obtained from multiple diagnostic methods. The vector Z is generated by augmenting vectors A to B, C, D and E one after another. The concrete stages are described below:

(1) Feature Normalization: The individual feature values of particular vectors, such as a_{11} and b_{m2}, may exhibit significant variations both in their range and distribution. The goal of feature normalization is to modify the location (mean) and scale (variance) of the values to ensure that the contribution of each vector to the final vector Z is comparable. Min-max normalization techniques were used in this work. It computes the value x' after normalization using the formula,

$x' = \dfrac{x - \min(Fx)}{\max(Fx) - \min(Fx)} /$, where x and x' denote respectively a feature value

before and after normalization and Fx is the feature value set that contains all value of a specific feature. Normalize all feature value via this method and we get the modified feature vectors $A', B, C', D', and E'$.

(2) Feature Concatenation: Augment the five feature vectors, which results in a new feature vector, $Z' = \{a_1', \ldots, a_n', b_1', \ldots, b_m', \ldots, e_1', \ldots, e_l'\}$.

As illustrated in Sect. 1, multi-label learning model is believed to be more suitable classification model for TCM clinical data. Specifically, we constructed models of the relationship between symptoms and syndrome by means of the multi-label k-nearest neighbor (ML-kNN) algorithm (Zhang and Zhou 2007) in this study. ML-kNN is a lazy multi-label learning algorithm developed on the basis of kNN algorithm, which regards an instance as a point in synthesis space. kNN's idea is to search for k training instances nearest to the testing instance, and then predict the label of the test instance according to the nearest instances' labels. Compared with other algorithms, advantage of kNN lies in its simpler training process, better efficiency, and competitive performance. Based on the theory of kNN, ML-kNN also aims to find k nearest instances for each test instance. But rather than judging labels directly by nearest instances, ML-kNN utilizes the "maximum a posteriori estimation" principle to determine the label set based on statistical information derived from the label sets of neighboring instances. The concrete steps are demonstrated below (Guo-Ping et al. 2010):

(1) Calculate the conditional probability distribution of each instance associated to each label;
(2) Calculate the distance between the x_i test instance and the training instances; then find k nearest instances for x_i. Repeat for each test instance;

(3) According to the labels of k training instances and the conditional probability associated to each label, forecast the probability of the x_i instance and then acquire the forecast results ($\geq$0.5 is taken here); Repeat for each test instance;

(4) Evaluate the forecast results according to multi label evaluation criteria.

3 Applications

3.1 Symptom Selection by Using RAD on the CHD Data Set

RAD performed better than MRMR in feature selection for machine learning to discover CM relationships among the symptoms, syndromes, and even between the symptoms and syndromes in a CHD data set. RAD analysis found one-way connections among symptoms and the syndromes that are consistent with CM theory. RAD not only improves prediction accuracy but also enhanced interpretability.

According to CM theory (Deng 1984; Wang 2004), a symptom is an expression of internal syndrome, and a syndrome is essential to symptom appearance. The RAD results (Table 1) calculated by Eq. 6 showed the one-way connections of symptoms to syndromes, whose connections could be viewed as the contributions of symptoms to syndromes.

Figure 7 illustrates the data in Table 2, where the x-axis represents the 63 symptoms and the y-axis represents the 10 syndromes. Red rectangles represent high RAD values, and the blue ones represent low RAD values. From Fig. 7, the correlations between symptoms and syndromes were determined. As shown in Fig. 7, the symptoms of palpitation, chest distress, short breath, weakness, soreness, and weakness of waist and knees were related to most of the syndromes. At the same time, chills and some other symptoms showed strong connections to some syndromes, such as heart kidney yang deficiency and yang asthenia. Table 3 lists the symptoms and syndromes with high and low RAD values. In Table 3, chills showed a low relation to most of the syndromes except for heart-yang insufficiency and heart-kidney yang deficiency, indicating that chills were closely related to the latter syndromes.

Table 1 Part of the RAD values of symptoms to syndromes

Syndromes	Symptoms					
	Chills	Cold limbs	Night sweat	Palpitation	Chest distress	Chest pain
Heart-*qi* deficiency	0.260	0.127	0.367	0.627	0.790	0.441
Heart-*yang* deficiency	0.592	0.437	0.310	0.684	0.782	0.546
Heart-*yin* deficiency	0.294	0.182	0.509	0.696	0.827	0.453
Heart-blood deficiency	0.250	0.250	0.250	0.625	0.750	0.250
Turbid phlegm	0.354	0.239	0.373	0.701	0.802	0.522
Blood stasis	0.348	0.216	0.344	0.652	0.787	0.512
Qi stagnation	0.374	0.235	0.400	0.670	0.739	0.522

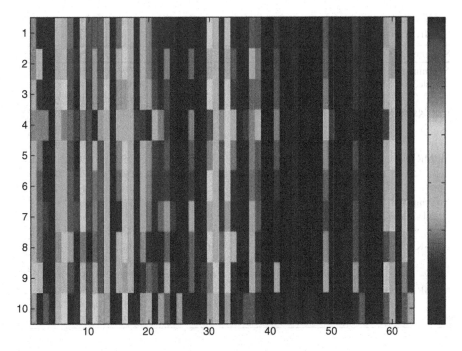

Fig. 7 The correlations between symptoms and syndromes

Table 2 Symptoms with relative high and low RAD values to syndromes

Symptoms	Syndromes
Strong relation	
Chills	Heart-*yang* deficiency syndrome, Heart-kidney *yang* deficiency syndrome
Night sweat	Heart-*yin* deficiency syndrome, Cardiopulmonary-*qi* deficiency syndrome
Cough	Cardiopulmonary-*qi* deficiency syndrome
Soreness and weakness of waist and knees	Heart-blood deficiency syndrome
Constipation	Heart-blood deficiency syndrome
The frequent and increased urination at night	Heart-kidney *yang* deficiency syndrome
Edema	Cardiopulmonary-*qi* deficiency syndrome
Chest pain	Heart-blood deficiency syndrome
Weak relation	
The frequent and increased urination at night	Heart-blood deficiency syndrome, Cardiopulmonary-*qi* deficiency syndrome
Edema	Heart-blood deficiency syndrome

CM theory (Deng 1984; Wang 2004) holds that weakness of yang and qi and lack of warmth may cause chills. The high RAD values of night sweats to insufficiency of heart-yin did confirm the CM theory that yang cannot be restricted by yin asthenia, and then deficiency fire will be an internal disturbance and cause night sweats

Table 3 Statistical results of TPR, TNR and G-means by using SVM and KNN with RAD and MRMR or without symptom selection

Syndromes		1	2	3	5	6	7	Average
No symptom	TPR	0.708	0.463	0.729	0.472	0.799	0.906	0.680
selection-SVM	TNR	0.411	0.770	0.535	0.602	0.516	0.667	0.583
	G-m	0.539	0.597	0.625	0.533	0.642	0.777	0.630
RAD-SVM	TPR	0.723	0.518	0.786	0.588	0.796	0.771	0.713
	TNR	0.429	0.781	0.547	0.536	0.592	0.865	0.609
	G-m	**0.557**	0.636	**0.656**	0.561	0.686	**0.817**	**0.652**
MRMR-SVM	TPR	0.955	0.337	0.131	0.412	0.955	0.020	0.468
	TNR	0.070	0.893	0.970	0.704	0.027	0.970	0.606
	G-m	0.259	0.549	0.356	0.539	0.161	0.141	0.334
No symptom	TPR	0.757	0.553	0.439	0.461	0.826	0.534	0.595
selection-KNN	TNR	0.380	0.795	0.732	0.657	0.673	0.784	0.670
	G-m	0.536	0.663	0.567	0.550	0.746	0.647	0.631
RAD-KNN	TPR	0.749	0.670	0.509	0.485	0.887	0.522	0.607
	TNR	0.391	0.712	0.729	0.663	0.704	0.851	0.706
	G-m	0.541	**0.691**	0.601	**0.567**	**0.790**	0.667	0.643
MRMR-KNN	TPR	1.000	0.401	0.170	0.354	0.942	0.161	0.505
	TNR	0.146	0.901	0.981	0.783	0.018	0.897	0.621
	G-m	0.382	0.601	0.409	0.526	0.130	0.379	0.405

(Deng 1984; Wang 2004). Constipation and insufficiency of heart blood showed a strong connection. Inner Canon of Yellow Emperor points out that "people over 40 years old may lose half of the yin qi", and CM theory (Deng 1984; Wang 2004) holds that insufficiency of the heart blood causes body fluid deficiency, which in turn causes insufficient lubrication of the colon, leading to constipation. The strong connections between nocturnal frequent micturition and heart-kidney yang deficiency can be explained by the lack of yang in the heart and kidney which resulted in a decrease of the controlling and qi transformation functions, bladder retention failure, and then nocturnal frequent micturition.

The weak connections (Table 3) of chest pain and insufficiency of the heart blood, nocturnal frequent micturition and insufficiency of the heart blood, and edema and insufficiency of the heart blood were also significant and consistent with CM theory (Deng 1984; Wang 2004).

In this study, RAD was used for symptom selection, and then SVM (Yuan et al. 1998) and K-nearest neighbors (KNN) (Bernardini et al. 1999) were used for the prediction.

Table 2 shows individual contributions of symptoms to the syndromes.

The predictions were not sound as the syndromes 4, 8, 9, and 10 in this data set showed serious imbalance; therefore, we omitted these results. For syndromes 1, 2, 3, 5, 6, and 7, (Table 3), the results were much better. Table 3 indicates that the prediction results with MRMR favoured either the positive class or the negative class. In the G-means results of the syndromes, these maximum values were obtained by the RAD method, indicating that RAD achieved a good balance between the positive class and the negative class. Although for some syndromes, the prediction results of RAD and MRMR were close when the TPR, TNR, and G-means values were all considered. In general, the results obtained by RAD were more reasonable.

3.2 Feature Selection by Using HOML on the CHD Data Set

(a) Settings

In this chapter, several state-of-the-art multi-label learning algorithms including ML-KNN (Zhang and Zhou 2007), BP-MLL (Zhang and Zhou 2006), Rank-SVM (Elisseeff and Weston 2002) and MLNB-BASIC (Zhang et al. 2009) are adopted by HOML as base classifiers and compared on the dataset of CHD in TCM. We compare HOML with the following benchmark algorithms: SA (Ronen and Jacob 2006), GA (Yang and Honavar 1998), sequential floating forward selection (SFFS) (Pudil et al. 1994), sequential floating backward selection (SFBS) (Pudil et al. 1994), Multi-label Dimensionality reduction via Dependence Maximization (MDDM) (Zhang et al. 2010) and Embedded Feature Selection for Multi-Label Learning (Ge et al. 2009). The target dimensionality d of MDDM is decided by thr = 99 % (Zhang Y et al. 2010). The inner product of label matrix Y is set as the kernel function (Zhang et al. 2010).

Parameters of the multi-label classifiers are set as follows: (1) For ML-KNN, the best parameter k and smoothing factor in (Zhang and Zhou 2007) are used, which are 10 and 1. (2) For BP-MLL, the number of hidden neurons is set to eight after which its performance does not significantly change. (3) For Rank-SVM, the type is set to linear SVM. (4) For MLNB-BASIC, the smoothing factor is set to 1.

Tenfold cross-validation is carried out to compute the fitness value. In each fold, the time simulated annealing (SA), genetic algorithm (GA) and hill-climbing are allocated 5 h, 3 h and 2 h, respectively. SA adopts the same mutation probability and selective acceptance strategy as in HOML when SA is used as independent optimization techniques. GA adopts the same selection operator, crossover probability and mutation probability as they are in HOML when it is used as independent optimization techniques. When simulated annealing (SA) and genetic algorithm (GA) are used as independent optimization techniques, in each fold, they are allocated 10 h, which is the same time duration for SFFS, SFBS, MDDM, and MEFS. In the training process, 2/3 of the training data are taken as training set, 1/3 as validation.

We also made paired t test on the experimental result on the base classifiers to compare the performance of the feature selection/feature reduction algorithms.

(b) Evaluation metrics

The following multi-label evaluation metrics proposed in (Gheyas and Smith 2010) are used in this paper: (1) Hamming loss evaluates how many times an instance-label pair is misclassified. (2) One error evaluates how many times the top-ranked label is not in the set of proper labels of the instance. (3) Coverage evaluates

Table 4 Comparison of HOML and other feature selection/reduction methods on the TCM CHD dataset: Hamming loss, one-error, and coverage. For each criteria, the less the better

| FS \ CRI | Hamming loss↓ | | | | |
	ML-KNN	BP-MLL	Rank-SVM	MLNB-BASIC	AVE
ORI	0.3148	0.3733	0.3809	0.3118	0.3452
SA	0.3000	0.3492	0.3370	0.2870	0.3183
GA	0.3051	0.3468	0.3235	0.3124	0.3220
SFFS	0.2897	0.3690	0.3421	0.2942	0.3237
SFBS	0.2876	0.3263	0.3845	0.3214	0.3300
MDDM	0.3009	0.3569	0.3012	0.2899	0.3122
MEFS	0.3006	0.3422	0.3265	0.2912	0.3151
HOML	**0.1964**	0.2577	0.2411	0.2246	**0.2295**

| FS \ CRI | One-error↓ | | | | |
	ML-KNN	BP-MLL	Rank-SVM	MLNB-BASIC	AVE
ORI	0.2536	0.2620	0.3559	0.3028	0.2936
SA	0.2391	0.2603	0.2885	0.2681	0.2640
GA	0.2410	0.3003	0.3609	0.3083	0.3026
SFFS	0.2356	0.2182	0.3746	0.2693	0.2744
SFBS	0.2458	0.2285	0.3638	0.2145	0.2631
MDDM	0.2111	0.2678	0.2111	0.2412	0.2328
MEFS	0.2464	0.2774	0.2484	0.2492	0.2553
HOML	0.2143	**0.1200**	0.1455	0.1986	**0.1696**

| FS \ CRI | Coverage↓ | | | | |
	ML-KNN	BP-MLL	Rank-SVM	MLNB-BASIC	AVE
ORI	2.8491	3.1236	3.4000	3.6691	3.2604
SA	2.7669	2.8688	2.9745	2.6473	2.8143
GA	2.8284	2.9675	3.0902	2.9545	2.9601
SFFS	2.6334	3.9107	3.2929	2.8188	3.1639
SFBS	2.6537	2.9864	3.2105	3.1764	3.0067
MDDM	2.8556	3.0700	3.8667	3.3944	3.2967
MEFS	2.7190	2.9976	2.2863	2.4630	2.6164
HOML	2.3750	2.5214	2.5179	**2.1421**	**2.3891**

how far we need, on the average, to go down the list of labels in order to cover all the proper labels of the instance. (4) Ranking loss evaluates the average fraction of label pairs that are reversely ordered for the instance. (5) Average precision evaluates the average fraction of labels ranked above a particular label y∈Y which actually are in Y.

(c) Results

After the TCM CHD dataset is preprocessed, we made experiment on it and the experimental results are shown in Tables 4 and 5. FS represents feature selection/reduction method, CRI represents performance criteria, and ORI represents the original classification results. Average means the average value of the four classifiers under the same condition.

Tables 4 and 5 show that compared to the original classification results, predication accuracy have been improved after feature selection/feature reduction for all the five evaluation criteria: hamming loss, one-error, coverage, ranking loss,

Table 5 Comparison of HOML and other feature selection/reduction methods on the TCM CHD dataset: Ranking loss and average precision. For each criteria, "ÿ" indicates "the smaller the better" while the "ÿ" indicates "the bigger the better"

CRI / FS	Ranking loss↓				
	ML-KNN	BP-MLL	Rank-SVM	MLNB-BASIC	AVE
ORI	0.2271	0.2728	0.3724	0.2209	0.2733
SA	0.2139	0.2365	0.2623	0.2072	0.2300
GA	0.2236	0.2627	0.3028	0.2399	0.2572
SFFS	0.1957	0.1786	0.3251	0.2294	0.2322
SFBS	0.1876	0.2402	0.3368	0.2018	0.2416
MDDM	0.2178	0.2566	0.2207	0.2124	0.2268
MEFS	0.2063	0.2397	0.3294	0.1875	0.2407
HOML	**0.1193**	0.1536	0.2672	0.1642	**0.1760**

CRI / FS	Average precision↑				
	ML-KNN	BP-MLL	Rank-SVM	MLNB-BASIC	AVE
ORI	0.7754	0.7651	0.6985	0.5194	68.96%
SA	0.7940	0.7727	0.7583	0.7994	78.11%
GA	0.8055	0.7960	0.7289	0.7418	76.80%
SFFS	0.8027	0.7842	0.7254	0.7890	77.53%
SFBS	0.8146	0.7882	0.7235	0.7087	75.87%
MDDM	0.7856	0.7529	0.7842	0.7746	77.43%
MEFS	0.7933	0.7318	0.7456	0.8231	77.35%
HOML	**0.8819**	0.8533	0.8604	0.7443	**83.50%**

average precision. On the other hand, we can see that the corresponding feature selection/feature reduction methods of the optimal value of the five evaluation criteria are all HOML. The optimal values of the five evaluation criteria, which are the corresponding values of HOML, are as follows: hamming loss 0.2295, 0.1157 lower than the original result 0.3452; one-error 0.1696, 0.1240 lower than the original result 0.2936; coverage 2.3891, 0.8713 lower than the original result 3.2604; ranking loss 0.1760, 0.0913 lower than the original result 0.2733; average precision 83.50 %, significantly increased by 14.54 % than the original result 68.96 %.

HOML outperforms all the other six feature selection/feature reduction methods (SA, GA, SFFS, SFBS, MDDM, and MEFS): HOML is significantly lower than the six feature selection/reduction methods in terms of hamming loss, one-error, coverage and ranking loss, and has significantly outperformed the six methods in terms of average precision: SA by 5.44 %, SFFS by 5.52 %, SFBS by 7.63 %, MDDM by 6.07 %, and MEFS by 6.15 %

Excluding the average value, the separate corresponding classifiers of the optimal values of the five evaluation criteria are as follows: the corresponding classifier of the optimal value of hamming loss (0.1964) is ML-KNN; the corresponding classifier of the optimal value of one-error (0.1200) is ML-KNN; the corresponding classifier of the optimal value of coverage (2.1421) is MLNB-BASIC; the corresponding classifier of the optimal value of ranking loss (0.1193) is ML-KNN; the corresponding classifier of the optimal value of average precision (88.19 %) is ML-KNN.

CHD belongs to the scope of heart diseases family in TCM. The main physiological functions of the heart are to control the blood vessels and govern the mind. In TCM, heart diseases result in dysfunction of blood vessels and bring on symptoms such as chest pain, choking sensation in chest, palpitation and numb of hands or feet. Dysfunction of "governing the mind" results in symptoms such as insomnia, anxiety and amnesia. In the TCM, heart is the monarch organ: it pumps blood to warming the body, and thereby it pertains to fire. Therefore, heart diseases may lead to decreased function of warm, presenting chilly or cold limb, soreness and weakness of waist and knees and night-time frequency or nocturia. Heart dominates sweat in secretion, so heart diseases may lead to self-sweating and night sweat. If the heart-fire flames up with liver-fire, it may cause irritability, impatience and bitter taste. Heart and spleen have a mother-child relationship, so heart disease may result in spleen disease and bring on the symptoms like anorexia, decreased appetite, abdominal fullness and distension.

The duration, inducing (or aggravating) factors and relieving factors of chest pain are the main factors to determine the feature of CHD. Basically, most of the information about general pathology of CHD is listed in the table, and these items comprise the optimal symptom subset. Our results suggest that combination of symptom feature selection with classification algorithms could simplify symptom information and further improve both the comprehension and forecast accuracy of the syndromes of CHD.

(d) Discussions

Tables 4 and 5 reveal that of the seven feature selection/feature reduction methods (SA, GA, SFFS, SFBS, MDDM, MEFS and HOML); HOML outperforms all the other six methods in terms of hamming loss, one-error, coverage, ranking loss and average precision. Whether for the average predication or for the optimal value of the single evaluation criterion, the corresponding feature selection/feature reduction method is HOML. As mutation operator is introduced in SA and each newly generated feature subset is selectively accepted, the better feature subset is retained with a greater probability. On the other hand, genetic diversity is maintained in GA since unbiased tournament selection is adopted. Finally, feature subset is further optimized by hill-climbing greedy algorithm based on the optimization by SA and GA. Therefore, HOML has greatly increased the effectiveness of feature selection. It can be observed from Table 4 that HOML is optimal among the seven feature selection/feature reduction methods (SA, SFFS, SFBS, MDDM, MEFS, and HOML). As for the yeast dataset, compared to the original results, hamming loss, one-error, coverage, ranking loss were decreased by 0.0429, 0.1312, 1.0900, and 0.0635, and the average precision was increased by 10.62 %; As for the TCM CHD dataset, hamming loss, one-error, coverage, ranking loss were decreased by 0.1157, 0.1240, 0.8713, and 0.0913, and the average precision was particularly significantly increased by 14.54 %.

3.3 Multi-Value Classification by Using MAPLSC on the IOS and Liver Data Sets

(a) Settings

MAPLSC is compared with six other multi-class classification methods. APLSC_PWC is similar to MAPLSC. It is also based on APLSC classifier for binary classification, but when combining the posterior probability output from APLSC, pairwise coupling described in Fig. 5 is employed instead of the Eq. 11. APLSC_Vote is based on one-vs-one combination strategy, and uses APLSC as the binary classifier. SVM_PWC includes SVM as the binary classifier, and adopts pairwise coupling when combining. Posterior probability calculation in Eq. 10 is also used by SVM_PWC before pairwise coupling. SVM_Prob refers to posterior probability output and voting combination in Eq. 11, with SVM binary classifier. SVM_Vote refers to the one-vs-one multi-class SVM, which is widely applied. J48 is an implementation for Decision Tree. KNN implemented in TCM clinical data set stands for K-Nearest-Neighbor, in which parameter K is set to 1.

SVM computes a decision plane to separate the training samples belonging to different classes and use this plane to predict the class labels for test samples. There are a number of kernels used in SVM for decision plane computing. RBF kernel is used, and the parameter c and σ are carefully selected in the range of $c \in \{1.0e-3, \cdots, 1.0e+3\}$ and $\sigma^2 \in \{1.0e-3, \cdots, 1.0e+3\}$ respectively by elaborated experiments.

To compare the results of different methods, we have conducted stratified fivefold cross-validation. The folds are stratified so that the training set contains approximately the same proportions of class labels as the original data set. The whole process is repeated 20 times and the average result of them is taken as the fivefold cross-validation classification result.

(b) Evaluation Criterion

In order to measure the performance of MAPLSC, multiple evaluation criterions are included. Marco-average accuracy, micro-average accuracy and macro-average F1-measure are inspected. The macro-average weights equally all the classes, regardless of how many examples belong to it. The micro-average weights equally all the examples, thus favoring the performance on major classes. F1-measure is calculated based on precision and recall, which are defined as follows:

$$precision = \frac{|\{correct\_labels\} \cap \{predicted\_labels\}|}{|predicted\_labels|} \quad (14)$$

$$recall = \frac{|\{correct\_labels\} \cap \{predicted\_labels\}|}{|correct\_labels|} \quad (15)$$

$$F1 - measure = \frac{2 \cdot precision \cdot recall}{precision + recall} \quad (16)$$

In multi-class classification task, prediction result of every class is important. All of them should be inspected carefully. *precision* and *recall* are calculated for every class. If none of the examples are predicted into some class, in other words, *predicted_labels* = 0 in the Equations above, we set *precision* to 0. If *precision* + *recall* = 0, *precision* and *recall* all equal to 0, *F*1 − *measure* is set to 0.

(c) Results

In the following subsection, experimental comparison and more related results are presented and analyzed. After evaluating the performance of MAPLSC on publicly available microarray data sets, MAPLSC is applied to analyzing the TCM clinical data. Tables 6 and 7 demonstrate the comparison results. From the two tables, we can observe that:

- On macro_average accuracy and macro_average F1-measure, MAPLSC outperforms other algorithms in both two TCM data sets. On micro_average accuracy, SVM_Vote is better.
- On TCM clinical data sets, APLSC_PWC is worse than MAPLSC on all the measurement rules.
- APLSC_Vote is slightly better than APLSC_PWC, but still loses to the proposed algorithm MAPLSC.
- SVM related methods get more poor performance than APLSC related techniques on macro_average accuracy and macro_average F1-measure. However, SVM_Vote gets higher micro_average accuracy values on both of the TCM clinical data sets.
- Similar to the results got on microarray data sets described above, SVM_Vote is still stronger than SVM_Prob and SVM_PWC here.
- On macro_average accuracy and macro_average F1-measure, KNN is superior to J48. The micro_average accuracy values achieved by J48 are usually higher than that of MAPLSC, but it is worse on macro_average accuracy and macro_average F1-measure.
- The accuracies of TCM clinical data sets are all dissatisfactory.
- An interesting phenomenon should be mentioned in Table 7, the variance of SVM_Vote is zero for all the three measures.

(d) Discussions

As we have observed, there is a parameter k in the APLSC algorithm (Qu et al. 2010), which refers to the number of components used in PLS. Does the value of k influence the performance of APLSC? Out of curiosity, we record the variation F1-measure with different k on all the six data sets involved in the experimental results above. Figure 8 plots the variation curve.

From Fig. 8, we find out that APLSC achieves similar performance with different k. APLSC is insensitive to the parameter choice. In addition, k = 3 may be a suitable choice on all six data sets, which is actually adopted in the comparison experiments presents in the subsections above.

Table 6 Comparative results on Mr. Wang Qiaochu's TCM clinical data set

Methods	APLSC_Vote	MAPLSC	APLSC_PWC	SVM_Vote	SVM_Prob	SVM_PWC	J48
Macro avg_acc	32.15±2.66	**33.09±2.16**	30.95±3.20	25.45±1.52	18.39±0.88	18.92±1.23	19.86±1.31
Micro avg_acc	49.38±2.19	50.99±2.24	49.52±2.21	**57.47±1.58**	56.96±0.99	57.23±1.11	52.24±1.65
Macro avg_f1meas	32.03±2.40	**32.38±2.52**	30.84±3.13	26.55±1.83	16.04±1.47	16.93±2.03	19.27±1.72

Table 7 Comparative results on Mr. Zhang Yunpeng's TCM clinical data set

Methods	APLSC_Vote	MAPLSC	APLSC_PWC	SVM_Vote	SVM_Prob	SVM_PWC	J48
Macro avg_acc	38.33±6.81	**40.07±6.69**	38.74±7.22	33.33±0.00	32.79±0.32	32.79±0.32	30.11±2.06
Micro avg_acc	45.78±5.00	52.42±5.49	51.8±5.42	**71.88±0.00**	70.70±0.69	70.70±0.69	62.73±3.49
Macro avg_f1meas	34.73±5.19	**38.14±5.57**	37.13±5.72	27.88±0.00	27.61±0.16	27.61±0.16	27.36±2.27

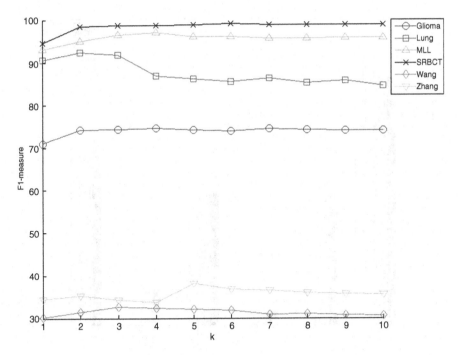

Fig. 8 F1-measure variations with different k in MAPLSC

After studying into the experimental results summarised in Subsections 5.1 and 5.2, some ideas and discussions can be aroused.

- Hastie and Tibshirani (1998) proposed that pi is inferior to pi for multiple binary classes' combination. In our results presented, pi is mostly superior to pi for SVM combination, but inferior to pi for APLSC combination. The combination strategy should be selected according to the attribute of the binary classifier. At the same time, calculation of pi is more complicated.
- For APLSC combination, posterior probability output is more suitable than the vote technique. It may be because that in APLSC_Vote, some classes get the same number of votes and the decision is partly arbitrary.
- SVM_Vote seems better than SVM_PWC in all cases. It disagrees to the evaluation results reported in Duan and Keerthi (2005). With detailed comparison, Duan and Keerthi (2005) adopt test set error as the evaluation criterion, which may be similar to the micro_average accuracy in our paper. In our idea, test set error or micro_average accuracy favours over the majority class and is unsuitable for the evaluation on imbalanced data sets. More experiments on macro_average measures in more data sets listed in Duan and Keerthi (2005) should be conducted in the future work for sophistic ranking of SVM_Vote and SVM_PWC.
- Performances of SVM on Lung and MLL data sets are dissatisfactory. A most possible reason is that the parameters of SVM are not set to appropriate values. The search range for the parameters proposed in Sect. 4.2 should be wider.

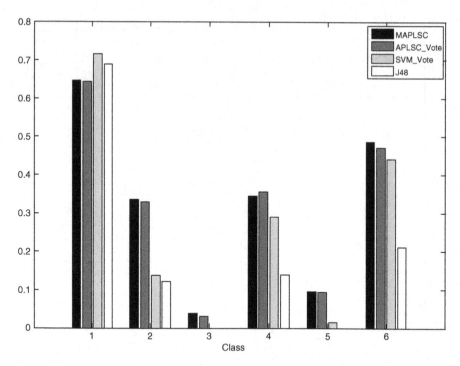

Fig. 9 F1-measure of each class in Mr. Wang's clinical data

- While losing on macro_average measures, SVM related methods always win on micro_average ones, especially in TCM clinical data sets. It is because SVM does not take the imbalanced problem in data sets into consideration. They usually classify all the examples into majority class. In addition, this result is unacceptable in real world applications.
- MAPLSC has the ability of balancing performance among classes. In imbalanced TCM clinical data sets, MAPLSC sometimes sacrifices the accuracy of majority class and save that of minority class. Balanced performance leads to higher macro_average measure. Performance distributions on different classes in TCM clinical data sets are demonstrated in Figs. 9 and 10. From the figures, we can find out that on some difficult classes, SVM_Vote and J48 cannot correctly identify any of the examples, and their diversity among classes is huge. MAPLSC successfully recognise some examples of the difficult class, although the accuracy remains poor. At the same time, MAPLSC tries to balance the performances among the classes, which is required in the future applications.
- APLSC is insensitive to different choice of parameter k in its algorithm and its calculation is simpler. SVM is very sensitive to the decision of parameters c and σ and has a complicated calculation process.
- Comparing with the microarray data sets, accuracies achieved in TCM clinical data sets are very low. It may be attribute to the imperfect data pre-process for TCM clinical data sets. Moreover, insufficient data may be another important reason. More analysis should be considered in the next work.

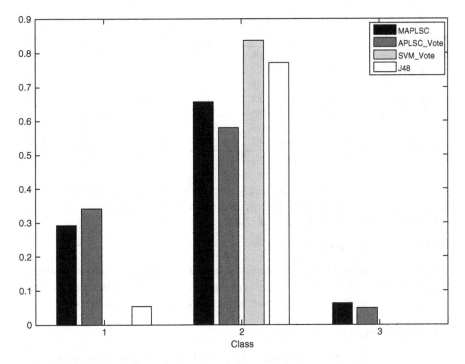

Fig. 10 F1-measure of each class in Mr. Zhang's clinical data

3.4 Diagnosis by Using Fusion-MLKNN on the Hypertension Data Set

(a) Settings

Firstly, five single-diagnosis datasets are retrieved from LEVIS Hypertension TCM Database. Secondly, data preprocessing is conducted on all the five datasets. Thirdly, feature-level information fusion is applied to the single-diagnosis datasets and yield fusional-diagnosis dataset. There are five single diagnosis datasets and one fusional-diagnosis dataset. Fourthly, ML-kNN is used to train models and test models on all the six datasets with parameter k set to be 10; to better reveal performance of models, 10-fold cross-validation is conducted, and the average results of each fold are taken as the final results.

3.4.1 Evaluation Criterion

In order to measure and compare effectively and comprehensively the performance of ML-kNN, multiple evaluation criterions are computed, including Precision, Macro-Average F1-Measure, Micro-Average F1-Measure, Coverage, Hamming

Table 8 Experimental results of ML-kNN on six datasets

Dataset type	Face	Tongue	Inquiry	Palpation	Others	Fusional
AveragePrecision	0.84	0.7905	0.7814	0.7627	0.7674	0.8623
Coverage	−0.5236	−0.6527	−0.6532	−0.7005	−0.7084	−0.4462
HammingLoss	−0.2595	−0.3098	−0.3186	−0.3526	−0.3163	−0.2493
macroF1Measure	0.4569	0.3184	0.2879	0.3554	0.2448	0.5256
microF1Measure	0.6273	0.5385	0.5357	0.5101	0.4583	0.6475
OneError	−0.2704	−0.3476	−0.3753	−0.4109	−0.3876	−0.2451
RankingLoss	−0.2153	−0.2808	−0.2806	−0.3159	−0.3102	−0.1739

Loss, One Error and Ranking Loss. Each criterion has its own characteristic which display one aspect of a model's performance. More information about these criterions can be found on (Tsoumakas et al. 2009).

(b) Results and Discussions

Table 8 summarizes the experimental results on the five single-diagnosis datasets and the one fusional-diagnosis dataset. All the seven evaluation criterions are configured to be the bigger the better, even for negative number (the closer to zero, the better).

From the Table 8, we can find that:

(1) The model built on face-diagnosis dataset perform the best in all the evaluation criterions, among the five models built on single-diagnosis datasets, which demonstrates that inspection of face may be the best way to differentiate syndrome about hypertension.
(2) For all evaluation criterions, performance of fusional-diagnosis model are the best, which may prove strongly the TCM theory that "Fusion use of the four classical diagnostic methods" is essential and help improve the accuracy of syndrome differentiation.

4   Data Sets

4.1   Coronary Heart Disease

In this chapter, a heart system inquiry diagnosis scale is designed, in which the symptoms are defined clearly, and the detailed collecting methods are listed.

The patients with coronary heart disease are selected in Cardiology Department of Longhua Hospital Affiliated to Shanghai University of Traditional Chinese Medicine, Shuguang Hospital Affiliated to Shanghai University of Traditional Chinese Medicine, Shanghai Renji Hospital and Shanghai Hospital of Chinese Medicine. The cases with incomplete information or inconformity with the diagnosis criteria of CHD are removed. This work has been approved by the Shanghai

Society of Medical Ethics. All the patients have signed the informed consent form. Finally, a total of 555 cases were obtained in the study.

Three senior chief TCM physicians performed diagnosis individually for the 555 cases by referring to the diagnosis criteria established in the study, and the data with consistent results between two physicians are recorded; as for the inconsistent results, the data was not recorded until the result was consistent after discussion with the other experts.

Among the 555 patients, 265 patients were male (47.7 %, with mean ages of 65.15 ± 13.17), and 290 patients are female (52.3 %, with mean ages of 65.24 ± 13.82). The symptoms collected for inquiry diagnosis include eight dimensions: cold or warm, sweating, head, body, chest and abdomen, urine and stool, appetite, sleeping, mood, and gynecology, a total of 125 symptoms. There are 15 syndromes in differentiation diagnosis, of which six commonly-used patterns are selected in our study, including: z1 Deficiency of heart qi syndrome; z2 Deficiency of heart yang syndrome; z3 Deficiency of heart yin syndrome; z4 Qi stagnation syndrome; z5 Turbid phlegm syndrome and z6 Blood stasis syndrome.

The data had been preprocessed in [shao12]. Experimental results show that the predication accuracy was the highest on the set of 52 symptoms. We made experiments based on the set with 52 syndromes, three redundant features like "edema" were manually removed before the experiments, and then we got a dataset with 49 symptoms, which may be downloaded at http://levis.tongji.edu.cn/gzli/data/chd-data.zip. The minimum number of labels for each instance is 0, and the maximum number of labels for each instance is 5. The average number of labels of the sample is 2.58. The attributes of the sample are all discrete.

4.2 IOS and Liver

TCM clinical records from veteran practitioners not only embody the theory understanding and clinical practice of the experienced TCM doctor but also reveal their personalised diagnostic thought. As most of the famous TCM practitioners are getting older, preserving and researching into their clinical records, books or publications become urgent and important. In our previous work, we set up a personalised online system (PTCMS) for preserving the precious materials of TCM veteran practitioner (You et al. 2008). After 3 years' cooperation with 11 old TCM practitioners, we have collected more than three thousand clinical records. In this paper, we report our analytic results on the diagnostic data of two specialists from the 11 ones. Zhang Yunpeng is a famous TCM liver specialist. In all, 64 clinical records on fatty liver from Zhang are gathered here for syndrome differentiation. A total of 137 symptoms (called feature in data mining) are recorded in the collected clinical data and totally three syndromes (called objective class in data mining) are taken into consideration. In all, 137 symptoms are illustrated in Table 9. The number of clinical data belonging to each syndrome class is shown in Table 10. Another TCM veteran

Table 9 TCM symptoms collected in Mr. Zhang Yunpeng's clinical records

S1 wake up early	S2 normal sleep	S3 hard to sleep
S4 profuse dreaming	S5 soreness of waist	S6 hypochondriac during menstruation
S7 hypochondriac caused by diet	S8 hypochondriac caused by spirit	S9 hypochondriac caused by weather
S10 hypochondriac caused by overexertion	S11 paroxysmal hypochondriac	S12 spasm hypochondriac
S13 persistent hypochondriac	S14 distending hypochondriac	S15 no hypochondriac
S16 hypochondriac	S17 oppressive hypochondriac	S18 oppressive pain
S19 stabbing pain	S20 yellow urine	S21 purple tongue with wet
S22 red center purple margins of the tongue	S23 ecchymotic tongue	S24 bluish purple tongue
S25 moist tongue	S26 bluish purple tongue	S27 blue tongue
S28 white withered tongue	S29 crimson wollen tongue	S30 crimson tongue
S31 red tip of the tongue	S32 mirror tongue	S33 red dry tongue
S34 red prickly tongue	S35 red tongue	S36 dry tongue
S37 pale red tongue	S38 pale white tongue	S39 pale tongue
S40 red tip and margins of the tongue	S41 gray tongue	S42 dark tongue
S43 wollen tongue	S44 normal tongue body	S45 thin tongue
S46 spontaneous bleeding of the tongue	S47 boil tongue	S48 luxuriant tongue
S49 enlarged tongue	S50 tender-soft tongue	S51 fissured tongue(nature)
S52 fissured tongue(disease)	S53 tough tongue	S54 withered tongue
S55 spotted tongue	S56 pale tongue	S57 trembling tongue
S58 few fur	S59 gray slimy fur	S60 yellow slimy fur
S61 slippery fur	S62 thick fur	S63 filthy fur
S64 curdy slimy fur	S65 pale yellow slimy fur	S66 rough fur
S67 thin fur	S68 white slimy fur	S69 dark red fur
S70 depression	S71 vomiting	S72 nausea vomiting
S73 poor appetite	S74 yellow eyes	S75 sallow complexion
S76 lusterless complexion	S77 vacuous pulse	S78 small pulse
S79 string-like pulse	S80 fine pulse	S81 faint pulse
S82 rapid pulse	S83 replete pulse	S84 rough pulse
S85 weak pulse	S86 soggy pulse	S87 weak pulse
S88 pulse without vitality	S89 forceful pulse	S90 pulse with little vitality
S91 hollow pulse	S92 tight pulse	S93 bound pulse
S94 racing pulse	S95 moderate pulse	S96 slippery pulse
S97 surging pulse	S98 floating pulse	S99 hidden pulse
S100 short pulse	S101 intermittent pulse	S102 large pulse
S103 skipping pulse	S104 slow pulse	S105 sunken pulse
S106 long pulse	S107 bitter taste in mouth	S108 thirst
S109 no dry mouth	S110 dry mouth no thirst	S111 lassitude of spirit
S112 accidie	S113 lack of strength	S114 liver pain during menstruation

(continued)

Table 9 (continued)

S115 liver pain caused by diet	S116 liver pain caused by spirit	S117 liver pain caused by weather
S118 liver pain caused by overexertion	S119 paroxysmal liver pain	S120 liver spasm
S121 persistent liver pain	S122 distending liver pain	S123 distending pain
S124 dull pain	S125 fine	S126 oppressive pain
S127 stabbing pain	S128 abdomen distend	S129 acid regurgitation
S130 nausea	S131 mushy excrement	S132 overcast and rainy at first visit
S133 freezing at first visit	S134 thunderstorm at first visit	S135 high temperature at first visit
S136 constipation	S137 bletching	

Table 10 TCM syndrome classes and their number in Mr. Zhang Yunpeng's clinical records

Syndrome classes	Number
Intermingled phlegm and blood stasis and retained dampness heat toxin	46
Intermingled phlegm and blood stasis	13
Intermingled phlegm and blood stasis and ascendant hyperactivity of liver yang	5

practitioner, Wang Qiaochu is a well-known specialist in insomnia. A total of 217 clinical data on insomnia from Wang are assembled. In all, 122 symptoms and six syndromes are focused. The information of the data from Wang is declared in Tables 11 and 12.

4.3 Hypertension

4.3.1 Data Source

The hypertension datasets used in this paper are from LEVIS Hypertension TCM Database. The data are from the in-patient, out-patient cases of Cardio Center, Cardiovascular Internal Department, Nerve Internal Department, and Medical Examination Center, etc. in Guangdong Provincial Hospital of TCM in China during November 2006 to December 2008, as well as some cases from on-the-spot investigation in Li Wan District Community in Guangzhou of China during March 2007 to April 2007. With strict control measures, 775 reliable TCM hypertension clinical cases are recorded in this database. 148 features, including 143 TCM symptoms from inspection, auscultation and olfaction, inquiry and palpation, and five common indexes including gender, age, hypertension duration, SBPmax, and DBPmax, are investigated and collected in this

Table 11 TCM symptoms collected in Mr. Wang Qiaochu's clinical records

s1 thin fur	s2 fine pulse	s3 fiddle
s4 scatterbrained	s5 Joggled muscle	s6 early wake
s7 menstrual irregularities	s8 scant menstruation	s9 profuse menstruation
s10 scant menstruation	s11 seminal emission	s12 sleep 6–8 h per day
s13 sleep 5–6 h per day	s14 sleep 3–5 h per day	s15 sleep 2–3 h per day
s16 frequent nocturia	s17 antipyretic and analgesic	s18 lumbago pain
s19 soreness of waist	s20 eyes bulge	s21 angina dry in the throat
s22 lockjaw	s23 distending pain in hypochondrium	s24 oppression in chest and shortness of breath
s25 oppression in chest	s26 slump in interest	s27 palpitations
s28 flusteredness	s29 vexation and fiery	s30 limp and numb of lower limb
s31 edema of lower extremity	s32 stomach distention	s33 stomach dull pain
s34 stomach distending pain	s35 distention and fullness	s36 gastric discomfort
s37 poor appetite	s38 fair appetite	s39 torpid intake
s40 take no sleeping pill	s41 phalacrosis	s42 stretching headache
s43 dizziness	s44 headache	s45 insomnia
s46 hearing lose	s47 arouse	s48 handshaken
s49 hoarse	s50 lassitude of spirit	s51 red center purple margins of the tongue
s52 crimson tongue	s53 red tip of the tongue	s54 red tongue
s55 pale red tongue	s56 pale tongue	s57 red tip and margins of the tongue
s58 dark tongue	s59 normal form of the tongue	s60 macroglossia
s61 few fur	s62 yellow slimy fur	s63 pale yellow slimy fur
s64 rough fur	s65 white slimy fur	s66 hard to sleep
s67 breast pain	s68 in low spirits	s69 dry cough
s70 general itching	s71 fear of cold	s72 sound in head
s73 poor appetite	s74 eye bulge	s75 dry eye
s76 lusterless complexion	s77 face heat sore	s78 face rash
s79 lactation	s80 string-like pulse	s81 soggy pulse
s82 dental ulcer	s83 bitter taste in mouth	s84 dry mouth
s85 painful neck	S86 hard neck	s87 scared
s88 unhappy	s89 mental fatigue	s90 heel pain
s91 discontinuity sleep	s92 weakening of the memory	s93 disease in body
s94 mental disease	s95 work at night	s96 work in three shifts
s97 poor hoursing conditions	s98 environment change	s99 nightlife
S100 foreign body sensation in threat	S101 phlegm in threat	S102 arthralgia
S103 no desire to speak	S104 fullness in the abdominal and hypochondrium	S105 abdominal pain
S106 taken sleeping pill	S107 tinnitus	S108 nausea
S109 profuse though	S110 profuse dreaming	S111 sweating when acting
S112 nervous	S113 profuse vaginal discharge	S114 vaginal discharge
S115 sloppy stool	S116 normal stool	S117 diluted stool
S118 dry stool	S119 dry bound stool	S120 hectic fever and sweating
S121 numbness of hands	S122 bletch acid vomiting	

Table 12 TCM syndrome classes and their number in Mr. Wang Qiaochu's clinical records

Syndrome classes	Number
Ascendant hyperactivity of liver yang	124
Liver constraint with Qi stagnation	34
Liver constraint transforming into fire (wind)	5
Liver constraint invading the stomach	15
Liver constraint invading the heart	11
Hyperactivity of liver yang with kidney deficiency	28

database. It also stores the 13 labels (TCM syndrome) of each case. Academic and noncommercial users may access it at http://levis.tongji.edu.cn/datasets/index_en.jsp.

4.3.2 Data Preprocessing

According to the theory of TCM, the characteristics of the LEVIS Hypertension TCM Database, and our research target that evaluation of the performance of multi-label classification model on datasets with information from particular diagnostic methods only (we call them single diagnosis datasets later) and on dataset with fusional information of all diagnostic methods (called fusional-diagnosis dataset), five single-diagnosis datasets are retrieved from the LEVIS Hypertension TCM Database. The information contained in each datasets is shown in Tables 13, 14, 15, 16 and 17, which comes respectively from face diagnosis, tongue diagnosis, inquiry diagnosis, palpation diagnosis and other diagnosis. Analyzing the 775 cases, four cases are found to have empty value in one of the features mentioned above in the five tables. Thus, these four cases are removed from all the five single-diagnosis datasets to ensure smooth progress of the following tasks -information fusion and classification model building.

In the above data sets, we find some labels occur rarely, which will severely hurt performance of classification methods. We randomly choose part of the data set in this work. Firstly, labels are selected to decrease the degree of imbalance. In this case, we chose label 6, 10, and 12, as they have the largest number of positive cases and multi-label method should predict at least three labels simultaneously. Secondly, cases are selected that are marked negative on all the selected labels to be the pending removable set, so that the entire positive cases in any label are preserved. Finally, remove randomly enough cases from the pending removable set. Here, we removed 500 cases and retain 271 cases. The final used data set may be downloaded from: http://levis.tongji.edu.cn/datasets/htn-ecam.zip.

Table 13 Information from face diagnosis

Pale whit complexion	Lusterless complexion	Sallow complexion	Reddened complexion	Bleak complexion	Facial hot flashes	Flushed complexion
Hot eyes	Blue lips	Dark purple lips	Lusterless lips	Red ear	Reddish urine	Yellow urine
Clear abundant urine	Lassitude of spirit	No desire to speak	Listlessness	Palptate with fear	Impatient	Irritability

Table 14 Information from tongue diagnosis

Pale tongue	Red tongue	Dark red tongue	Pale red tongue	Crimson tongue	Teeth-marked tongue	Tender tongue
Tender and red tongue	Bluish purple tongue	Enlarged and pale tongue	Red margins and tip of the tongue	Petechia on tongue	Enlarged tongue	Dark tongue body
Sublingual collateral vessels tongue	Thin fur	Yellow fur	White slimy fur	Few fur	White fur	Thin yellow fur
Yellow slimy fur	No fur	Thin white fur	Slimy fur	Thick slimy fur	White slippery fur	

Table 15 Information from inquiry diagnosis

Headache	Dizzy	Swelling pain of head-eye	Vertigo	Wrapped head	Heavy-headedness	Stretching
Empty pain	Dizzy vision	Visual deterioration	Blurred vision	Dry	Eyes bulge	Deaf
Tinnitus	Chest pain	Distending pain in hypochondrium	Soreness of waist	Weakness of knees	Oppression in chest	Stuffiness in chest
Weakness of limb	Abdominal distention	Numbness	Anorexia	Dry mouth	Insomnia	Dreamy
Bitter taste in mouth	Bland taste in the mouth	Somnolence	Constipation	Short urine	Frequent nocturia	Sloppy stool
Heat in the palms and soles	Torrid	Cold body	Cold limbs	Fear of cold	Vexinf heat in the chest palms and soles	

Table 16 Information from palpation diagnosis

Fine	Rough	Fine rapid	Slippery wiry	Fine rapid wiry	Slippery	Weak
Fine wiry	Rough wiry	Slippery rapid	Rapid	Intermittent bound	Soggy slippery	Rapid wiry
Wiry	Fine weak	Rough sunken	Fine wiry	Soggy	Fine rough	Fine sunken

Table 17 Information from other diagnosis

Night sweating	Palpitate	Muscular twitching and cramp	Sputum	Facial paralysis	Spermatorrhoea	Palpitation
Nausea vomiting	Dry in the throat	Stiffness of the neck	Fogettery	Short breath	Lusterless of hair	Luxated tooth
Heavy body	Impotence	Shortness of breath	Retch nausea sputum	Fat		

References

S. Bernardini, S. Bertolini, A. Pastore, C. Cortese, C. Motti, R. Massoud, G. Federici, Homocysteine levels are highly predictive of CHD complications in subjects with familial hypercholesterolemia. Clin. Chem. Lab. Med. 255 (1999)

T. Blickle, L. Thiele, A comparison of selection schemes used in evolutionary algorithms. Evol. Comput. **4**(4), 361–394 (1996)

C. Cortes, V. Vapnik, Support-vector networks. Mach. Learn. **20**(3), 273–297 (1995)

T.T. Deng, *Diagnostics of TCM* (Shanghai Scientific and Technology Press, Shanghai, 1984)

T.T. Deng, *Practical TCM Diagnostics* (People's Medical Publishing House, Beijing, 2004)

K. Duan, S.S. Keerthi, Which is the best multi-class SVM method? An empirical study, in *Proceedings of the Sixth International Workshop on Multiple Classifier Systems* (2005), pp. 278–285

A. Elisseeff, J. Weston, A kernel method for multi-labelled classification. Adv. Neural Info. Process. Syst. **14**, 681–687 (2002)

I.A. Gheyas, L.S. Smith, Feature subset selection in large dimensionality domains. Pattern Recognit. **43**(1), 5–13 (2010)

L. Guo-Ping, L. Guo-Zheng, W. Ya-Lei, W. Yi-Qin, Modelling of inquiry diagnosis for coronary heart disease in traditional Chinese medicine by using multi-label learning, BMC Complementary and Alternative Medicine, **10**, 37 (2010)

I. Guyon, A. Elisseeff, An introduction to variable and feature selection. J. Mach. Learn. Res. **3**, 1157–1182 (2003)

T. Hastie, R. Tibshirani, Classification by pairwise coupling. Ann. Stat. **26**(2), 451–471 (1998)

H. He, E.A. Garcia, Learning from imbalanced data. IEEE Trans. Knowl. Data Eng. **21**(9), 1263–1284 (2009)

I.S. Helland, PLS regression and statistical models. Scand. J. Stat. **17**, 97–114 (1990)

X.H. Hu, D. Wu, Data mining and predictive modeling of biomolecular network from biomedical literature databases. IEEE/ACM Trans. Comput. Biol. Bioinform. **4**, 251–263 (2007)

S.W. Ji, J.P. Ye, Linear dimensionality reduction for multi-label classification, in *Proceedings of the 21st International Conference on Artificial Intelligence*, Pasadena (2009), pp. 1077–1082

I.T. Jolliffe, *Principal Component Analysis* (Springer, New York, 1986)

D. Kerstin, N. Wolfgang, How valuable is medical social media data? Content analysis of the medical web. Inform. Sci. **179**, 1870–1880 (2009)

G. Lei, L. Guo-Zheng, Y. Ming-Yu, Embedded feature selection for multi-label learning. J. Nanjing Univ. (Nat. Sci.) **45**(5), 671–676 (2009) (in Chinese)

G.-Z. Li, H.-L. Bu, M.Q. Yang, X.-Q. Zeng, J.Y. Yang, Selecting subsets of newly extracted features from PCA and PLS in microarray data analysis. BMC Genomics **9**(S2), S24 (2008)

H.T. Lin, C.J. Lin, R.C. Weng, A note on Platt's probabilistic outputs for support vector machines. Mach. Learn. **68**(3), 267–276 (2007)

G.P. Liu, G.Z. Li, Y.L. Wang, Y.Q. Wang, Modeling of inquiry diagnosis for coronary heart disease in traditional Chinese medicine by using multi-label learning. BMC Complement. Altern. Med. **10**, 4–37 (2010)

X.M. Lu, Z.L. Xiong, J.J. Li, S.N. Zheng, T.G. Huo, F.M. Li, Metabonomic study on 'Kidney-Yang Deficiency syndrome' and intervention effects of Rhizoma Drynariae extracts in rats using ultra performance liquid chromatography coupled with mass spectrometry. Talanta **15**, 700–708 (2011)

J. Moody, J. Utans, Principled architecture selection for neural networks: application to corporate bond rating prediction, in *Neural Information Processing Systems 4*, ed. by J.E. Moody, S.J. Hanson, R.P. Lippmann (Morgan Kauffmann,San Mateo CA, USA, 1992), pp. 683–690

T. Motoki, Calculating the expected loss of diversity of selection schemes. Evol. Comput. **10**(4), 397–422 (2002)

H.C. Peng, F. Long, C. Ding, Feature selection based on mutual information: criteria of max-dependency, max-relevance, and min-redundancy. IEEE Trans. Pattern Anal. Mach. Intell. **8**, 1226–1238 (2005)

J.C. Platt, Probabilistic outputs for support vector machines and comparisons to regularized likelihood methods. in *Advances in large margin classifiers* (MIT Press, Cambridge, MA, USA 1999), pp. 61–74

J.C. Platt, N. Cristianini, J. Shawe-Taylor, Large margin DAGs for multi-class classification, in *Proceedings of Neural Information Processing Systems*, NIPS'99 (Denver, CO, USA, 2000), pp. 547–553

P. Pudil, J. Novovicov, J. Kittler et al., Floating search methods in feature selection. Pattern Recognit. Lett. **15**(11), 1119–1125 (1994)

H.N. Qu, G.Z. Li, W.S. Xu, An asymmetric classifier based on partial least squares. Pattern Recognit. **43**(10), 3448–3457 (2010). Elsevier

J.R. Quinlan, *C4.5: Programs for Machine Learning* (Morgan Kaufmann, San Mateo, 1993)

M. Ronen, Z. Jacob, Using simulated annealing to optimize feature selection problem in marketing applications. Eur. J. Oper. Res. **171**, 842–858 (2006)

A. Ross, A. Jain, Information fusion in biometrics. Pattern Recognit. Lett. **24**, 2115–2125 (2003)

A. Ross, R. Govindarajan, Feature level fusion using hand and face biometrics, in *Proceedings of SPIE Conference on Biometric Technology for Human Identification II*, (Orlando, USA, 2005), pp. 196–204

R.E. Schapire, Y. Singer, Improved boosting algorithms using confidence-rated predictions. Mach. Learn. **37**(3), 297–336 (1999)

H. Shao, G.Z. Li, G.P. Liu, Y. Wang, Symptom selection for multi-label data of inquiry diagnosis in traditional Chinese medicine. Sci. China Info. Sci. 56, 052118(13) (2011) (DOI: 10.1007/s11432-011-4406-5)

A. Sokolov, D. Whitley, Unbiased tournament election, in *Proceedings of the 2005 Conference on Genetic and Evolutionary Computation* (ACM, Washington, DC, 2005), pp. 1131–1138

G. Tsoumakas, I. Katakis, I. Vlahavas, Mining multi-label data, in *Data Mining and Knowledge Discovery Handbook*, ed. by O. Maimon, L. Rokach (Springer, Boston, 2009), pp. 667–685

Y.Q. Wang, *Diagnostics of TCM* (Chinese Medicine Science and Technology Press, Beijing, 2004)

Y. Wang, Progress and prospect of objectivity study on four diagnostic methods in traditional Chinese medicine, in *Bioinformatics and Biomedicine Workshops (BIBMW), 2010 IEEE International Conference on* (Hongkong, China, 2010)

J. Wang, Q.Y. He, K.W. Yao, W. Rong, Y.W. Xing, Z. Yue, Support vector machine (SVM) and traditional Chinese medicine: syndrome factors based an SVM from coronary heart disease treated by prominent traditional Chinese medicine doctors, in *Fifth International Conference on Natural Computation: 14–16 August 2009; Tianjian*, ed. by H.Y. Wang, K.S. Low, K.X. Wei, J.Q. Sun (IEEE Computer Society, Los Alamitos, 2009a), pp. 176–180

Y.Q. Wang, Z.X. Xu, F.F. Li, H.X. Yan, Research ideas and methods about objectification of the four diagnostic methods of traditional Chinese medicine. Acta Universitatis Traditionis Medicalis Sinensis Pharmacologiaeque Shanghai **23**, 4–8 (2009b)

H. Wold, Path models with latent variables: the NIPALS approach, in *Quantitative Sociology: International Perspectives on Mathematical and Statistical Model Building* (Academic, New York, 1975), pp. 307–357

J. Yang, V. Honavar, Feature subset selection using a genetic algorithm. IEEE Intell. Syst. Appl. **13**, 44–49 (1998)

M.Y. You, G.Z. Li, X.Q. Zeng, L. Ge, L. Bi, S. Huang, J.Y. Yang, M.Q. Yang, A personalized traditional Chinese medicine system in the case of Cai's gynecology. Int. J. Funct. Inform. Personal. Med. **1**(4), 419–438 (2008). Inderscience

K. Yu, S.P. Yu, V. Tresp, Multi-label informed latent semantic indexing, in *Proceedings of the 28th Annual International ACM SIGIR Conference on Research and Development in Information Retrieval*, ACM, New York, 2005, pp. 258–265

Z.K. Yuan, X.P. Huang, F.Y. Fan, Analysis of the tongue micro-indexes of qi-blood patterns of heart disorders. J. Tradit. Chin. Med. Univ. Hunan (1998-04)

X.-Q. Zeng, G.-Z. Li, G.-F. Wu, J.Y. Yang, M.Q. Yang, Irrelevant gene elimination for partial least squares based dimension reduction by using feature probes. Int. J. Data Min. Bioinform. **3**(1), 85–103 (2009). Inderscience

M. Zhang, MLA 2010. Grigorios Tsoumakas, Ioannis Katakis. *Multi-Label Classification: An Overview*. International Journal of Data Warehousing & Mining, 3(3), 1–13, July–September 2007

M.L. Zhang, Z.H. Zhou, Multilabel neural networks with applications to functional genomics and text categorization. IEEE Trans. Knowl. Data Eng. **18**(10), 1338–1351 (2006)

M.L. Zhang, Z.H. Zhou, ML-KNN: a lazy learning approach to multi-label learning. Pattern Recognit. **40**(7), 2038–2048 (2007)

M.L. Zhang, J.M. Pena, V. Robles et al., Feature selection for multi-label naive Bayes classification. Inform. Sci. **179**(19), 3218–3229 (2009)

Y. Zhang, Z.-H. Zhou. Multi-label dimensionality reduction via dependency maximization. ACM Transactions on Knowledge Discovery from Data (ACM TKDD), 4(3), Article 14 (2010)

Z.H. Zhou, X.Y. Liu, Training cost-sensitive neural networks with methods addressing the class imbalance problem. IEEE Trans. Knowl. Data Eng. **18**(1), 63–77 (2006)

X. Zhou, S. Chen, B. Liu, R. Zhang, Y. Wang, P. Li, Y. Guo, Development of traditional Chinese medicine clinical data warehouse for medical knowledge discovery and decision support. Artif. Intell. Med. **48**, 139–152 (2010)

Network Based Deciphering of the Mechanism of TCM

Yi Sun, Qi Liu, and Zhiwei Cao

Abstract Currently, there has been increased global interest in traditional herbal medicines because of the emerging systematic "multi-target" drug design strategy. The herbal ingredients, their corresponding protein targets, the biological processes its targets participate in, as well as the drug-target interactions and target-target interactions are necessary to understand the molecular mechanism of TCMs. Varieties of relevant databases have been set up. Additionally, the massive amounts of data produced by '-omics' technologies has also provided considerable support for the exploration of TCM mechanism. They would be more useful for depicting a global picture of the underlying mechanism of TCM, as network-based multi-targets drug design methodologies could integrate relevant information across different platforms. In this chapter, taking the study of herbal medicines against *Alzheimer's Disease* (AD) as an example, the value of the network-based integration of different data sources for TCM is exemplified by the study for clinically tested anti-AD herbs. Network-based integration of the various databases and '-omics' data are discussed, which will not only facilitate the holistic understanding of the disease pathogenesis, but also suggest new clues for the usage of TCMs in future drug discovery.

1 Motivations and Introduction

Traditional Chinese Medicine (TCM) has long been used for the treatment of a wide variety of complex diseases. A TCM formula is usually composed of several herbs with considerable amount of chemical ingredients which may have multiple targets. The "multi-component, multi-target" feature mainly leads to the unclear mechanism for TCM, especially their combination effects including pharmacodynamically

Y. Sun • Q. Liu (✉) • Z. Cao (✉)
School of Life Sciences and Technology, Tongji University,
1239 Siping Road, Shanghai 200092, People's Republic of China
e-mail: qiliu@tongji.edu.cn; zwcao@tongji.edu.cn

J. Poon and S.K. Poon (eds.), *Data Analytics for Traditional Chinese Medicine Research*,
DOI 10.1007/978-3-319-03801-8_4, © Springer International Publishing Switzerland 2014

synergistic, additive or antagonistic and pharmacokinetically potentiative or reductive effects. There raised the first question: **How to decipher herb mechanism comprehensively?**

Now, it is possible to explore the mode of action (MOA) for TCM from different views, as the various '-omics' technologies have shown the promise to be a powerful technical platform during the past decade. Experimental platforms including gene expression microarray, proteomic profiles and metabolomics analysis, as well in-silico platforms involving pathway analysis, docking and inver-docking programs have been widely employed for uncovering the molecular mechanism of TCM (Leung et al. 2012). Currently, '-omics' technologies have produced massive data, and it keeps growing. However, individual '-omics' platform is not informative enough to elucidate the MOA of TCM, while tighter integration across different platforms could facilitate to provide a global picture for the underlying mechanism of TCM. There raised the second question: **How to analysis the diverse data integratively?**

The newly developed network-based computational models can expand the capacity of '-omics' platforms by building tight correlations among them (Hopkins 2008; Wist et al. 2009). Thus, network-based methodologies could afford new possibilities to establish a multi-dimensional system for uncovering TCM mechanism from a systematic point of view.

2   Data Sources of Herb Ingredients and Targets

The essence of TCM is natural products which contains many chemical constitutes. Therefore, identifying the ingredients of TCM is very important for TCM pharmacology study. As drugs generally perform their functions by binding to target proteins, the target information is also necessary. Currently, several databases have been developed by text mining on literature and books, and they could provide useful data for TCM study (Table 1). The information derived from each database has its own focus and they could be complementary in application. **TCM-ID database** (Traditional Chinese Medicine Information Database) collects comprehensive information of TCM including prescriptions, constituent herbs, herbal ingredients, molecular structure and functional properties of active ingredients, therapeutic and side effects, clinical indication and application and related matters (Chen et al. 2006). **HIT** (Herb Ingredient's Target) contains information related to therapeutic targets for herbal ingredients from TCM, and a total of 221 direct targets of 586 herbal compounds are collected in the current version (Ye et al. 2011). **HICD** (Herbal ingredient and content database) stores content information of more than 15,000 ingredients, and includes all potential factors affecting ingredient content, e.g., collecting time and site, herb part, processing methods, method to measure the content, therapeutic effects, as well as diseases. **TTD** (Therapeutic target database) contains information related to therapeutic targets and has a user-friendly search interface (Zhu et al. 2012). Although these databases are not complete, data mining techniques could be employed to further expand them.

Table 1 Available data sources for herb study

Database_Type	Database_Name	Details
Herbal database	TCM-ID	Containing 1,197 formulas, 1,102 herbs, 12,120 compounds
	HIT	Containing 5,208 entries about 1,301 known protein targets (221 of them are described as direct targets) affected by 586 herbal compounds from more than 1,300 reputable Chinese herbs, overlapping with 280 therapeutic targets from Therapeutic Targets Database (TTD), and 445 protein targets from DrugBank corresponding to 1,488 drug agents
	HICD	Containing content information of more than 15,000 ingredients, and includes all potential factors affecting ingredient content, e.g., collecting time and site, herb part, processing methods, method to measure the content, therapeutic effects, as well as diseases
PPI database	HPRD	Containing information pertaining to domain architecture, post-translational modifications, interaction networks and disease association for each protein in the human proteome. All the information in HPRD has been manually extracted from the literature by expert biologists who read, interpret and analyze the published data
	Mint	Containing experimentally verified protein-protein interactions mined from the scientific literature by expert curators, and 235,000 binary interactions have been captured from over 4,750 publications
	Intact	Containing approximately 275,000 curated binary interaction evidences from over 5,000 publications
	BioGRID	Containing 347,966 interactions (170,162 genetic, 177,804 protein) curated from both high-throughput data sets and individual focused studies, as derived from over 23,000 publications in the primary literature, and 48,831 are human protein interactions that have been curated from 10,247 publications
	DIP	Containing the diverse body of experimental evidence on protein-protein interactions
	MIPS	Containing high-quality experimental protein interaction data in mammals

(continued)

Table 1 (continued)

Database_Type	Database_Name	Details
Pathway database	KEGG	Containing over 300 pathways partitioned into seven sections, and the pathways having four formats for download: KGML, BioPAX, SBML and GPML
	WikiPathways	Open, collaborative platform dedicated to the curation of biological pathways, and the download format is GPML
	BioCarta	Could be downloaded in BioPAX Level 2 format through NCI/Nature Pathway Interaction Database (Gilbert et al. 2010)
	PID	Aiming at the cancer research community and others interested in cellular pathways, such as neuroscientists, developmental biologists, and immunologists. The database focuses on the biomolecular interactions that are known or believed to take place in human cells. And data could be downloaded in PID XML and BioPAX Level 2 format
	Reactome	Providing an intuitive website to navigate pathway knowledge and a suite of data analysis tools to support the pathway-based analysis of complex experimental and computational data sets
	Pathway commons	A collection of publicly available pathway data from multiple organisms. The database aims to collect and integrate all public pathway data available in standard formats, and currently contains data from nine databases with over 1,400 pathways and 687,000 interactions

To understand the molecular mechanism of a drug, it is critical to know the biological processes its targets participate in, as well as the drug-target interactions and target-target interactions. With the development of high-throughput proteomics technology, various online databases containing experimental **information of protein-protein interaction (PPI)** have been set up, such as HPRD (Keshava Prasad et al. 2009), Mint (Licata et al. 2012), Intact (Kerrien et al. 2012), BioGRID (Stark et al. 2011), DIP (Salwinski et al. 2004), MIPS (Pagel et al. 2005), etc. In addition, some **cellular network or signaling pathway databases** have systematically collected pathways associated with biological processes (Table 1). For example, the KEGG database includes over three hundred pathways partitioned into seven sections, in which the section of human diseases consists of pathways concerning cancers, immune disorders, neuro-degenerative diseases, Substance dependence diseases, Cardiovascular Diseases, Endocrine and Metabolic Diseases, and infectious diseases, and the information is updated regularly (Kanehisa et al. 2012). Other available collection of curated and peer-reviewed pathways could be found in PID (Pathway Interaction Database) (Schaefer et al. 2009), Reactome (Matthews et al. 2009) etc.

3 Network-Based Deciphering of Herb Mechanisms

Complex diseases like cancers, cardiovascular diseases, and neurodegenerative disorders are regulated by complex biological networks and depend on multiple factors of genetic and environmental challenges to progress. Single-target drugs have been shown with limited efficacy or too many adverse effects for these systemic diseases. Drug discovery strategies show the favor for designing drugs to produce overall therapeutic synergy based on mutual complements and drugs could interfere with multiple avenues of pathological cross-talk. This new appreciation of the role of polypharmacology has significant implications for tackling the two major sources of attrition in drug development: efficacy and toxicity. Integrating network biology and polypharmacology holds the promise of expanding the current opportunity space for druggable targets. The concept of network pharmacology may establish the foundation for the development of multi-target interventions.

TCM formulas and individualized treatment concept may provide the major sources for developing multi-target intervention. They have been used to treat complex diseases for thousands of years. Compared with the western drugs, TCM often treats the function and dysfunction of living organisms in a more holistic way.

The development of **'-omics' technologies** has produced massive amounts of data, and it has provided considerable support for the exploration of TCM mechanism (Table 2). These data would be even more useful for the understanding of the holistic, complementary and synergic essence of TCM in the context of molecular networks, if we have computational tools that could integrate relevant information across genomics, transcriptomics, proteomics, metabolomics, microbiome, pharmacogenomics and clinical samples. Currently, there are lots of **computational and mathematical models** available for network-based multi-targets drug design (Table 3). The conceptual diagram of integrating multiple "-omics" platforms using computational tools for network-based drug discovery is shown in Fig. 1 (Leung et al. 2012).

4 Case Study: Target Network Based Anti-AD Herbal Mechanism

Here, we present the case study on applying TCM-related databases and various high-throughput data sources to understand the anti-AD MOA for TCM from a target network perspective (Sun et al. 2012). (i) We systematically collected and reviewed anti-AD herbs, their ingredients, and the target proteins from public databases and literatures; (Paez et al. 2004) We studied the anti-AD mechanism with the application of network analysis (Fig. 2).

We performed a large-scale text mining of PubMed and the clinical trial database (www.Clinicaltrials.gov), and extracted the available promising anti-AD herbs from the English literatures (from 1995 to 2011) (Table 4). Then, the ingredients

Table 2 Current "-omics" techniques applied for drug discovery

Platforms	Techniques	Applications	Findings	References
Genomic platform	Array comparative genomic hybridization arrays	Analysis of DNA copy number gain or loss	Global analysis of DNA copy number change across chromosomes between normal and pathological samples	Shinawi and Cheung (2008)
	Single cell exome sequencing	Analysis the mutational profiles of the whole exome of intratumoral cells	Spectrumsclear cell renal cell carcinoma (ccRCC) tumor did not contain any significant clonal subpopulations and mutations that had different allele frequencies within the population also had different mutation	Xu et al. (2012)
RNAi platform	Multiplex RNAi screening	Analyzing accumulated genetic alternation of loss-of-function phenotypes in vitro	Profiling essential genes in human mammalian cells by multiplex RNAi screening	Silva et al. (2008)
Transcriptomic platform	Gene expression array	Discovery of whole genome gene expression profile of a disease	Rheumatoid Arthritis (RA) patients diagnosed with TCM heat or cold pattern	van der Greef et al. (2010)
	Gene expression array	Examining the action of Si-Wu-Tang in treating women menstrual discomfort, climacteric syndrome, peri- or postmenopausal syndrome and other ostrogen-related diseases	Identify the nuclear factor erythroid 2-related factor 2 (Nrf2) cytoprotective pathway is the most significantly affected by Si-Wu-Tang (SWT)	Wen et al. (2011)
Clinical sample platform	Tissue arrays/ Cellular arrays	Identifying specific cellular components within tissue or single cells	Identifying the proteomic profiles of preeclampsia tissue and normal placenta tissue using recombinant antibody microarrays.	Dextlin-Mellby et al. (2010)
Proteomic platform	2D gel-MS/MS	Detecting global targets and candidate proteins	Identifying proteomic profiles of human pathogenesis for molecular targeting	Qiao et al. (2010)
	2D gel-MS/MS	Detecting network targets response to drug	Identifying of a network of 21 differentiated regulated core proteins response to Ganoderic acid D	Yue et al. (2008)

Platform	Method	Application	Description	References
Metabolomic platform	GC-MS/MS	Studying the effect of drugs from metabolites	Identifying of the differential metabolic profiles of the Xiaoyaosan-treated chronic unpredictable mild stress rats and control rats	Gao et al. (2011)
	LC-MS/MS	Detecting metabolomics marker from serum	Identifying pentol glucuronide as relevant serum biomarkers of epithelium ovarian cancer	Chen et al. (2011)
Microbiome platform	Large scale sequencing-based analysis of microbial genomes	Global genomic analysis of human microbiome and earth microbiome	Identification of specific contribution of symbiotic-pathogen in human and earth to host's pathology and drug metabolism	Gilbert et al. (2010), Clemente et al. (2012), Ichinohe et al. (2011), Kane et al. (2011), Kostic et al. (2012), Peterson et al. (2009)
	Gut-Microbiota-mediated drug metabolism	Gut-Microbiota-Drug interaction analysis	Identification of new compound K, which is a gingseng metabolite metabolized by human gut microbiota, possess significant stronger cancer prevention activity	Qi et al. (2011)
Pharmacogenomics platform	SNP analysis	Identification of subgroup of patients receiving particular types of treatment or drug dosage	Determination of maintenance dose for warfarin based on the CYP2C9 and VKORC1 genotypes	Sconce et al. (2005)
	SNP analysis	Identification of SNP that is associated to drug treatment outcome	Identification of BIM polymorphic deletion is associated with shorter progression-free survival in NSCLC patients with EGFR activating mutation after TKI therapy	Cheng and Sawyers (2012)

(continued)

Table 2 (continued)

Platforms	Techniques	Applications	Findings	References
Chemical screening platform	High-throughput screening of natural products for cancer therapy and data collection	High-throughput screening of useful biological active small molecules from natural products	Discovering drugs for cancer therapy and screening bioactive components from medicinal herbs	Harvey and Cree (2010), Zhu et al. (2010)
	Herbalomic	Identifying potential benefit and toxicity of the components in herbals	Herbalome chips in which arrays of compounds are screened for their binding to key peptides as well as doing the multi-component multi-target coordination research	Kang (2008), Stone (2008)

Table 3 Available computational tools for multi-targets drug discovery

Computational tools	Models	Application	Findings	References
Algorithm-based	Systematic combination screening	Combination optimization	Statically analyze drug efficacy by denoting matrix of scores across 435 possible two-component combinations of 30 compounds, three optimized drug combinations were found	Borisy et al. (2003)
	Stochastic search algorithm using Gur Game	Combination optimization	Closed-loop control of cellular functions using combinatory drugs	Wong et al. (2008), Yoon (2011)
	Medicinal Algorithmic Combinational Screen (MACS)	Combination optimization	Identifying a combination of four drugs from 72 combinations that are the most effective to kill 8 non-small cell lung cancer	Zinner et al. (2009)
	Extensive search algorithm model for examining the quantitative composition-activity relationship (QCAR) of herbal formulae	Combination optimization	Optimizing a combination regimen of three components of TCM formula Shenmai and Qi-Xue-Bing-Zhi-Fang	Wang et al. (2010), Wang et al. (2006)
	Algorithm-based computational program link with Steiner Tree method	Multi-layer correlation analysis of trans-omics	Linking the gene expression array and proteomic data to expand the understanding of the underlying cellular mechanism	Huang and Fraenkel (2009), Lan et al. (2011)

(continued)

Table 3 (continued)

Computational tools	Models	Application	Findings	References
Network-based	Network-based study on three drug combinational analysis using combination index	Multi-target mechanistic study	Identifying six core proteins from a protein network which responds to the Chinese herbal preparation, Realgar-Indigo Naturalis Formula-RIF	Wang et al. (2008)
	Integrative multiple systems biology platforms	Multi-target mechanistic study	Identifying the key pathways underlying the synergistic effects of combined imatinib and arsenic sulfide	Zhang et al. (2009)
	Network target-based identification of multicomponent synergy (NIMS) model	Solving a stochastic relationship of drugs and combination optimization	Transferring the relations between drugs to the interactions among their targets of a specific disease network and prioritizing synergistic pairs from 63 manually collected agents for a disease instanced by angiogenesis	Li et al. (2011a)
	Network-based multi-target estimation by combining docking scores	Combination optimization	Screening anticoagulant activities of a series of argatroban intermediates and eight natural products based on affinity predictions	Li et al. (2011b)
	Systematically target network analysis	Disease crosstalk and herbal mechanism of action analysis	Ingredients of anti-Alzheimer's disease (AD) herbs interact closely with therapeutic targets that showed crosstalk with multiple diseases. Furthermore, pathways of Ca2t equilibrium maintaining, upstream of cell proliferation and inflammation were densely targeted by the herbal ingredients	Sun et al. (2012)

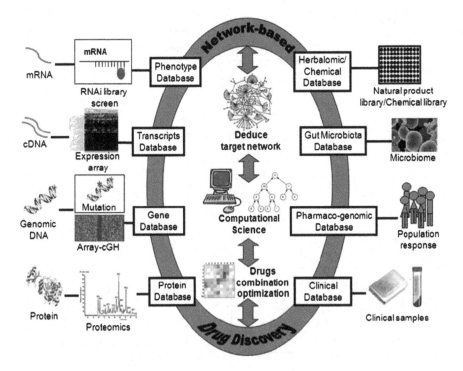

Fig. 1 Integrating "-omics" platform to network-based drug discovery

contained in each herb were collected from Traditional Chinese Medicine Information Database (TCM-ID), "Pharmacopoeia of People's Republic of China" and PubMed (Table 4).

The information of target proteins for herbal ingredients was identified from HIT, and 34 target proteins were retrieved. And, we found three of the herbal ingredients are successful therapeutic targets against AD, and the majority of the herbal targets (74 %) are either successful or research targets for AD-related diseases, including cancer, inflammation, diabetes, ischemia reperfusion injuries and Parkinson. These results imply that anti-AD herbs are primarily interacting with tens of important proteins critical to disease treatment. Although the relationship between these diseases is not fully understood, these targets are serving as the material basis for the therapeutic effects of the anti-AD herbs, as well as suggesting important cross-talks between AD and the other complex diseases.

To better elaborate the holistic modulation of the anti-AD herbal medicines, an integrated "*AD pathway*" was compiled based on the "Alzheimer's disease pathway" from KEGG Pathway database (Kanehisa et al. 2012), and human PPI data from online databases (Keshava Prasad et al. 2009; Licata et al. 2012; Kerrien et al. 2012; Stark et al. 2011; Salwinski et al. 2004; Pagel et al. 2005). Of the 34 target proteins, 28 can be mapped or connected to the pathway. As shown in Fig. 3, several AD-related processes were involved, including proliferation, Aβ degradation and cell death. The

Part I

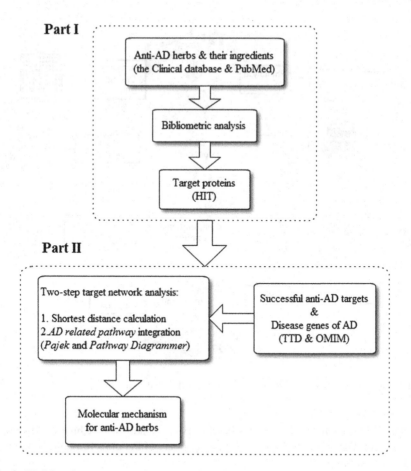

Part II

Fig. 2 Workflow for target network analysis of anti-AD herbal mechanism

Table 4 Anti-AD herbs and their ingredients

Herb	Ingredient
Ginkgo biloba	Quercetin, Kaempferol, Ginkgolide a, Ginkgolide b
Huperzia serrata	Huperzine A, Huperzine B
Melissa officinalis	Quercetin, Gallic acid
Salvia officinalis	Apigenin, b-Sitosterol, Ursolic acid

targets can be organized into the following pathways: AD symptoms-associated pathways, inflammation-associated pathways, cancer-associated pathways, diabetes mellitus-associated pathways, Ca^{2+}-associated pathways and cell proliferation pathways. Several possible anti-AD mechanisms for the herbal ingredients were suggested in Fig. 3. The herbal ingredients could produce their anti-AD effect not only by improving the symptom of AD patients, but also by targeting the fundamental of

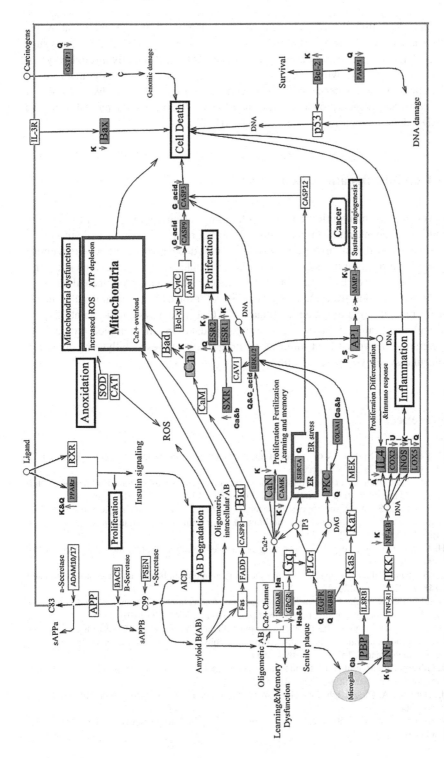

Fig. 3 Distribution of target proteins of herbs on compressed "*AD pathway*"

the disease pathophysiology such as the inflammation-associated pathways, cancer-associated pathways, diabetes-associated pathways and so on. And, it is suggested that *Huperzia serrata* might produce anti-AD effects mainly through a symptom-improving way, while targets of *Salvia officinalis* are mainly involved in inflammation and cancer-associated pathways. As for *Ginkgo biloba* and *Melissa officinalis*, their targets are more diversely distributed in these fundamental pathways of AD indicating their more extensive anti-AD effects.

5 Conclusions and Discussions

Network-based intervention has been a trend of curing complex diseases, and the "multi-component, multi-target" nature of herbal medicine may provide resources to network-based drug discovery. During the past decade, the rapid development of "-omics" platforms and systems biology has facilitated systems-level understanding of biological processes concerning the interactions of genes, proteins and environmental factors, thus affording new possibilities for uncovering the molecular mechanisms related to the therapeutic efficacy of TCM from a systematic point of view. Through integrating various high-throughput data, in-silico models could help accelerating network-based multi-target drug discovery, especially for optimizing molecular synergy of herbal formulas.

References

A.A. Borisy et al., Systematic discovery of multicomponent therapeutics. Proc. Natl. Acad. Sci. U. S. A. **100**(13), 7977–7982 (2003)

X. Chen et al., Database of traditional Chinese medicine and its application to studies of mechanism and to prescription validation. Br. J. Pharmacol. **149**(8), 1092–1103 (2006)

J. Chen et al., Serum 27-nor-5beta-cholestane-3,7,12,24,25 pentol glucuronide discovered by metabolomics as potential diagnostic biomarker for epithelium ovarian cancer. J. Proteome Res. **10**(5), 2625–2632 (2011)

E.H. Cheng, C.L. Sawyers, In cancer drug resistance, germline matters too. Nat. Med. **18**(4), 494–496 (2012)

J.C. Clemente et al., The impact of the gut microbiota on human health: an integrative view. Cell **148**(6), 1258–1270 (2012)

L. Dexlin-Mellby et al., Tissue proteome profiling of preeclamptic placenta using recombinant antibody microarrays. Proteomics Clin. Appl. **4**(10–11), 794–807 (2010)

X. Gao et al., Metabonomic study on chronic unpredictable mild stress and intervention effects of Xiaoyaosan in rats using gas chromatography coupled with mass spectrometry. J. Ethnopharmacol. **137**(1), 690–699 (2011)

J.A. Gilbert et al., Meeting report: the terabase metagenomics workshop and the vision of an Earth microbiome project. Stand Genomic Sci. **3**(3), 243–248 (2010)

A.L. Harvey, I.A. Cree, High-throughput screening of natural products for cancer therapy. Planta Med. **76**(11), 1080–1086 (2010)

A.L. Hopkins, Network pharmacology: the next paradigm in drug discovery. Nat. Chem. Biol. **4**(11), 682–690 (2008)

S.S. Huang, E. Fraenkel, Integrating proteomic, transcriptional, and interactome data reveals hidden components of signaling and regulatory networks. Sci. Signal. **2**(81), ra40 (2009)

T. Ichinohe et al., Microbiota regulates immune defense against respiratory tract influenza A virus infection. Proc. Natl. Acad. Sci. U. S. A. **108**(13), 5354–5359 (2011)

M. Kane et al., Successful transmission of a retrovirus depends on the commensal microbiota. Science **334**(6053), 245–249 (2011)

M. Kanehisa et al., KEGG for integration and interpretation of large-scale molecular data sets. Nucleic Acids Res. **40**(Database issue), D109–D114 (2012)

Y.J. Kang, Herbogenomics: from traditional Chinese medicine to novel therapeutics. Exp. Biol. Med. (Maywood) **233**(9), 1059–1065 (2008)

S. Kerrien et al., The IntAct molecular interaction database in 2012. Nucleic Acids Res. **40**(Database issue), D841–D846 (2012)

T.S. Keshava Prasad et al., Human protein reference database – 2009 update. Nucleic Acids Res. **37**(Database issue), D767–D772 (2009)

A.D. Kostic et al., Genomic analysis identifies association of Fusobacterium with colorectal carcinoma. Genome Res. **22**(2), 292–298 (2012)

A. Lan et al., ResponseNet: revealing signaling and regulatory networks linking genetic and transcriptomic screening data. Nucleic Acids Res. **39**(Web Server issue), W424–W429 (2011)

E.L. Leung et al., Network-based drug discovery by integrating systems biology and computational technologies. Brief. Bioinform. **14**(4), 491–505 (2013)

S. Li, B. Zhang, N. Zhang, Network target for screening synergistic drug combinations with application to traditional Chinese medicine. BMC Syst. Biol. **5**(Suppl 1), S10 (2011a)

Q. Li et al., A network-based multi-target computational estimation scheme for anticoagulant activities of compounds. PLoS One **6**(3), e14774 (2011b)

L. Licata et al., MINT, the molecular interaction database: 2012 update. Nucleic Acids Res. **40**(Database issue), D857–D861 (2012)

L. Matthews et al., Reactome knowledgebase of human biological pathways and processes. Nucleic Acids Res. **37**(Database issue), D619–D622 (2009)

J.G. Paez et al., EGFR mutations in lung cancer: correlation with clinical response to gefitinib therapy. Science **304**(5676), 1497–1500 (2004)

P. Pagel et al., The MIPS mammalian protein-protein interaction database. Bioinformatics **21**(6), 832–834 (2005)

J. Peterson et al., The NIH Human Microbiome Project. Genome Res. **19**(12), 2317–2323 (2009)

L.W. Qi et al., Metabolism of ginseng and its interactions with drugs. Curr. Drug Metab. **12**(9), 818–822 (2011)

R.C. Yue, L. Shan, S.K. Yan et al., Utilization of the chemical proteomics for the study of Chinese medicines towards modernization. World SciTechnol. **12**, 502–510 (2010)

L. Salwinski et al., The database of interacting proteins: 2004 update. Nucleic Acids Res. **32**(Database issue), D449–D451 (2004)

C.F. Schaefer et al., PID: the pathway interaction database. Nucleic Acids Res. **37**(Database issue), D674–D679 (2009)

E.A. Sconce et al., The impact of CYP2C9 and VKORC1 genetic polymorphism and patient characteristics upon warfarin dose requirements: proposal for a new dosing regimen. Blood **106**(7), 2329–2333 (2005)

M. Shinawi, S.W. Cheung, The array CGH and its clinical applications. Drug Discov. Today **13**(17–18), 760–770 (2008)

J.M. Silva et al., Profiling essential genes in human mammary cells by multiplex RNAi screening. Science **319**(5863), 617–620 (2008)

C. Stark et al., The BioGRID interaction database: 2011 update. Nucleic Acids Res. **39**(Database issue), D698–D704 (2011)

R. Stone, Biochemistry. Lifting the veil on traditional Chinese medicine. Science **319**(5864), 709–710 (2008)

Y. Sun et al., Towards a bioinformatics analysis of anti-Alzheimer's herbal medicines from a target network perspective. Brief. Bioinform. (2012)

J. van der Greef et al., Systems biology-based diagnostic principles as pillars of the bridge between Chinese and Western medicine. Planta Med. **76**(17), 2036–2047 (2010)

Y. Wang, X. Wang, Y. Cheng, A computational approach to botanical drug design by modeling quantitative composition-activity relationship. Chem. Biol. Drug Des. **68**(3), 166–172 (2006)

L. Wang et al., Dissection of mechanisms of Chinese medicinal formula Realgar-Indigo naturalis as an effective treatment for promyelocytic leukemia. Proc. Natl. Acad. Sci. U. S. A. **105**(12), 4826–4831 (2008)

Y. Wang et al., A novel methodology for multicomponent drug design and its application in optimizing the combination of active components from Chinese medicinal formula Shenmai. Chem. Biol. Drug Des. **75**(3), 318–324 (2010)

Z. Wen et al., Discovery of molecular mechanisms of traditional Chinese medicinal formula Si-Wu-Tang using gene expression microarray and connectivity map. PLoS One **6**(3), e18278 (2011)

A.D. Wist, S.I. Berger, R. Iyengar, Systems pharmacology and genome medicine: a future perspective. Genome Med. **1**(1), 11 (2009)

P.K. Wong et al., Closed-loop control of cellular functions using combinatory drugs guided by a stochastic search algorithm. Proc. Natl. Acad. Sci. U. S. A. **105**(13), 5105–5110 (2008)

X. Xu et al., Single-cell exome sequencing reveals single-nucleotide mutation characteristics of a kidney tumor. Cell **148**(5), 886–895 (2012)

H. Ye et al., HIT: linking herbal active ingredients to targets. Nucleic Acids Res. **39**(Database issue), D1055–D1059 (2011)

B.J. Yoon, Enhanced stochastic optimization algorithm for finding effective multi-target therapeutics. BMC Bioinformatics **12**(Suppl 1), S18 (2011)

Q.X. Yue et al., Proteomics characterization of the cytotoxicity mechanism of ganoderic acid D and computer-automated estimation of the possible drug target network. Mol. Cell. Proteomics **7**(5), 949–961 (2008)

Q.Y. Zhang et al., A systems biology understanding of the synergistic effects of arsenic sulfide and Imatinib in BCR/ABL-associated leukemia. Proc. Natl. Acad. Sci. U. S. A. **106**(9), 3378–3383 (2009)

Y. Zhu et al., High-throughput screening for bioactive components from traditional Chinese medicine. Comb. Chem. High Throughput Screen. **13**(10), 837–848 (2010)

F. Zhu et al., Therapeutic target database update 2012: a resource for facilitating target-oriented drug discovery. Nucleic Acids Res. **40**(Database issue), D1128–D1136 (2012)

R.G. Zinner et al., Algorithmic guided screening of drug combinations of arbitrary size for activity against cancer cells. Mol. Cancer Ther. **8**(3), 521–532 (2009)

Prescription Analysis and Mining

Guang Zheng, Miao Jiang, Cheng Lu, and Aiping Lu

Abstract Prescription analysis is an important task in traditional Chinese medicine (TCM), both in theoretical development and clinical practices. However, with the rapid development of TCM researches, massive literature collected in databases blocks end users from acquiring general knowledge of prescriptions. Fortunately, with the rapid development of text mining technology, now, it is possible to extract associated networks focused on prescriptions. In this chapter, focused on Liuwei-Dihuang formula as an example, by executing discrete derivative algorithm in the text mining process, prescription associated networks are mined out. These networks include prescription-pattern-disease, prescription-disease-Chinese herbal medicine, prescription-pattern-Chinese herbal medicine, prescription-Chinese herbal medicine-symptom, and prescription-pattern-symptom. These networks might be good references for TCM research and clinical practices.

G. Zheng
School of Information Science & Engineering, Lanzhou University,
730000 Lanzhou, Gansu, People's Republic of China

Institute of Basic Research in Clinical Medicine, China Academy of Chinese Medical
Sciences, Beijing 100700, People's Republic of China
e-mail: forzhengguang@163.com

M. Jiang • C. Lu
Institute of Basic Research in Clinical Medicine, China Academy of Chinese Medical
Sciences, Beijing 100700, People's Republic of China

A. Lu (✉)
Institute of Basic Research in Clinical Medicine, China Academy of Chinese Medical
Sciences, Beijing 100700, People's Republic of China

School of Chinese Medicine, Hong Kong Baptist University,
Kowloon Tong, Hong Kong, People's Republic of China
e-mail: lap64067611@126.com

J. Poon and S.K. Poon (eds.), *Data Analytics for Traditional Chinese Medicine Research*,
DOI 10.1007/978-3-319-03801-8_5, © Springer International Publishing Switzerland 2014

1   Introduction

Over several thousand years of clinical research and theoretical thoughts, traditional Chinese medicine has developed into a stable period both in theoretical re-search and clinical practices. The therapeutic process in traditional Chinese medicine can be called as "Li-Fa-Fang-Yao" which is of critical importance in clinical practices (Deng 2008). Li-Fa-Fang-Yao, which means principles, methods, prescription/formula, and Chinese herbal medicines respectively, indicate the four basic steps of diagnosis and treatment: determining the cause, mechanism and location of the disease according to the medical theories and principles, then deciding the treatment principle and method, and finally selecting a prescription as well as proper Chinese herbal medicines.

In the history of traditional Chinese medicine, herbal prescription/formula has been adapted in the clinical practices over 2,000 years. It is an important means in the therapeutic system of traditional Chinese medicine. What's more, with rapid development on the research of traditional Chinese medicine, huge number of literature on prescriptions are published and collected in databases with electronic version. So, it is a meaningful task to analyze the prescriptions with text mining approach.

In the clinical practices of traditional Chinese medicine, the determination of prescription is based on the determination of two other processes: (1) pat-tern/syndrome differentiation, and (2) treatment principle and method. In the theory of traditional Chinese medicine, pattern/syndrome can be defined as sets of symptoms. As for the treatment principle and method, it is based on the analysis of pattern differentiation. Based on this, the analysis of prescription involves its connection with the symptom, disease, pattern, Chinese herbal medicine, treatment principle and method.

In this chapter, take description of "Liuwei-Dihuang Formula" for example. We explored the information or networks on several aspects within the framework of traditional Chinese medicine. These aspects focused on symptom, disease, pat-tern, Chinese herbal medicine, treatment principle and method.

2   Why Liuwei-Dihuang Formula?

In the textbook of Prescription of Chinese medicine (Fang-ji-xue in Pinyin, and 方劑學 in Chinese), there are 362 prescriptions (Deng 2008). Most of these descriptions are widely used in clinical practice, in the form of both decoction and patient medicine. Among them, Liuwei-Dihuang Tang is a famous one which has been intensively studied (Chang et al. 2006; Chen et al. 1994, 2010; Cheng et al. 2007; Deng et al. 2009; Fang et al. 2001; Gao et al. 2008; He et al. 2007; Hsiu et al. 2011; Huang et al. 2012; Jiang et al. 1984, 1989; Lee et al. 2005; Li et al. 2010a, b; Liu

Table 1 Top 10 prescriptions of traditional Chinese medicine mined from SinoMed

ID	Chinese herbal medicine		Frequency
	Chinese name	Pinyin name	
1	補陽還五湯	Buyang-Huangwu Tang	3,302
2	生脈散	Shengmai San	3,036
3	血府逐瘀湯	Xuefu-Zhuyu Tang	2,825
4	逍遙散	Siaoyao San	2,685
5	補中益氣湯	Buzhong-Yiqi Tang	2,676
6	六味地黃湯	Liuwei-Dihuang Tang	2,592
7	小柴胡湯	Xiao-Chaihu Tang	2,587
8	四物湯	Siwu Tang	2,365
9	瀉心湯	Xiexin Tang	2,204
10	桂枝湯	Guizhi Tang	1,821

et al. 2010, 2012; Mao et al. 1993; Qian et al. 2008; Song et al. 2006; Xue et al. 2005; Zhao et al. 2007). By scanning the literature database of SinoMed (http://sinomed.imicams.ac.cn/index.jsp) which is focused on biological and medical publications, Liuwei-Dihuang formula is the 6th formula among the top 10 which can be demonstrated in Table 1.

Liuwei-Dihuang was invented by famous doctor Qian Yi who wrote a book named Xiaoer-Yaozheng-Zhijue (小兒藥證直訣 in Chinese) in Song dynasty (Deng 2008; Xu 2011; Zheng et al. 2011a). This formula is the basic description on treating the pattern of kidney-yin deficiency by tonifying kidney yin. It is composed by six Chinese herbal medicines, i.e., Shudidhuang (Radix Rehmanniae Preparata in Latin, and 熟地黃 in Chinese), the chief medicinal for supplementing the kidney yin and is combined with the flash of Shanzhuyu (Fructus Corni in Latin, and 山茱萸 in Chinese) and Shanyao (Dioscorea opposita in Latin, and 山藥 in Chinese), as the deputy medicinals for addressing liver and spleen yin; it is assisted by Zexie (Rhizoma Alismatis in Latin, and 澤瀉 in Chinese), Mudanpi (Cortex Moutan Radicis in Latin, and 牡丹皮 in Chinese) and Baifuling (Chinaroot Greenbrier Rhizome in Latin, and 白茯苓 in Chinese) for clearing and removing fire in the liver and kidney and concurrently dispelling dampness and turbidity, thus achieving a famous formula for supplementing yin with the function of mainly supplementing yin and draining while supplementing. These six Chinese herbal medicines form the "three tonify and tree purge" of this description (Deng 2008).

Based on description of Liuwei-Dihuang formula, some other descriptions (Qiju-Dihuang-Wan, Zhibai-Dihuang-Wan, and etc.) are composed by adding some other Chinese herbal medicines into this description. Studied by modern medical experiments, Liuwei-Dihuang formula shows many more functions under the framework of western medicine. These functions are strengthen the immune system, anti-aging, anti-fatigue, anti-freezing, hypoxia tolerance, reducing blood fat, reducing blood pressure, reducing blood sugar, improve kidney's function, improve the metabolism.

3   Data and Methods

3.1   Source Data

The data sets used in this chapter were downloaded from SinoMed (http://sinomed.imicams.ac.cn/index.jsp). Our data sets were separated into different ones with respect to different topics. For example, the primary data set is for Liuwei-Dihuang formula which contains 3,046 records of literature on July 12, 2012. When it came to the situation of analyzing the network of Liuwei-Dihuang formula with diseases and patterns, in order to get a complete understanding of the whole network, data sets of patterns and diseases were also required. By filtering the data set on Liuwei-Dihuang formula, we got the network of diseases and patterns which are associated with it. When it came to these diseases, it is natural to check whether the patterns primarily associated with Liuwei-Dihuang formula are also the patterns associated with diseases primarily. In order to fulfill this requirement, we downloaded the data sets on these five diseases.

3.2   Methods

3.2.1   Principle

The text mining process on Liuwei-Dihuang formula is based on the principle of co-occurrence which is a typical method in biomedical text mining (Zheng et al. 2011a, b, c).

4   Result

4.1   Aspects Focused

As Liuwei-Dihuang formula is a famous prescription in traditional Chinese medicine, and we planned to get an overall view on it, so, the text mining process filtered the disease, pattern/syndrome, symptom, Chinese herbal medicine, and treatment principle.

4.2   Simple Networks

When these aspects were done, we built the one group of networks which are associated with Liuwei-Dihuang formula directly. These directly associated networks are:

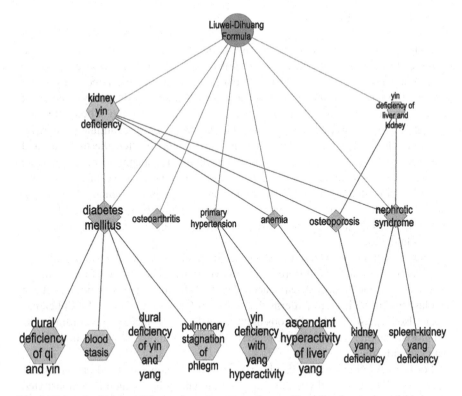

Fig. 1 Network of Liuwei-Dihuang formula-pattern-disease. The full color version of this image may be viewed in the eBook edition

Liuwei-Dihuang formula-disease, Liuwei-Dihuang formula-pattern, Liuwei-Dihuang formula-symptom, Liuwei-Dihuang formula-Chinese herbal medicine. Then, we built the networks which are not associated with Liuwei-Dihuang formula directly, i.e., disease-pattern, disease-symptom, disease-Chinese herbal medicine, pattern-symptom, pattern-Chinese herbal medicine, symptom-Chinese herbal medicine, and pattern-symptom.

4.3   Merged Networks

When these two groups of the networks were ready, we merged them with respect to different topics. For example, in order to get a comprehensive network of disease and pattern associated with Liuwei-Dihuang formula, we merged the networks of Liuwei-Dihuang formula-disease, Liuwei-Dihuang formula-pattern, and disease-pattern. When these three networks are merged, disease and pattern information about Liuwei-Dihuang formula are demonstrated clearly (in Fig. 1).

4.3.1 Disease and Pattern

Although both are focused on the healthy service, western medicine and traditional Chinese medicine are two different systems rooted from different culture foundations. For western medicine, doctors often make an accurate diagnosis by using advanced medical equipment and laboratory examinations. Also, they diagnose a disease by comprehensive and systematic examine the patient's body through inspection, palpation, percussion, auscultation and olfactory examination or with the aid of the stethoscope, reflex hammer, sphygmomanometer, thermometer and other simple tools. For traditional Chinese medicine, the diagnosis process can be taken as four diagnostic methods i.e., inspection, auscultation and olfaction, inquiry as well as pulse-taking and palpation. The human body is an organic whole. Local pathological changes may affect the viscera and the whole body and can be detected from the manifestations of the sensory organs, limbs and surface of the body (Xu 2011; Zhou 2008).

Thus, based on the disease names coined in the framework of western medicine, they can be classified into different pattern/syndromes in traditional Chinese medicine. Even for one specific disease, according to different patient's symptoms, it can be classified into different patterns in traditional Chinese medicine. This phenomena is also the case for prescriptions in traditional Chinese medicine according to its diagnosis, one prescription can be prescribed to different diseases yet with the same pattern/syndrome.

For Liuwei-Dihuang formula, this prescription is mainly focused on patterns of kidney yin deficiency and yin deficiency of liver and kidney which is demonstrated in Fig. 1.

By filtering the dataset of Liuwei-Dihuang formula, disease list associated with it can also be found. For significant and simplicity, top six diseases are demonstrated in light purple diamonds in Fig. 1.

For these six diseases, text mining algorithm was also executed, and their associated patterns were also filtered out. Although Liuwei-Dihuang formula can regulate a large list of disease names, it is not the primary pattern associated with the diseases listed. Take diabetes mellitus for example, it main pattern associated are dual deficiency of qi and yin, and dual deficiency of yin and yang. That is to say, although Liuwei-Dihuang formula is adopted, also, it is focused on the pattern of kidney yin deficiency, yet it is not the most popular formula reported in the literature of diabetes mellitus. In the clinical practice, it may also be used together with other prescriptions or western medicines. This phenomenon is also commonly existed in other diseases associated with Liuwei-Dihuang formula, i.e., anemia also associated with kidney yang deficiency, nephrotic syndrome also associated with spleen-kidney yang deficiency, primary hypertension also associated with yin deficiency with yang hyperactivity and ascendant hyperactivity of liver yang.

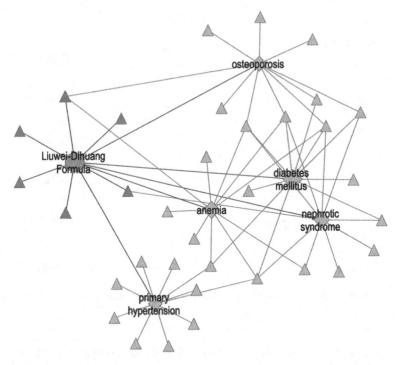

Fig. 2 Network of Liuwei-dihuang formula-disease-Chinese herbal medicine. The full color version of this image may be viewed in the eBook edition

4.3.2   Disease and Chinese Herbal Medicine

By filtering the data set on Liuwei-Dihuang formula, we can mine out the disease list associated with it. Although there are about 58 diseases associated with it, based on the principle of significant and simplicity, only five outstanding diseases are demonstrated in Figure. They are osteoporosis, diabetes mellitus, anemia, primary hypertension, and nephrotic syndrome.

In this figure, dark green triangle nodes represent the six Chinese herbal medicines which are composed in the prescription of Liuwei-Dihuang formula. Light green triangle nodes represent Chinese herbal medicines which are associated with outstanding five diseases which Liuwei-Dihuang formula regulates.

For grey diamond nodes, they represent five significant diseases associated with Liuwei-Dihuang formula. Around them are light green triangles represent Chinese herbal medicines. These Chinese herbal medicines are filtered out from different data sets of five diseases. Together with the dark green triangle nodes, they form the sub networks of disease-Chinese herbal medicine. Just like the merged network of pattern-disease-Liuwei-Dihuang formula in Fig. 1, kidney yin deficiency is just one pattern associated with those diseases, and because prescriptions are tightly associated with pattern. What's more, different prescriptions have different sets of Chinese herbal medicines according. Then, in Fig. 2, it is natural and clear that different

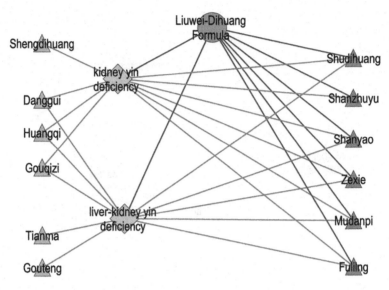

Fig. 3 Network of Liuwei-Dihuang formula-pattern-Chinese herbal medicine

diseases have different sets of Chinese herbal medicines. However, as all of them are associated with Liuwei-Dihuang formula, so, it is also natural for them to have intersections between Chinese herbal medicine sets. That is why there are also lines connecting dark green triangle nodes with diseases.

4.3.3 Pattern and Chinese Herbal Medicine

As we have known that pattern and prescription are tightly connected, and prescriptions are also have their kernel composition of Chinese herbal medicines, together with the knowledge that prescriptions can be modified in clinical practice when situations are complex, then, it is natural come to the question of constructing the network which merging the network of pattern-Chinese herbal medicine and Liuwei-Dihuang formula-Chinese herbal medicine. Based on this, we constructed the network of Liuwei-Dihuang formula-pattern-Chinese herbal medicine in Fig. 3.

In Fig. 3, dark triangles on the right are six Chinese herbal medicines in prescription of Liuwei-Dihuang formula. Two blue diamond nodes representing patterns of kidney yin deficiency and liver-kidney yin deficiency. Light green triangles on the part are Chinese herbal medicines tightly associated with pattern kidney yin deficiency and pattern liver-kidney yin deficiency.

In this figure, it is easy to understand that six Chinese herbal medicines on the right are tightly connected with Liuwei-Dihuang formula, kidney yin deficiency, and liver-kidney yin deficiency because they composed the prescription of Liuwei-Dihuang formula and this prescription is also tightly associated with these two patterns.

As for the light green triangles representing other Chinese herbal medicines associated with patterns, they also have their reasons. These light green triangles can be classified into three groups:

1. Group one are three Chinese herbal medicines which associated with both two patterns of kidney yin deficiency and liver-kidney yin deficiency. They are Danggui (Radix Angelicae Sinensis in Latin, and 當歸 in Chinese), Huangqi (Radix Astragali in Latin, and 黃芪 in Chinese), and Gouqizi (Fructus Lycii in Latin, and 枸杞子 in Chinese). Among them, Guoqizi tonifies liver and kidney, Danggui tonnifies blood, and Huangqi tonifies qi. Taking them together, they can nourish yin and tonify qi which are commonly used in clinical practice. As for the five diseases demonstrated in Fig. 2, they all have the therapeutic effect.

2. Group two has only one Chinese herbal medicine called Shengdihuang which is associated with pattern kidney yin deficiency. Shengdihuang (Radix Rehmanniae Recens in Latin, and 生地黃 in Chinese) can nourish yin and clearing heat. Thus, Shengdihuang can be used in the treatment of kidney yin deficiency pattern.

3. Group three has two Chinese herbal medicines and they are associated with pattern liver-kidney yin deficiency. They are Tianma (Rhizoma Gastrodiae in Latin, and 天麻 in Chinese), and Gouteng (Ramulus Uncariae cum Uncis in Latin, and 鉤藤 in Chinese). Tianma and Gouteng can pacify the liver, suppresses exuberant yang. So, they can be adopted in the treatment of pattern ascendant hyperactivity of liver yang which can be caused by pattern liver-kidney yin deficiency.

Based on the analysis above, Fig. 3 demonstrates clear and reasonable relationships among Liuwei-Dihuang formula, pattern, and Chinese herbal medicine.

4.3.4 Symptom and Chinese Herbal Medicine

In the theory of Chinese herbal medicine, each Chinese herbal medicine has its individual therapeutic effect(s). To be composited into prescriptions, they all contribute to the main therapeutic effects of these prescriptions according to the theory of ingredients in a prescription that have different roles, i.e., sovereign, minister, assistant and courier.

According to the textbook, symptoms of soreness and weakness of waist and knees, hot flash, dizzy, spermatorrhea, night sweat, and tinnitus. Through text mining the data set on Liuwei-Dihuang formula, we got the network of Liuwei-Dihuang formula-Chinese herbal medicine-symptom which is demonstrated with darker lines connecting to the red node of Liuwei-Dihuang Formula. Apart from these darker lines, there are also light gray lines connecting symptoms and Chinese herbal medicines.

4.3.5 Pattern and Symptom

In the theory of traditional Chinese medicine, pattern is a set of symptoms. Different patterns include different sets of symptoms. More interesting, even for one particular pattern, it can also be determined by different sets of symptoms. That is to say, pattern can verify. However, no matter how symptoms verify in patterns, they all are associated with diseases and cannot exist independent of the diseases. So, it is the pathogenesis and etiology that form the core of the pattern.

For prescription of Liuwei-Dihuang formula, it is tightly associated with patterns of kidney yin deficiency and liver-kidney yin deficiency. By mining the symptoms associated with Liuwei-Dihuang formula, kidney yin deficiency, and liver-kidney yin deficiency, their associated network with symptom are listed in Figure.

In this figure, symptoms associated with Liuwei-Dihuang can be classified into two groups. One group consists of dizzy, tinnitus, night sweat, lost sleep, and soreness and weakness of waist and knees. These symptoms are also connected with pattern liver-kidney yin deficiency and pattern kidney yin deficiency. The other group consists of fever, spermatorrhea, ulcer, aphtha, and hot flash. These symptoms are associated with Liuwei-Dihuang formula yet not so tightly associated with pattern liver-kidney yin deficiency and pattern kidney yin deficiency.

5 Conclusion

By mining the literature data sets about prescription of Liuwei-Dihuang formula, several merged networks were constructed and interpreted. Examining these networks, there are several interesting points which might be good references for TCM researches and clinical practices.

1. Liuwei-Dihuang formula can affect a wide variety of diseases.
   By filtering the dataset of Liuwei-Dihuang, we found that about 58 diseases can be regulated with this formula. In traditional Chinese medicine, Liuwei-Dihuang formula has its specific pattern/syndrome. However, as western medicine is another different medical system, then, the pattern/syndrome of Liuwei-Dihuang formula can scatter among different disease names in western medicine. Based on this, we have the point of one formula for many diseases. The major diseases are demonstrated in Fig. 1.
2. Liuwei-Dihuang formula can be modified for personalized medicine.
   Personalized medical practice can also be demonstrated in the analysis of Liuwei-Dihuang formula. Figure 2 demonstrates the network of disease and Chinese herbal medicine associated with Liuwei-Dihuang formula. Figure 4 demonstrates the network of disease and symptoms associated with Liuwei-Dihuang formula. These two figures reveal a fact that in clinical practices, Liuwei-Dihuang formula can be modified according to different disease and symptoms which are also personalized medicine.
3. Liuwei-Dihuang formula can be modified for different TCM pattern/syndromes together with other Chinese herbal medicines.
   In traditional Chinese medicine, treatments based on formulae are flexible according to different pattern/syndrome. Even under the same pattern/syndrome, different symptoms can also cause the change in prescriptions. This can be demonstrated in Figs. 3 and 4.

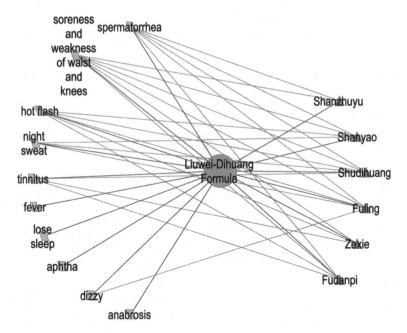

Fig. 4 Network of Liuwei-Dihuang formula-Chinese herbal medicine-symptom

4. Literature reports may have different emphasizes compared with textbooks.
   Checking networks demonstrated in Figs. 1, 2, 3, 4, and 5, and comparing them with textbooks, they are not quite consistent. For contents described in textbooks, they cover most the possible situations. However, in current situations, as traditional Chinese medicines at the complementary positions, some serious conditions might be prevented and some further treatments described in textbook have no chance to be executed in clinical practice. So, the results demonstrated in networks have their current emphasis and cannot be complete consistent with the textbook.

5. Merged networks of different aspects about prescription demonstrate meaningful information.
   In this chapter, every network (Figs. 1, 2, 3, 4, and 5) is composed by merging two networks associated with Liuwei-Dihuang formula. Take Fig. 1 for example, this figure demonstrates the connection among the pattern/syndrome and diseases associated with Liuwei-Dihuang formula. In this network, it is clear that different diseases and different pattern/syndrome are associated with Liuwei-Dihuang formula. Besides the pattern/syndromes associated with Liuwei-Dihuang formula, there are also some other pattern/syndromes associated with these diseases associated with Liuwei-Dihuang formula. That is to say, one disease can be regulated by different Chinese herbal formulae according to different pattern/syndromes associated with this disease. On the other side, one Chinese herbal formula can also regulate different diseases based on the same pattern/syndromes.

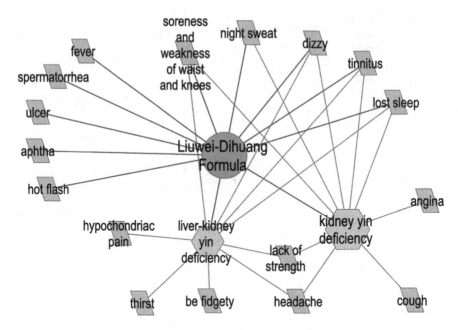

Fig. 5 Network of Liuwei-Dihuang formula-pattern-symptom

Acknowledgments This chapter is partially supported by National Science Foundation of China (No. 30825047, 30902003, 30973975, and 81072982). China Postdoctoral Science Foundation (No. 20110940553).

References

Y.L. Chang, B. Liu, Supercritical fluid extraction of paeonol from Liuwei Dihuang pill. Zhongguo Zhong Yao Za Zhi **31**(8), 653–655 (2006)

Y. Chen et al., Effects of liuwei dihuang wan [symbol: see text:bd and some other TCM drugs on bone biomechanics and serum 25 (OH)D3 content in rats. J. Tradit. Chin. Med. **14**(4), 298–302 (1994)

B. Chen et al., Analysis method of the fingerprint of LiuWei DiHuang pills by near infrared spectroscopy. Guang Pu Xue Yu Guang Pu Fen Xi **30**(8), 2124–2128 (2010)

X.R. Cheng, W.X. Zhou, Y.X. Zhang, The effects of Liuwei Dihuang decoction on the gene expression in the hippocampus of senescence-accelerated mouse. Fitoterapia **78**(3), 175–181 (2007)

Z. Deng, *Formulae of Chinese Medicine*, China Press of Traditional Chinese Medicine, (2008), (in Chinese)

Y. Deng et al., Effects of Liuweidihuang Decoction on cell proliferation and melanin synthesis of cultured human melanocytes in vitro. Nan Fang Yi Ke Da Xue Xue Bao **29**(4), 701–703 (2009)

J. Fang et al., Effect of liuwei dihuang decoction, on the cytokine expression in splenocytes in AA rats. Zhongguo Zhong Yao Za Zhi **26**(2), 128–131 (2001)

D. Gao et al., Experimental study on effect of Liuwei Dihuang Pill on HSC from mouse marrow. Zhong Yao Cai **31**(2), 251–254 (2008)

H. He et al., Protective effect of Liuwei Dihuang decoction on early diabetic nephropathy induced by streptozotocin via modulating ET-ROS axis and matrix metalloproteinase activity in rats. J. Pharm. Pharmacol. **59**(9), 1297–1305 (2007)

H. Hsiu et al., Assessing the microcirculatory response following oral administration of Liuwei Dihuang formula by spectral analysis of skin-surface laser Doppler signals. Zhong Xi Yi Jie He Xue Bao **9**(10), 1101–1109 (2011)

Y. Huang et al., Liuwei Dihuang decoction facilitates the induction of long-term potentiation (LTP) in senescence accelerated mouse/prone 8 (SAMP8) hippocampal slices by inhibiting voltage-dependent calcium channels (VDCCs) and promoting N-methyl-d-aspartate receptor (NMDA) receptors. J. Ethnopharmacol. **140**(2), 384–390 (2012)

T.L. Jiang et al., Effect of "liuwei dihuang decoction" on prevention and treatment of tumor. J. Tradit. Chin. Med. **4**(1), 59–68 (1984)

T.L. Jiang, S.C. Yan, L.F. Zhao, Preventing effect of "liuwei dihuang decoction" on esophageal carcinoma. Gan To Kagaku Ryoho **16**(4 Pt 2–2), 1511–1518 (1989)

K.S. Lee et al., Liuweidihuang-tang improves spatial memory function and increases neurogenesis in the dentate gyrus in rats. Fitoterapia **76**(6), 514–519 (2005)

J. Li et al., Effects of Liuweidihuang pills on pancreatic islet structure in OLETF rats. Nan Fang Yi Ke Da Xue Xue Bao **30**(6), 1407–1409 (2010a)

W. Li et al., Preventing steroid-induced osteonecrosis of the femoral head with Liuwei dihuang pills and molecular mechanism. Zhongguo Xiu Fu Chong Jian Wai Ke Za Zhi **24**(4), 446–451 (2010b)

W. Liu et al., Human osteoblast-like cells OS-732 intervened with alcohol and treated with liuwei-dihuang pill medicated serum. Zhong Yao Cai **33**(2), 249–252 (2010)

Y. Liu et al., The regulatory effect of liuwei dihuang pills on cytokines in mice with experimental autoimmune encephalomyelitis. Am. J. Chin. Med. **40**(2), 295–308 (2012)

P. Mao et al., Effect of liuweidihuang decoction on the changes in metal elements inside the internal organs of "yin-deficiency" mice models. Zhongguo Zhong Yao Za Zhi. **18**(11), 690–2, 704 (1993)

Y. Qian, Y.M. Xue, J. Li, Effects of Liuweidihuang pills on plasma adiponectin level in OLETF rats. Nan Fang Yi Ke Da Xue Xue Bao **28**(1), 34–36 (2008)

L.L. Song et al., Determination of ursolic acid of Liuwei Dihuangwan simulation samples by NIR. Zhongguo Zhong Yao Za Zhi **31**(19), 1590–1593 (2006)

R. Xu, *Internal Medicine*, China Press of Traditional Chinese Medicine, (2011), (in Chinese)

Y.M. Xue et al., Effects of liuwei dihuang pills on expressions of apoptosis-related genes bcl-2 and Bax in pancreas of OLETF rats. Zhong Xi Yi Jie He Xue Bao **3**(6), 455–458 (2005)

X. Zhao, Y. Wang, Y. Sun, Quantitative and qualitative determination of Liuwei Dihuang tablets by HPLC-UV-MS-MS. J. Chromatogr. Sci. **45**(8), 549–52 (2007)

G. Zheng, H. Guo, Y. Guo, X. He, Z. Li, A. Lu, Two dimensions data slicing algorithm, a new approach in mining rules of literature in traditional Chinese medicine, in *2011 International Conference on Artificial Intelligence and Computational Intelligence, AICI 2011*, Taiyuan, 23–25 Sept 2011, pp. 161–174

G. Zheng, M. Jiang, X. He, J. Zhao, H. Guo, G. Chen, Q. Zha, A. Lu, Discrete derivative: a data slicing algorithm for exploration of sharing biological networks between rheumatoid arthritis and coronary heart disease. BioData. Min. **4**, 18 (2011b)

G. Zheng, M. Jiang, C. Lu, H. Guo, J. Zhan, A. Lu, Exploring the biological basis of deficiency pattern in rheumatoid arthritis through text mining, in *2011 IEEE International Conference onBioinformatics and Biomedicine Workshops, BIBMW 2011*, Atlanta, 12–15 Nov 2011, pp. 811–816

Z. Zhou, *Internal Medicine of Traditional Chinese medicine*, China Press of Traditional Chinese Medicine, (2008), (in Chinese)

Statistical Validation of TCM Syndrome Postulates in the Context of Depressive Patients

Yan Zhao, Nevin L. Zhang, Tianfang Wang, Qingguo Wang, and Tengfei Liu

Abstract

Objective: Traditional Chinese medicine (TCM) has many postulates that explain the co-occurrence of symptoms using syndrome factors such as YANG DEFICIENCY and YIN DEFICIENCY. A fundamental question is whether the syndrome factors have verifiable scientific contents in them or they are pure subjective notions. We investigate the issue in the context of depressive patients.

Design: In the past, researchers have tried to show that TCM syndrome factors correspond to real entities by means of laboratory tests, but there has been little success. An alternative approach called latent tree analysis has recently been proposed. The idea is to discover latent variables behind unlabeled symptom data based on statistical principles and compare them with TCM syndrome factors. If there is good match, then one obtains statistical evidence in support of the validity of the relevant TCM postulates. We use latent tree analysis in our investigation.

Setting: TCM symptom data of 604 depressive patients were collected from nine hospitals from several regions of China in 2005–2006.

Results: Latent tree analysis of the data yielded a model with 29 latent variables. Many of them correspond to TCM syndrome factors.

Conclusions: The results provide statistical evidence for the validity of TCM postulates in the context of depressive patients. In other words, they show that TCM postulates are applicable to depressive patients. This is significant because it is a precondition for the TCM treatment of those patients.

Y. Zhao • T. Wang • Q. Wang
Beijing University of Chinese Medicine, Beijing, People's Republic of China

N.L. Zhang (✉) • T. Liu
The Hong Kong University of Science and Technology, Hong Kong, People's Republic of China
e-mail: lzhang@cse.ust.hk

J. Poon and S.K. Poon (eds.), *Data Analytics for Traditional Chinese Medicine Research*, 111
DOI 10.1007/978-3-319-03801-8_6, © Springer International Publishing Switzerland 2014

1 Introduction

TCM diagnosis starts with an overall observation of symptoms (including signs) using four diagnostic methods, namely inspection, listening, inquiry, and palpation. Based on the information collected, patients are classified into various categories that are collectively known as *ZHENG* (WHO 2007). The Chinese term ZHENG is usually translated as *TCM syndrome*. The process of classifying patients into various syndrome classes is known as *syndrome differentiation*.

TCM syndrome classes such as YANG DEFICIENCY and YIN DEFICIENCY come from TCM postulates where they are used to explain the co-occurrence of signs and symptoms. For example, TCM asserts that YANG QI and YIN FLUID are essential materials of human body and have the functions of warming and nourishing the body respectively. Deficiency of YANG QI can lead to the co-occurrence of, among others, 'fear of cold' and 'cold limbs'. Hence patients with those symptoms are often classified into the YANG DEFICIENCY class. Similarly, deficiency of YIN FLUID may lead to the co-occurrence of, among others, 'dry mouth and throat' and 'heat in the palms and soles'. Hence patients with those symptoms are often classified into the YIN DEFICIENCY class.

Western Medicine divides patients into various classes according to disease types or subtypes and treats them accordingly. In contrast TCM divides patients into various classes according to syndrome types and treats them accordingly. Syndrome-oriented treatment, rather than disease-oriented treatment, is regarded as the key characteristic and strength of TCM.

Two fundamental questions are often asked of TCM syndrome classes. Do they correspond to real-world entities or are they pure subjective notions? Is TCM syndrome differentiation a completely subjective matter or can it be based on objective evidence? For more than half a century, researchers have been seeking answers to those questions by means of laboratory tests (Wang and Xu 1999; Feng et al. 2004). However, the questions still remain open today (Liang et al. 1998).

A different approach has recently been proposed by Zhang et al. (2008a, b). They distinguish between two kinds of variables in TCM. Symptoms such as 'fear of cold' and 'dry mouth and throat' can be directly observed clinically and hence are called *observed variables*. Syndrome types such as YANG DEFICIENCY and YIN DEFICIENCY, on the other hand, cannot be directly observed and must be indirectly determined based on symptoms. Hence they are called *latent factors*.

Zhang et al. conjecture that specific syndrome notions such as YANG DEFICIENCY and YIN DEFICIENCY originated from patterns of symptom co-occurrence observed in clinic practice. They propose a new approach to TCM syndrome research where a researcher: (1) Collects data about the occurrence of symptoms on patients while excluding the diagnostic judgments by doctors, and (2) tries to, from the unlabelled data collected, re-extract the latent factors postulated in TCM. Diagnosis results are not collected in the first step because the very purpose of the method is to provide objective evidence for TCM diagnosis. The second step is done using a new class of probabilistic models called latent tree models that they have developed specifically for TCM syndrome research (Zhang et al. 2008b). As such the approach is known as latent tree analysis.

Zhang et al. (2008a, b) have tested the latent tree analysis method on a KYDNEY DEFICIENCY data set. The latent variables they discovered do match the relevant TCM latent factors well.[1] This provides statistical validation to the relevant TCM postulates and is a breakthrough. Although they have not proved that TCM syndrome classes correspond to real entities, their results have confirmed that the symptom co-occurrence patterns implied by TCM syndromes do exist in data. It is a breakthrough. A similar study has recently been carried out on patients of cardiovascular disease (Xu et al. 2013).

In this work we use latent tree analysis to study a data set of 604 depressive patients, henceforth referred to as the depression data set. The latent variables we discovered also match TCM latent factors well. This provides evidence for the validity of the relevant TCM postulates in the context depressive patients, and consequently offers justifications for dividing depressive patients according into TCM syndrome classes.

2　Methods

2.1　Data Collection

The data were collected in 2005–2006. The subjects were inpatients or outpatients aged between 19 and 69 from nine hospitals from several regions of China. They were selected using the Chinese classification of mental disorder clinic guideline CCMD-3 (Chen 2002). CCMD-3 is similar in structure and categorization to the ICD and DSM manuals, though includes some variations on their main diagnoses and around 40 culturally related diagnoses.

Excluded from the study were subjects who took anti-depression drugs within 2 weeks prior to the survey, women in the gestational and suckling periods, patients suffering from other mental disorders such as mania, and those suffering from other severe diseases or having had operations recently.

The symptoms (and signs) were extracted from the TCM literature on depression between 1994 and 2004. We searched with the phrase "抑郁 and 证" (Depression and ZHENG) on the CNKI (China National Knowledge Infrastructure) database. Among the articles returned by CNKI, we kept only those on studies where patients were selected using the ICD-9, ICD-10, CCMD-2, or CCMD-3 guidelines. This resulted in 65 articles and they contain totally 198 distinct symptoms. The symptoms that appear only one time or two times were removed. We finally ended up with 143 symptoms.

---

[1] Note that we use 'latent factors' to refer to unobserved factors in TCM, and 'latent variables' to refer to unobserved variables in statistical models.

An epidemiologic survey was conducted on the 143 symptoms. Six hundred and four patient cases were collected. Each patient case contains information about which symptoms occurred on the patient and which ones did not. Various measures were taken to ensure data quality. Examples include staff training, site visit by principal investigators, and dual data entry.

In the 604 patient cases, 57 symptoms occur fewer than 10 times. They were removed from the data set and the remaining 86 symptoms were included in further analysis.

2.2 Latent Tree Analysis

The data were analyzed using latent tree analysis. In the following, we first briefly review latent tree analysis and explain how and in what sense it can provide statistical validation to postulates about latent factors.

Latent tree analysis refers to the analysis of data using latent tree models. An example latent tree model is shown in Fig. 1a. It asserts that a student's Math grade (MG) and Science grade (SG) are influenced by his analytical skill (AS); his English grade (EG) and History grade (HG) are influenced by his literal skill (LS); and the two skills are correlated. Here, the grades are *observed variables*, while the skills are *latent variables*.

For simplicity, assume all the variables have two possible values 'low' and 'high'. The dependence of MG on AS is characterized by the conditional distribution P(MG|AS), which is also shown in Fig. 1. It says that a student with high AS tends to get high MG and a student with low AS is tends to get low MG. Similarly the dependence of other grade variables on the skill variables are characterized by P(SG|AS), P(EG|LS) and P(HG|LS) respectively. They are not shown to save space. The quantitative relationships between AS and LS are described by the distributions P(AS) and (LS|AS). Alternatively, they might also be described by P(LS) and P(AS|LS).

In Fig. 1, correlation strength between variables is visually shown as edge (line) width. For example, the dependence of MG on AS is stronger than that of SG on AS, and the dependence of EG on LS is stronger than that of HG on LS. Technically, the width of an edge represents the mutual information between the two variables that it connects. The mutual information is computed from the probability distributions of the model.

The input to latent tree analysis is a table where each column represents an observed variable and each row consists of the values of the observed variables for an individual. It does not contain values for latent variables. Many different latent tree models can be constructed for the observed variables that appear in the data. A model selection criterion is used to pick one of the models as the output. Latent tree analysis uses the Bayes information criterion (BIC) (Schwarz 1978) for this purpose. The BIC score consists of two terms, a likelihood term and a penalty term. The likelihood term requires that the model fits the data as closely as possible, while the penalty term ensures that the model is not overly complicated.

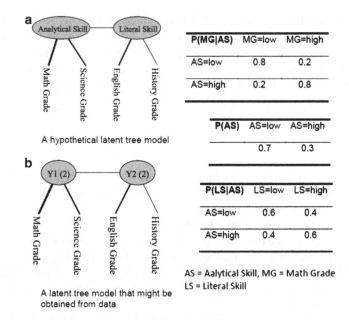

P(MG|AS)	MG=low	MG=high
AS=low	0.8	0.2
AS=high	0.2	0.8

P(AS)	AS=low	AS=high
	0.7	0.3

P(LS|AS)	LS=low	LS=high
AS=low	0.6	0.4
AS=high	0.4	0.6

AS = Aalytical Skill, MG = Math Grade
LS = Literal Skill

Fig. 1 The first subfigure and the tables illustrate the concept of latent tree models using an example that involves two latent variables (the skill variables) and four observed variables (the grade variables). The second subfigure shows a model that might be obtained from data on the four observed variables. The numbers next to the latent variables *Y1* and *Y2* indicate that they both have two possible values

There usually are too many possible latent tree models to enumerate exhaustively. An algorithm called Expand-Adjust-Simplify-Termination (EAST) (Chen et al. 2011) is used to deal with this computational difficulty.[2] It has empirically been shown to be efficient enough to handle data with up to 100 observed variables and is able to find high quality models.

Now assume that we want to provide, with respect to a student population, statistical validation for the following postulates:

(1) MG and SG are influenced by the latent factor AS, and
(2) EG and HG are influenced by the latent factor LS.

The first step would be to sample a subset of students and survey their grades on the four subjects. The next step would be to perform latent tree analysis on the survey data. Suppose, in the data, high MG is frequently accompanied by high SG while high EG is frequently accompanied by high HG. Further suppose that the correlation between the two groups {MG, SG} and {EG, HG} is not as strong as those between the group members. Then latent tree analysis is likely to yield the model shown in Fig. 1b. If this turns out to be the case, we draw this conclusion: It fits to the data to

---

[2] A Java implementation of EAST that is available at http://www.cse.ust.hk/~lzhang/ltm/index.htm.

hypothesize that there is latent factor which influences MG and SG, and there is another latent factor that influences EG and HG. In this sense, we have provided statistical evidence that supports the two postulates. Although we have not proved that AS and LS correspond real entities, we have shown that postulating the existence of AS and LS would explain the correlations among four grade variables well.

3 Results

The result of the analysis is a latent tree model, which will be referred to as the depression model. The structure of the model is shown in Fig. 2. In the model, the nodes labeled with English phrases represent symptom variables. Each of them has two possible values, representing the presence or absence of the symptoms. The symptom variables come from the data set. The nodes labeled with the capital letter 'Y' and integer subscripts are the latent variables. They are not from the data set. Rather they were introduced during data analysis to explain patterns in the data. There is an integer next to each latent variable. It is the number of possible values of that latent variable.

The edges in the model represent probabilistic dependence. Each edge is characterized by a conditional probability distribution. The widths of the edges denote the strength of correlations between variables. For example, Y29 is strongly correlated with 'cold limbs', moderately correlated with 'fear of cold', and weakly correlated with 'rough pulse'. In this paper, we will mainly focus on the links between variables and the strength of those links. The conditional probability distributions contain quantitative information that can be used as evidence for syndrome differentiation. We will discuss them in future work.

4 Discussions

4.1 Latent Variables as Evidence for TCM Postulates

In a latent tree model, the collection of observed variables directly connected to a particular latent variable is called a *sibling cluster*. The sibling cluster together with the latent variable forms a *family*. For example, the three symptom variables under Y28 'aching lumbus', 'lumbar pain liking pressure' and 'lumbar pain liking warmth' make up a sibling cluster. Together with Y28, they form a *family*, which is said to be *headed* by Y28.

Why some symptom variables are grouped to form sibling clusters during latent tree analysis? Why are latent variables introduced? An examination of the model (both qualitative and quantitative information) reveals that there are three cases with regard to this question. First, some symptom variables are grouped into one sibling cluster because they tend to co-occur. One example is 'baking heat' and 'heat in

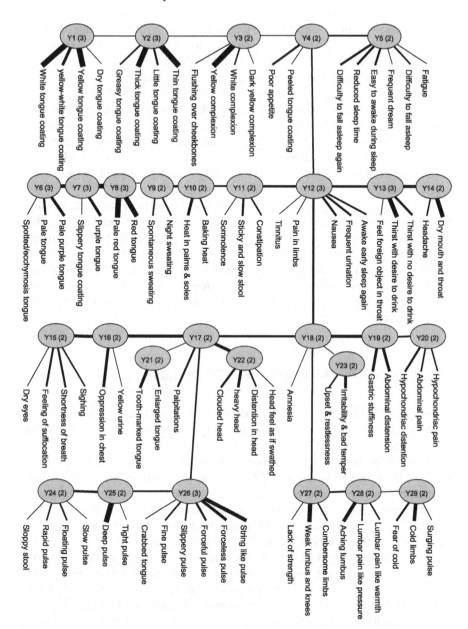

Fig. 2 The structure of the latent tree model learned from the depression data set

palms & soles' in the family headed by Y10. In this case, the latent variable is introduced to explain the co-occurrence of the symptoms. Second, some symptom variables are grouped into one sibling cluster because they are mutually exclusive. One
example is 'red tongue' and 'pale red tongue' in the family headed by Y8. In this

case, the latent variable is introduced to represent a partition of the patients based on those symptoms. The third case is a mixture of the first two cases. One example is in the family headed by Y26, where 'forceful pulse' and 'forceless' are mutually exclusive, whereas they both co-occur with 'string like pulse'.

Latent variables of the first case are evidence for the validity of TCM postulates. For example, TCM posits that YIN DEFICIENCY may lead to 'baking heat' and 'heat in palms & soles'. An implication of this postulate is that the two symptoms would tend to co-occur in clinic practice. The introduction of Y10 during latent tree analysis has confirmed that 'baking heat' and 'heat in palms & soles' indeed tend to co-occur in the data. In other words, it has verified an implication of the postulate. In this sense, it provides support for the TCM postulate.

Note that several symptom variables in the model seem to be out of place. They include 'somnolence' under Y11, 'tinnitus' and 'pain in limbs' under Y12, 'dry eyes' under Y15, 'yellow urine' under Y16, 'sloppy stool' under Y24, and 'rough pulse' under Y29. Those symptoms occur rarely in the data and hence there is not sufficient information to determine appropriate locations for them in the model. As a matter of fact, those symptoms variables are only weakly related to the latent variables to which they are directly connected. We will ignore those variables in subsequent discussions.

4.2   Evidence for the Validity of TCM Postulates

Having explained how latent tree analysis can provide evidence for the validity of TCM postulates, we now set out to systematically examine the depression model for such evidence.

Starting from the bottom right corner of the model, we notice that 'fear of cold' and 'cold limbs' are grouped under Y29. This and relevant quantitative information indicate that the two symptoms tend to co-occur in the data. On the other hand, the co-occurrence of the two symptoms is an implication of the postulate that YANG DEFICIENCY leads to 'fear of cold' and 'cold limbs'. So, Y29 has verified the implication and is hence evidence for the validity of the postulate.

The family headed by Y28 indicates the three symptoms 'aching lumbus', 'lumbar pain like pressure' and 'lumbar pain like warmth' tends to co-occur in the data. It is evidence in support of the postulate that KINDNEY DEPRIVED OF NOURISHMENT may lead to 'aching lumbus', 'lumbar pain like pressure' and 'lumbar pain like warmth'. The family headed by Y27 indicates that 'weak lumbus and knees' and 'cumbersome limbs' tends to co-occur in the data. It is evidence in support of the postulate that KINDNEY DEFICIENCY may lead to 'weak lumbus and knees' and 'cumbersome limbs'. The close proximity of Y27 and Y28 to each other is consistent with the postulate that KINDNEY DEPRIVED OF NOURISHMENT and KINDNEY DEFICIENCY are closely related.

The family headed by Y23 indicates that 'upset and restlessness' and 'irritability & bad temper' tend to co-occur in the data. It is evidence in support of the postulate

STAGNANT QI TRANSFORMING INTO FIRE leads to 'upset and restlessness' and 'irritability & bad temper'. The family headed by Y21 indicates that 'enlarged tongue' and 'tooth-marked tongue' tend to co-occur in the data. It is evidence in support of the postulate SPLEEN DEFICIENCY AND INTERNAL ACCUMULATION OF EXCESSIVE DAMPNESS leads to 'enlarged tongue' and 'tooth-marked tongue'.

The family headed by Y20 indicates that the three symptoms 'hypochondriac distention', 'hypochondriac pain' and 'abdominal pain' tend to co-occur in the data. It is evidence in support of the postulate that LIVER QI FAILING TO FLOW FREELY leads to 'hypochondriac distention', 'hypochondriac pain' and 'abdominal pain'. The family headed by Y19 indicates that 'gastric stuffiness' and 'abdominal distention' tends to co-occur in the data. It is evidence in support of the postulate that IMPAIRED HARMONIOUS DOWNBEARING OF STOMACH leads 'gastric stuffiness' and 'abdominal distention'. The close proximity of Y20 and Y19 to each other is consistent with the TCM notion of LIVER-STOMACH DISHARMONY.

The latent variables Y15, Y16 and Y17 are strongly correlated with each other. Collectively, they are strongly correlated with 'feeling of suffocation', 'shortness of breath', 'sighing', 'oppression in chest' and 'palpitation'. Those support the postulate that STAGNATION OF QI ACTIVITY IN THE CHEST leads to those five symptoms.

The family headed by Y22 indicates that the three symptoms 'clouded head', 'heavy head' and 'distention in head' tend to co-occur in the data. It is evidence in support of the postulate that QI STAGNATION IN HEAD leads to 'clouded head', 'heavy head' and 'distention in head'.

The family headed by Y11 indicates that 'constipation' and 'sticky and slow stool' tend to co-occur in the data. It is evidence in support of the postulate that SPLEEN DEFICIENCY AND INTERNAL ACCUMULATION OF EXCESSIVE DAMPNESS leads to 'constipation' and 'sticky and slow stool'. The family headed by Y10 indicates that 'baking heat' and 'heat in palms & soles' tend to co-occur in the data. It is evidence in support of the postulate that YIN DEFICIENCY leads to 'baking heat' and 'heat in palms & soles'. Finally, the family headed by Y9 indicates that 'spontaneous sweating' and 'night sweating' tend to co-occur in data. It is evidence in support of the postulate that QI-YIN BOTH IN DEFICIENCY can lead to 'spontaneous sweating' and 'night sweating'.

A summary of the foregoing discussion is given in Table 1. We see that latent variables Y23, Y22, Y20, Y17, Y16, Y15 are all related to QI-STAGNATION. They capture different aspects of the TCM syndrome factor. Similarly, Y21 and Y11 capture different aspects of SPLEEN DEFICIENCY AND INTERNAL ACCUMULATION OF EXCESSIVE DAMPNESS.

The other sibling clusters in the model are also clearly meaningful. The variables under Y1 are mostly about the color of tongue coating; The variables under Y2 are mostly about the thickness of tongue coating; The variables under Y3 are mostly about facial complexions; The variables under Y5 are mostly about sleep disorders; The variables under Y6, Y7 and Y8 are mostly about the color of tongue; The variables under Y13 are about thirst; The variables under Y24, Y25 and Y26 are mostly about

Table 1 Summary of evidence for the validity of TCM postulates: The first column shows TCM syndrome factors. The second column shows some of the symptoms that the syndrome factor might bring about according to TCM postulates. An implication of the postulates is that the symptoms tend to co-occur in clinic practice. The third column shows that latent variables that confirm the co-occurrence patterns in data. They are evidence in support of the postulates

TCM syndrome factors	Symptoms	Latent variables
YANG DEFICIENCY	fear of cold, cold limbs	Y29
KINDNEY DEPRIVED OF NOURISHMENT	aching lumbus, lumbar pain like pressure, lumbar pain like warmth	Y28
KINDNEY DEFICIENCY	weak lumbus and knees, cumbersome limbs	Y27
STAGNANT QI TRANSFORMING INTO FIRE	upset and restlessness, irritability & bad temper	Y23
QI STAGNATION IN HEAD	clouded head, heavy head, distention in head	Y22
SPLEEN DEFICIENCY AND INTERNAL ACCUMULATION OF EXCESSIVE DAMPNESS	enlarged tongue, tooth-marked tongue	Y21
LIVER QI FAILING TO FLOW FREELY	hypochondriac distention, hypochondriac pain, abdominal pain	Y20
IMPAIRED HARMONIOUS DOWNBEARING OF STOMACH	gastric stuffiness, abdominal distention	Y19
STAGNATION OF QI ACTIVITY IN THE CHEST	feeling of suffocation, shortness of breath, sighing, oppression in chest, palpitation	Y17, Y16, Y15
SPLEEN DEFICIENCY AND INTERNAL ACCUMULATION OF EXCESSIVE DAMPNESS	constipation, sticky and slow stool	Y11
YIN DEFICIENCY	baking heat, heat in palms & soles	Y10
QI-YIN BOTH IN DEFICIENCY	spontaneous sweating, night sweating	Y9

pulse. Like the latent variables discussed above, those latent variables identify patterns in the data. However, those patterns do not correspond to TCM latent factors. Rather they represent simple partitions of patients. For example, Y1 represents a partition of the patients into three groups: 'white tongue coating', 'yellow tongue coating' and 'yellow-white tongue coating'.

5 Conclusions

We have performed latent tree analysis on the symptom data of 604 depressive patients. We present the resulting model and explain how to understand and appreciate the qualitative aspect of the model. In particular we discuss how and in what sense the data analysis provides evidence in support of TCM postulates. We identify all the evidence contained the model in support of the relevant TCM postulates through a systematic examination of the model. This work has shown that TCM postulates are applicable to depressive patients. Consequently, it is justified to classify depressive patients using TCM syndrome factors.

Acknowledgments Research on this paper was supported by China National Basic Research 973 Program under project No. 2011CB505101, 2011CB505105, Guangzhou HKUST Fok Ying Tung Research Institute, Innovative Team Project of Beijing University of Chinese Medicine (2011-CXTD-08), and Research Base Development Project of Beijing University of Chinese Medicine (2011-JDJS-09). We thank the anonymous reviewers for useful comments.

References

Y.F. Chen, Chinese classification of mental disorders (CCMD-3): towards integration in international classification. Psychopathology **35**(2–3), 171–175 (2002)

T. Chen, N.L. Zhang, T.F. Liu, Y. Wang, K.M. Poon, Model-based multidimensional clustering of categorical data. Artif. Intell. **176**(1), 2246–2269 (2011)

Y. Feng, Z. Wu, X. Zhou, Z. Zhou, W. Fan, Knowledge discovery in traditional Chinese medicine: state of the art and perspectives. Artif. Intell. Med. **38**, 219–236 (2004)

M.X. Liang, J. Liu, Z.P. Hong, Y.Y. Xu, *Perplexity of TCM Syndrome Research and Countermeasures* (People's Health Press, Beijing, 1998)

G. Schwarz, Estimating the dimension of model. Ann. Stat. **6**(2), 461–464 (1978)

H.X. Wang, Y.L. Xu, *The Current State and Future of Basic Theoretical Research on Traditional Chinese Medicine* (Military Medical Sciences Press, Beijing, 1999)

WHO, *WHO International Standard Terminologies on Traditional Medicine in the Western Pacific Region* (World Health Organization, Manila, 2007)

Z.X. Xu, N.L. Zhang, Y.Q. Wang, G.P. Liu, J. Xu, T.F. Liu, A.H. Liu, Statistical validation of traditional Chinese medicine syndrome postulates in the context of patients with cardiovascular disease. J. Altern. Complement. Med. **18**, 1–6 (2013)

N.L. Zhang, S.H. Yuan, Y. Chen, Y. Wang, Latent tree models and diagnosis in traditional Chinese medicine. Artif. Intell. Med. **42**, 229–245 (2008a)

N.L. Zhang, S.H. Yuan, Y. Chen, Y. Wang, Statistical validation of TCM theories. J. Altern. Complement. Med. **14**(5), 583–587 (2008b)

Artificial Neural Network Based Chinese Medicine Diagnosis in Decision Support Manner and Herbal Ingredient Discoveries

Wilfred Lin and Jackei Wong

Abstract Artificial neural network (ANN) for fast and trusted herbal ingredient discoveries is proposed. It is fast, because different ANN modules can be executed in parallel, and the ANN results are trustworthy, because they can be verified by TCM domain experts in real clinical environments in Hong Kong, Nanning, GuangXi, China and New York, United States of America. The ANN is able to learn the relationship between herbal ingredients and the set of information given (e.g. symptoms and illnesses). The ANN output is called the relevance index (RI), which conceptually associates two TCM entities.

1 Introduction

We propose a novel approach of applying the artificial neural network (ANN) based on backpropagation for Chinese Medicine Diagnosis in decision support manner and for fast, trusted herbal ingredient discoveries. The approach will be verified in a real TCM (Traditional Chinese Medicine) clinical environment. Firstly, the ANN modules will be trained with real patient cases, and secondly domain experts will be enlisted to confirm the discoveries to make them trustworthy. If the relevance between two TCM entities (e.g. an herbal ingredient and an illness) was never explicitly defined/annotated but is revealed by the trained named ANN module (e.g. named after an herbal ingredient or illness), it is a potential discovery in the context of the proposed ANN approach.

W. Lin (✉) • J. Wong
HerbMiners Informatics Limited, Unit 209A, Photonics Centre,
Hong Kong Science Park, Hong Kong
e-mail: wlin@herbminers.com; jwong@herbminers.com

J. Poon and S.K. Poon (eds.), *Data Analytics for Traditional Chinese Medicine Research*, 123
DOI 10.1007/978-3-319-03801-8_7, © Springer International Publishing Switzerland 2014

The proposal of the novel ANN approach is inspired for the following reasons:

(a) Our previous research and development experience in the area of clinical TCM ontology (Wong et al. 2008) indicates that ontological constructs can be huge and complex. Fast herbal discovery may therefore be quickened by parallel processing (Wong et al. 2010). In this light, many trained named ANN modules could be invoked at the same time for parallelism and thus speedup.

(b) The same basic ANN construct can be trained by different datasets to become specialized ANN modules, named after the specific TCM entities (e.g. an illness); for example the ANN_{Flu} module is dedicated to Flu analysis.

(c) The relevance between two TCM entities (e.g. an herbal ingredient U and an illness (or a set of illness) V) can be computed to indicate the likelihood of a discovery. The computed value is called the relevance index (RI) between U and V, to explicitly show their association. The algorithm to compute the specific RI should be already consensus-certified by domain experts.

2   Related Work

The HerbMiners Cloud Computing Platform, Chinese Medicine Clinical Data Warehouse architecture is illustrated in Fig. 1.

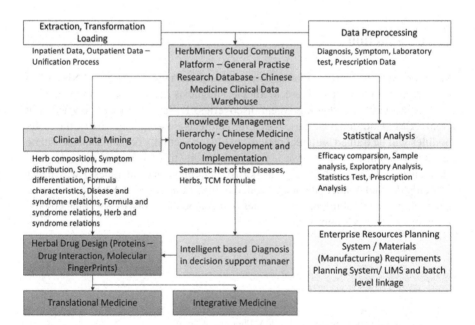

Fig. 1 The HerbMiners Cloud Computing Platform, Chinese Medicine Clinical Data Warehouse architecture

Our literature review of soft computing techniques (Lin et al. 2006; Ghosh and Tsutsui 2003; Wong et al. 2008; Yann et al. 1998; Zhao et al. 2003) indicates that the artificial neural network (ANN) based on backpropagation is suitable for fast, trusted herbal ingredient discoveries. The reasons are: (i) reusability – the same ANN construct can be trained to become named ANN modules that assume different roles; (ii) simplicity – it is easy to program and less error-prone than the traditional algorithmic programming approach; (iii) data-orientation – the logical points inside an ANN construct will converge to the required logical operation with respect to the given training dataset; (iv) versatility – an ANN construct can be combined with its clones or other constructs to form larger, more complex ANN configurations; (v) adaptability – the neuron's activation function can be replaced any time, and the input parameters to a neuron can be weighted and normalized according to the needs; (vi) optimization – an ANN can be effectively optimized or pruned for a particular operation (Wong et al. 2008); (vii) commodity – many ANN constructs in the form of freeware are available in the public domain with rich user experience, (viii) accuracy – as long as the number of the hidden neurons is twice that of the input neurons the ANN output is accurate (Hagan 1996; Gallant and White 1992); and (ix) parallelism – many named ANN constructs can be invoked to work in parallel for speedup. The ANN configuration by propagation has a three-layer architecture: (i) a layer of input neurons; (ii) a layer of hidden neurons interconnected with the input neurons; and (iii) one output neuron interconnected with the hidden neurons. The behavior of every neuron is governed by its activation function (e.g. Sigmoid) (Lin et al. 2006).

If O_i^n is the output of nth neuron in the ith stratum of the hidden layer in the ANN module, then $O_i^n = f(O_{i-1}{}^j | j = 1, 2, ..., m)$ indicates that O_i^n is the function of the m neurons in the $(i-1)^{th}$ stratum. If the activation function is Sigmoid, which is memoryless, then $O_i^n = f(O_{i-1}{}^j | j = 1, 2, ..., m)$ is simply $O_i^n = \sum_{j=1}^{j=m} O_{i-1}$. This is the obvious result from the rule of superposition that can be applied to any memoryless distribution. According to the Hessian minima concept (Wong et al. 2008), those ANN arcs (i.e. $O_{i-1}{}^j$ in $f(O_{i-1}{}^j | j = 1, 2, ..., m)$) of the lowest values may be pruned (i.e. optimized) on the fly to reduce the ANN computation time for higher speedup (e.g. Lin et al. 2004). That is, the impact by ANN arcs of the lowest weights on O_i^n is insignificant.

3   ANN by Backpropagation

The generic ANN configuration has three layers: (i) input neurons; (ii) hidden neurons; and (iii) one output neuron. The value computed by the output neuron, when training has completed, in the proposed approach is the relevance index (RI). Training is completed (i.e. the ANN has learned) with respect to the given dataset if the root mean square error (RMSE) has stabilized. In the proposed ANN approach every ANN is named after a specific TCM entity (e.g. an herbal name or an illness).

The RI conceptually indicates the relevance of two chosen entities; for example, the specific herbal ingredient that the trained ANN module is named after (e.g. GanCao) and the named illness (e.g. WindHeat in Fig. 6). If this relevance was not explicitly recorded in the original TCM ontology, it is a potential discovery in the context of this paper (Wong et al. 2010). The training process is also called supervised learning, which is an equitable scheme, for the ANN inputs can be weighted according to their degree of significance to the target result by the domain experts.

The RI concept is based on the IT (information technology) formalism, which is represented by the following logical expression, $P(U \cup V)$; that is, $P(U \cup V) = P(U) + P(V) - P(U \cap V)$. P is for probability; $\cup$ for union; $\cap$ for intersection; U and V are two entities defined separately by two sets of parameters/attributes; $P(U \cap V)$ is the degree of similarity or relevance between U and V. The $P(U \cap V)$ value, which can be computed by the predefined algorithm, is the relevance index (RI) in the proposed ANN approach for herbal ingredient discoveries. Figure 3 puts the RI formal basis into perspective. The three entities in this case are defined by attributes in the brackets $\{\}$, $E1 = \{x1, x2, x3, x4\}$, $E2 = \{x1, x2, x3, x6\}$ and $E3 = \{x1, x2, x3, x5, x7, x8\}$. Simply based on the number of common attributes and the angle of the referential entity (RC), the RI may be calculated. For example, if Entity 1 is the RC, the degree of similarity of Entity 2 (to Entity 1) is 3/4 or 0.75 (i.e. 75 %); same for Entity 3. If Entity 3 is the RC, however, the similarity of Entity 1 is only 3/7 (i.e. less than 45 %). The RC concept can be applied to entities of the same or different classes. In TCM, the three entities in Fig. 3 may be all herbal ingredients, all illnesses or a mix of herbal ingredient(s) and illness(es). Yet, the measurement of the RIs in this case is simply based on a common set of attributes (e.g. symptoms). For example, if Entity 1 is an herbal ingredient that can treat the symptoms in $\{x1, x2, x3, x4\}$ and Entity 3 is the illness defined by the set of symptoms in $\{x1, x2, x3, x5, x7, x8\}$, using E3 as the RC then by the "SAME/SIMILARITY" TCM formalism (Wong et al. 2008; Wong et al. 2010) E1 has a logical treatment efficacy of 3/7 for E3. This efficacy is usually consensus-certified beforehand, with the due adjustment for specific environments if necessary, by a sufficient number of TCM domain experts.

The SAME/SIMILARITY TCM formalism is a formal diagnostic principle enshrined (consensus-certified) in the TCM classics: "同病異治, 異病同治"; SAME and "同" are translational synonyms. In English this principle is defined as: "*If the symptoms are the same or similar, different conditions could be treated in the same way medically, independent of whether they come from the same illness or different ones* (World Health Organization 2007)." Consensus certification is a process to agree upon a concept, the semantics of an entity, or a set of procedures by a sufficient number of experts from a domain or community. The agreement creates the standard vocabulary/lexicon that serves as the communal ontology that embeds the body of knowledge to be passed on or adhered to in practice.

The ANN operation can be a 2-D or 3-D (D for dimension) relationship. For example, a 3-D relationship can be realized by combining elements from three major sets: (i) illnesses, $I = \{i_1, i_2, \ldots, i_n\}$; (ii) herbal ingredients for treatment, $H = \{h_1, h_2, \ldots, h_m\}$; and (iii) recognizable symptoms, $S = \{s_1, s_2, \ldots, s_k\}$. Thus, the diagnosis of an illness i_j is to identify S_j, which is a subset of S for $\{(i_j \in I)|(S_j \in S)\}$, where "|" means $(i_j \in I)$ satisfying $(S_j \in S)$. The set of treatments/prescriptions is then $T_j = \{(h_j \in H)|S_j\}$ for i_j conceptually. Therefore, training a dedicated ANN module, which is named after a herbal ingredient $h_x \in H$ (i.e. ANN_{h_x}), should involve a set of real T_j or patient cases C. If all the symptoms are identified from C and the training takes the symptoms of each case in C as input sequentially, then ANN_{h_x} would converge to a 2-D RI value that reflects the relevance of C or T_j (i.e. the set) to h_x as shown in Fig. 4.

A 3-D RI convergence that connects h_x and i_y can be created by pruning those cases other than i_y from C manually, to create the resultant trimmed subset C_{h_x,i_y}. If the symptoms of each patient case in C_{h_x,i_y} are fed as input to the ANN_{h_x} module during the training session, the resultant RI value has a 3-D implication conceptually. That is, the RI indicates how the herbal ingredient h_x associates with i_y. If this association or relevance was never explicitly and formally stated in the TCM environment of interest, it is a potential discovery, which has to be formally confirmed by domain experts (i.e. consensus-certified).

4 Experimental Results

Many experiments were conducted in the Nong's clinical environment (Wong et al. 2008) to verify the proposed ANN approach. These experiments involved real patient cases (i.e. T_j), and the results indicate that the proposed approach can indeed support effective herbal discoveries. In this section three sets of experimental results are presented as follows:

(a) 2-D training of three ANN modules named after the specific illnesses (i.e. ANN_{i_y}): In the experiments, each of these named modules is dedicated to an illness subtype formally classified in the TCM context under the illness Flu (感冒) (World Health Organization 2007) as: WindHeat Syndrome (風熱證), WindCold Syndrome (風寒證) and Summer-Heat Dampness Syndrome (暑濕證). The results, which are produced with the same training clinical dataset C or T_j (without pruning or trimming), are plotted in Fig. 4.

(b) 3-D training of the ten ANN modules named after the corresponding herbal ingredients (i.e. ANN_{h_x}): The same training dataset C was pruned first with respect to $\{h_x$ and $i_y\}$ so that the trimmed C_{h_x,i_y} was produced to train each distinct ANN_{h_x} (e.g. ANN_{GanCao}). For example, for the case of $\{h_x = GanCao, i_y = WindHeat\}$ only the trimmed subset $C_{GanCao,WindHeat}$ would be used to train the dedicated ANN_{GanCao} module. Figure 5 is the 3-D dimensional plot in which all the 3-D RI convergences from the ten dedicated ANN modules are superimposed for comparison.

(c) Example of an herbal ingredient discovery: A substantial number of fresh clinical records were added to the original training dataset C first before it was pruned to produce the new trimmed C_{h_x,i_y}^{new} subset that drove the training of a named module ANN_{h_x}. The training process is the same as for Fig. 5, except C_{h_x,i_y}^{new} would drive the new training process. Figure 6 shows that the new clinical knowledge included in C_{h_x,i_y}^{new} led to the discovery that involves the herb HeHuanPi. The old training data in C_{h_x,i_y} (Fig. 5) did not indicate the relevance between HeHuanPi and the two Flu subtypes: WindHeat and WindCold. Yet, the new knowledge included in C_{h_x,i_y}^{new} reveals that HeHuanPi can treat the two Flu subtypes as well, and this is a potential herbal ingredient discovery instance.

The training of a named ANN module (e.g. ANN_{h_x}) is based on the ambit/amount of knowledge embedded in the training dataset. The named ANN module is considered trained or learned if it has settled down to a stable RMSE (root means square error) after a sufficient number of training episodes; a training repetition with the same dataset is an episode. In Fig. 4 the RMSE (Y axis) for the three Flu subtypes have settled down to their stable values after roughly 100 training episodes (X axis).

In Fig. 5, the actual RI scores are not so important; the significance is the fact that the RI values indicate relevance between the herbs and the Flu subclasses. The result in this plot shows that there is no relevance between the herb HeHuanPi and the two Flu subtypes: WindHeat and WindCold. This is true because this relevance was not embedded in the knowledge in the given training dataset C and thus the trimmed subset C_{h_x,i_y}.

The plot in Fig. 6 differs from Fig. 5 by revealing the relevance between HeHuanPi and the two Flu subtypes WindHeat and WindCold. The difference is that the module ANN_{h_x} in this case was trained by a new trimmed data subset C_{h_x,i_y}^{new}, which had included newly added fresh T_j knowledge.

In fact, the results shown in Figs. 2, 3 and 4 were obtained at the same time because the corresponding named ANN modules were activated in parallel. The RI scores in Figs. 2, 3 and 4 are symptom-based because the inputs to the named ANN modules are symptoms from each patient record. They simply indicate the 2-D (Fig. 4) and 3-D (Figs. 5 and 6) relationship between two TCM entities, and their actual scores are not important in the herbal discovery process. Yet, the RI scores have huge potentials to be tapped to aid effective real-time diagnosis and treatment in the future. This can be shown by a scenario in a mobile clinic (MC) (Lin et al. 2008). The MC physician may have never come across an illness that has the following set of symptoms $S_x = \{S_s \in S; Z_k \notin S\}$. S_J is a subset of all the formally recorded symptoms S derived from the TCM classics, and Z_k are symptoms outside S. If the MC physician wants to know how to treat his patient quickly (i.e. in a time-critical or real-time sense), then he/she can activate all the named ANN modules dedicated to illness analysis (i.e. ANN_i for $i \in I$) in a remote manner via the Internet, assuming all the named ANN modules are located in the central high-speed node. The assumption is reasonable because a MC is usually far away from the central control and is connected only via the mobile Internet. Every ANN_i would process the S_x input and produce a 2-D RI score with respect to i (i.e. the RC). If all the 2-D RIs are sorted in descending order, two important suggestions would surface: (i) the highest RIs

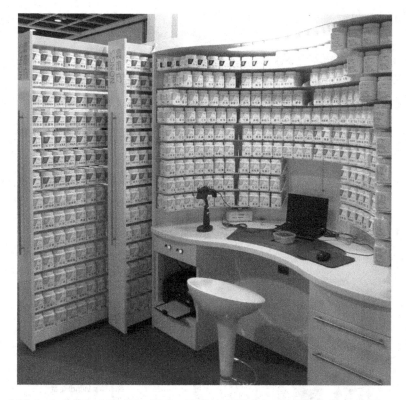

Fig. 2 Modernized Chinese Medicine Clinic with Chinese Medicine Granules for better quality control

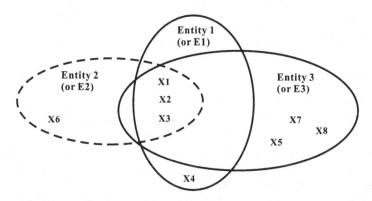

Fig. 3 Formal basis for computing the RI value

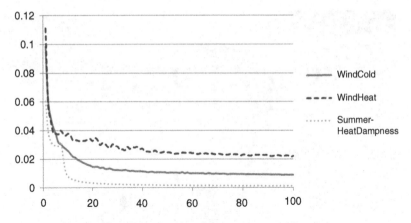

Fig. 4 Three examples (3 Flu subtypes) of 2-D training results

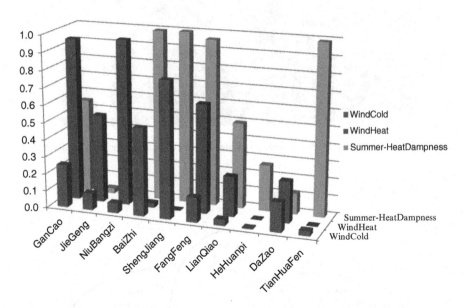

Fig. 5 3-D plot (X axis – 10 herbs; Y axis – 3 Flu subtypes; and Z axis – RI)

indicate the closer similarity between the unknown illness I_x defined by S_x and the corresponding RCs because the RI value is the quantification of $P(U \cap V)$; and (ii) from the TCM SAME/SIMILARITY principle that matches $P(U \cap V)$ in a commutable fashion there is an indication that the prescriptions for treating RCs of higher RI scores would be more usable for treating I_x as well. Then, the physician can make a quick, sound decision on which RC prescriptions would be more suitable for treating the unknown illness I_x.

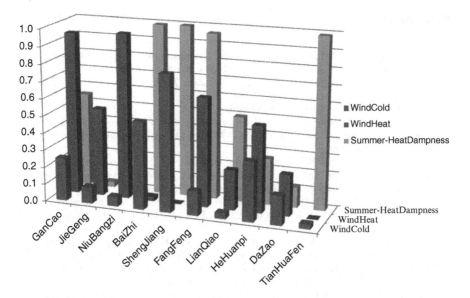

Fig. 6 3-D plot to show a potential herbal ingredient discovery (i.e. HeHuanPi)

5 Conclusion

In this paper, we propose a novel ANN (artificial neural network) based approach for herbal ingredient discovery. Each ANN is named after the specific TCM entity and trained by a set of real patient records. The output from the named ANN is the relevance index, which is associated with the name of the ANN with another TCM entity in either a 2-D or 3-D fashion. If the RI between the two entities was not observed before, it is a potential discovery to be formally confirmed by domain experts.

The main contributions by the proposed ANN based approach are as follows: (i) it can produce quick discoveries due to parallelism; and (ii) it produces trusted discoveries because it involves real clinical records and domain experts for confirmation. The trustworthiness comes from the fact that the RI computation is based on IT formalism, which is matched with the corresponding TCM formalism, for example the SAME/SIMILARITY principle, in a seamless and commutable manner. All the experimental results so far show that the proposed ANN based approach can indeed support potential herbal discovery effectively. The fringe benefit from the proposed ANN approach is in aiding physicians to find a treatment when the set of symptoms is difficult to decipher. The next immediate step in the research is to study how the ANN configuration can be safely pruned on the fly for faster execution and accurate results, based on the Hessian minima concept.

Acknowledgement The authors thank the anonymous reviewers for the positive comments.

References

A.R. Gallant, H. White, On learning the derivatives of an unknown mapping and its derivatives using multiplayer feedforward networks. Neural Netw. **5**, 129–138 (1992)

A. Ghosh, S. Tsutsui, *Advances in Evolutionary Computing: Theory and Applications* (Springer, Berlin, 2003)

M. Hagan, *Neural Network Design* (PWS Publishing, Boston, 1996)

International Standard Terminologies on Traditional Medicine in the Western Pacific Region (World Health Organization, 2007) ISBN 978-92-9061-248-7, http://www.wpro.who.int/publications/docs/WHO

W.W.K. Lin, A.K.Y. Wong, T.S. Dillon, HBP: an optimization technique to shorten the control cycle time of the Neural Network Controller (NNC) that provides dynamic buffer tuning to eliminate overflow at the user level. Int. J. Comput. Syst. Sci. Eng. **19**(2), 75–84 (2004)

W.W.K. Lin, A.K.Y. Wong, T.S. Dillon, Application of soft computing techniques to adaptive user buffer overflow control on the internet. IEEE Trans. Syst. Man Cybern. Part C **36**(3), 397–410 (2006)

W.W.K. Lin, J.H.K. Wong, A.K.Y. Wong, Applying Dynamic Buffer Tuning to Help Pervasive Medical Consultation Succeed, in *Proceedings of the 1st International Workshop on Pervasive Digital Healthcare (PerCare), – The 6th IEEE International Conference on Pervasive Computing and Communications*, Hong Kong, Mar 2008, pp. 675–679

J.H.K. Wong, W.W.K. Lin, A.K.Y. Wong, Real-time enterprise ontology evolution to aid effective clinical with text mining and automatic semantic aliasing support, in *Proceedings of the 7th International Conference on Ontologies, Databases, and Applications of Semantics (ODBASE 2008)*, Monterey, 11–13 Nov 2008a, pp. 1200–1214

A.K.Y. Wong, T.S. Dillon, W.W.K. Lin, *Harnessing the Service Roundtrip Time Over the Internet to Support Time-Critical Applications – Concept, Techniques and Cases* (Nova, New York, 2008b)

J.H.K. Wong, *Web-Based Data Mining and Discovery of Useful Herbal Ingredients* (WD^2UHI), Ph.D Thesis, Department of Computing, Hong Kong Polytechnic University, May 2010

L. Yann, B. Leon, G.B. Orr, K. Muller, Efficient BackProp, Neural Networks: Tricks of the Trade. Lect. Notes Comput. Sci. **1524**, 9–50 (1998), http://link.springer.com/chapter/10.1007%2F3-540-49430-8_2

W. Zhao, R. Chellappa, P.J. Phillips, A. Rosenfeld, Face recognition: a literature survey. ACM Comput. Surv. **35**(4), 339–458 (2003)

Chromatographic Fingerprinting and Chemometric Techniques for Quality Control of Herb Medicines

Zhimin Zhang, Yizeng Liang, Peishan Xie, Footim Chau, and Kelvin Chan

Abstract Chromatographic fingerprinting is commonly used for the instrumental inspection of herbal medicines. This chapter has reviewed the chromatographic techniques, especially by hyphenated chromatographies, to obtain chemical fingerprints which can represent appropriately the "chemical integrities" of the herbal medicines and therefore be used for authentication and identification of the herbal products. In order to extract useful information from fingerprints for the authentication and identification purpose, several recently proposed chemometric methods can be utilized for evaluating the fingerprints of herbal medicines, including Shannon information contents, Whittaker smoothing, air-PLS baseline correction, MSPA peak alignment, Haar wavelet peak detection, multivariate resolution, similarity analysis and pattern recongnition. It has been showed that the combination of chromatographic fingerprints and the chemometric methods might be a powerful tool for quality control of herbal medicines.

Z. Zhang • Y. Liang (✉)
College of Chemistry and Chemical Engineering, Research Center of Modernization of Chinese Medicines, Central South University, Changsha 410083, China
e-mail: yizeng_liang@263.net

P. Xie
Zhuhai Chromap Institute of Herbal Medicine Research, Zhuhai, People's Republic of China

F. Chau
Department of Applied Biology and Chemical Technology,
The Hong Kong Polytechnic University, Hung Hom, Kowloon, Hong Kong

K. Chan
Faculty of Pharmacy, University of Sydney, Science Road, Sydney, NSW 2006, Australia

National Institute of Complementary Medicine, University of Western Sydney,
Richmond, NSW 2560, Australia

J. Poon and S.K. Poon (eds.), *Data Analytics for Traditional Chinese Medicine Research*,   133
DOI 10.1007/978-3-319-03801-8_8, © Springer International Publishing Switzerland 2014

1 Introduction

Fingerprints obtained by chromatographic techniques, especially by hyphenated chromatographies, are strongly recommended for the purpose of quality control of herbal medicines, since they can represent appropriately the "chemical integrities" of the herbal medicines and therefore be used for authentication and identification of the herbal products (Liang et al. 2004; Xie et al. 2006; Liang et al. 2010; Tistaert et al. 2011). For example, Gas chromatography (GC) is successfully used to analysis volatile components in herbal medicines, and Liquid chromatography (LC) technique with electrospray ionization (ESI) can be complementary to GC for nonvolatile compounds (Drasar and Moravcova 2004; Fuzzati 2004). Chromatographic separation system hyphenated with a UV–vis or a mass spectrometer can provide structural information at an unprecedented level for analysis of herbal medicines (Tseng et al. 2000; Li et al. 2006; Xie et al. 2007; Li et al. 2009; Zhao et al. 2009; Kim et al. 2010; Zhu et al. 2010; Heaton et al. 2011; Xue et al. 2012). With the help of chromatographic fingerprinting techniques, We will definitely get more chance to deal with the difficult problems the problems in quality control of herbal medicines (Liang et al. 2004).

However, quality control of herbal medicines usually involves massive experiments and dataset collection, and these datasets usually are generated through experiments performed on different samples. Deviations in chromatographic datasets are inevitable when involving massive dataset, such as noise, baseline, shift in peaks and etc. It is not easy to extract meaningful quality control information from the datasets when there exists deviations. Hence, great efforts have been made by chemometricians to provide researchers in quality control of herbal medicines with chemometrics toolbox and method to cope, analyze and interpret these complex datasets. Shannon information content was introduced to evaluate the information of chromatographic fingerprints, which can be used as an index for optimizing the experimental conditions (Gong et al. 2003). Penalized least squares, adaptive iteratively reweighted procedure and sparse matrix techniques are adopted for smoothing (Eilers 2003), baseline correction of high-throughput chromatograms (Zhang et al. 2010a). Multi-scale peak alignment accelerated by fast fourier transform cross correlation is proposed to align the chromatograms automatically, accurately and rapidly (Zhang et al. 2012). These methods proposed by chemometrician may address the challenges of preprocess of massive dataset in quality control of herbal medicines, which enables researchers to preprocess, analyze, interpret and extract useful information from these datasets within an acceptable time. Multicomponent spectrum correlated chromatographic (MSCC) (Hu et al. 2004; Li et al. 2004) and Alternative moving window factor analysis (AMWFA) (Zeng et al. 2006) can be used to perform comparative analysis for chromatograms of herbal medicines, which can determine the same components in different fingerprints.

With the preprocessed chromatograms, similarity measurements, such as correlation coefficient, congruence coefficient, Kullback–Leibler divergence, can be used as standards identify the real herbal medicine and the false one, and further to

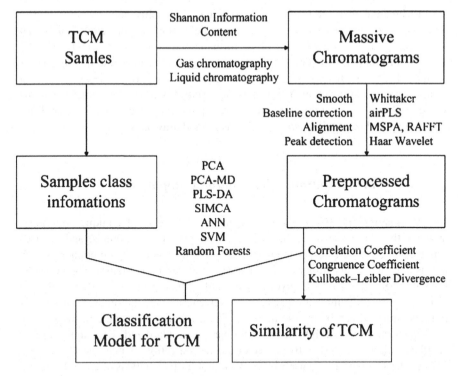

Fig. 1 Framework of quality control of herb medicines with chromatographic fingerprinting and chemometrics techniques

do quality control. Pattern recognition and machine learning methods, such as PCA-MD, PLS-DA (Matthew and William 2003), SIMCA (Wold 1976), SVM (Vapnik 1998), Random Forests (Breiman 2001) etc., can be taken into consideration for reasonable definition of the class of the herbal medicine.

The framework for quality control of herb medicines is shown in Fig. 1. It consists of fingerprinting techniques and chemometrics such as chromatographic experiments, preprocess of chromatograms, similarity calculation, pattern recognition and etc. The principle and theory will be explained as thoroughly and clearly as possible in the following sections.

2 Chromatographic Fingerprinting of Herbal Medicine

One or two markers or active components do not give a complete picture of a herbal product, which may contain up to hundreds of compounds. It seems to be necessary to determine most of the chemical constituents of herbal products in order to ensure the reliability and repeatability. Chromatographic techniques are commonly used as the instrumental inspection of herbal medicines for quality control, since finger-prints obtained by chromatography contain the "chemical integrities" of herbal medicines (Liang et al. 2004). High-performance liquid chromatography (HPLC) and gas chromatography (GC) are commonly applied to obtain the fingerprints of complex herbal medicines, since they can effectively separate complex chemical components in herbal medicines into many relatively simple sub-fractions. This section will describe the different chromatographic techniques used for herbal fin-gerprinting, and also will discusses their merits and drawbacks.

2.1 Gas Chromatography for Volatile Components

Gas chromatography (GC) is a well-established analytical technique commonly used for the characterization and identification volatile compounds, and most of active components in herbal medicines are volatile chemical compounds, which means that GC is very important in the analysis of herbal medicines. The powerful separation efficiency of GC gives a reasonable "fingerprint" of herbal medicine. Hence impurities, composition or relative concentration of the organic compounds in the volatile oil can be readily detected. The extraction procedure of the volatile oil is also relatively straightforward and can be standardized. By making use of capillary columns and sensitive detector (flame ionization or mass spectrometry), GC becomes a popular and useful analytical tool for the analysis of complex herbal products and essential oils. Despite its advantages, GC is unsuitable for analysis of polar, thermo-instable and non-volatile compounds, which make that GC analysis of herbal products is usually limited to the essentials oils. Therefore, liquid chroma-tography becomes an another necessary tool for us to apply the comprehensive analysis of the herbal medicines, which is complementary to GC.

2.2 Liquid Chromatography

High performance liquid chromatography (HPLC) is not limited by the volatility or stability of the sample compound, and it is possible to couple the technique to vari-ous detectors for different compounds, such as diode array detection for UV absorb-ing compounds, evaporative light scattering detection and chemiluminescence detection for non-chromophoric absorbing compounds, nuclear magnetic resonance and mass spectrometry for the qualitative analysis or structure elucidation. HPLC is also an easy to learn and use, fully automatable technique with high resolution, selectivity and sensitivity. These advantages make HPLC the most popular analyti-cal technique for analyzing herbal medicines. HPLC requires large volumes of envi-ronmentally unfriendly solvents, and current instrumentation of HPLC can withstand pressure up to 400 bar. Therefore, ultra-high performance liquid chromatography (UHPLC) (Du et al. 2010; Li et al. 2012) is emerging as a useful analytical tool to compensate the disadvantage of HPLC in herbal medicines. UHPLC brings liquid chromatographic analysis to another level by hardware modifications of the conventional HPLC machinery, which makes it possible to perform high resolution separations superior to HPLC analysis by using solid phase particles of sub-2 μm diameter to achieve superior sensitivity and resolution. As a smaller particle size leads to higher separation efficiency, shorter columns can be used for shorter analysis time with little solvent consumption.

2.3 Hyphenation Chromatographic System

Hyphenating chromatographic separation system with spectroscopic detector can obtain structural information on the analytes present in herbal samples, which becomes the most important approach for the identification and/or confirmation of the identity of target and unknown chemical compounds. Furthermore, the data obtained from hyphenated instruments are the so-called two-way data, say one way for chromatogram and the other way for spectrum, which could provide much more information than the classic one-way chromatography. With the help of chemometrics, we will definitely get more chance to deal with the difficult problems in the analysis of herbal medicines and also the problems in quality control of herbal medicines.

GC–MS was the first successful combination of chromatography with mass spectrometry. Mass spectrometry can yield information on the molecular weight as well as the structure of the molecule. With mass spectral databases from NIST and Wiley, the structure of the compounds of the herb could be identified by GC–MS and mass spectral databases. The capillary column can guarantee the good separation ability of GC–MS, which means that GC-MS can generate chemical fingerprint of high quality. The advantages make GC–MS the most preferable tool for the analysis of the volatile chemical compounds in herbal medicines (Li et al. 2009; Zhao et al. 2009; Kim et al. 2010; Zhu et al. 2010; Xue et al. 2012).

The hyphenated DAD detector can provide UV spectral information for peak purity check and unknown compound identification, which has make the qualitative analysis of complex samples in herbal medicines easier, and of course HPLC-DAD becomes a common technique in most analytical laboratories in the world (Li et al. 2006; Xie et al. 2007; Du et al. 2010; Heaton et al. 2011).

2.4 Other Chromatographic Techniques

Despite the low reproducibility and resolution disadvantages, thin layer chromatography (TLC) is still being used in quality control of herbal medicine as it is a readily available, easy to use and economical technique requiring few expensive machinery and solvents (Xie et al. 2006; Ciesla and Waksmundzka-Hajnos 2009). Hydrophilic interaction chromatography (HILIC) has gained more and more attention in herbal medicines, since majority of herbal medicines are extracted with aqueous solution and HILIC has good retention and separation of hydrophilic compounds (Alpert 1990; Koh et al. 2005; Hemstrom and Irgum 2006). Two-dimensional (2D) chromatography was also proposed to reveal all characteristics of complex biological samples. The main advantage of 2D chromatography is the increasing the peak capacity over conventional one dimensional chromatography (Bushey and Jorgenson 1990).

3   Chemometrics for Chromatograhpic Fingerprints

Modern chromatographic systems can generate massive datasets because of the evolution of chromatographic techniques, improvement in automation of instrument and rapid advancement in information techniques. Quality control of herbal medicines by chromatographic fingerprints usually involves massive experiments and dataset collection. In order to extract the information as much as possible from herbal medicines using chromatograph, the Shannon information content can be used to evaluate the information content of fingerprints. Commonly the herbal fingerprints are organized as a matrix X with dimension $n \times p$ with n being the number of samples (herbal fingerprints) and p the variables (scan points, peak areas, peak heights and etc.). Figure 2 is fingerprints of 38 Aurantii Immaturus Fructus samples.

One can see from Fig. 2 that noise, baseline and shift in peaks are inevitable when involving massive dataset. So preprocess methods should be applied to mitigate their influence for further analysis. After preprocess, pattern recognition and similarity measures should be used for extracting quality control information.

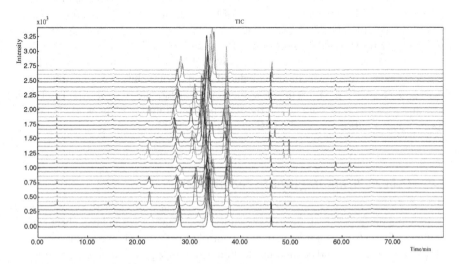

Fig. 2 Chromatographic fingerprints of 38 Aurantii Immaturus Fructus samples at wavelength $\lambda = 284$ nm

Depending on the applied chemometric method, only the information in X is used (unsupervised methods) or an additional $p \times 1$ response vector y containing additional information on the samples is needed (supervised methods). Commonly used methods are PCA, PLS-DA, SIMCA, SVM, Random Forests and etc. This section will explain chemometirc methods for analyzing the chromatographic fingerprints of herbal medicines.

3.1 Information Contents

Information contents of chromatograms should be calculated to optimize the experimental conditions, so the chromatograms will contain as much as possible information from herbal samples. The calculation burden of conventional methods based on signal intensity, retention time, peak area and/or peak height is rather heavy, besides the calculation of the information content of overlapped peaks will become complex and cause some errors using these methods. Here Shannon information content with modification based on the characteristics of chromatographic fingerprints can be applied to evaluate chromatographic fingerprints obtained. There is no need to detect peaks or obtain peak areas for calculating Shannon information content, so it is easy for us to select a chromatographic fingerprint with a high separation degree and uniform concentration distribution of all chemical components. Chromatographic fingerprint can be regarded as a concentration distribution curve of several peaks. According to information theory, the Shannon information content (Shannon 2001) of a continuous signal might be simply expressed as the following:

$$\Phi = -\sum(p_i)\log(p_i) \tag{1}$$

Here p_i is the positive real numbers of probability property, say $\sum p_i = 1$. Based on this idea, above equation should be modified to calculate the information content (Φ) for chromatographic fingerprints of herbal medicines as shown in the following equation, that is:

$$\Phi = -\sum\left(\frac{x_i}{\sum x_i}\right)\log\left(\frac{x_i}{\sum x_i}\right) \tag{2}$$

Where x_i is the real chromatographic response. The normalization of x_i divided by their sum is to make the chromatogram investigated be of probability property.

According to information theory, if and only if x_i with unchangeable variance is characterized by normal distribution can its information content Φ reach its maximum. A chromatographic fingerprint with all of peaks just completely separated should be featured by maximal information content. The maximal information content of chromatographic fingerprint will be achieved if and only if all of peaks just completely separated and each peak correspond to a normal distribution. So the modified version of Shannon information content can be applied to evaluation the information content of chromatographic fingerprints (Gong et al. 2003).

3.2 Smoothing

Smoothing is a preprocessing method that aims to capture important patterns in the chromatographic fingerprints, while leaving out noise. It can reduce the random noise and improve the signal to noise ratio (SNR) of fingerprints. The well-known and popular Savitzky-Golay Smoother (Savitzky and Golay 1964) has several disadvantages: (1) Programs for the SGS relatively complicated; (2) The SGS can also be slow, since it cannot exploit the speed of matrix and vector operations; (3) Need special treatment for the boundary. Penalized least squares is recommended for smoothing chromatographic fingerprint (Eilers 2003).

Assume x is vector of fingerprint, and z is the fitted vector. Lengths of them are both m. Fidelity of z to x can be expressed as the sum square errors between them:

$$F = \sum_{i=1}^{m}(x_i - z_i)^2 \tag{3}$$

Roughness of the fitted data z can be written as its squared and summed differences,

$$R = \sum_{i=2}^{m}(z_i - z_{i-1})^2 = \sum_{i=1}^{m-1}(\Delta z_i)^2 \tag{4}$$

The balance of fidelity and smooth can be then measured as the fidelity plus with penalties on the roughness, and it can be given by:

$$Q = F + \lambda R = \| \mathbf{x} - \mathbf{z} \|^2 + \lambda \| \mathbf{Dz} \|^2 \tag{5}$$

By finding for the vector of partial derivatives and equating it to 0 ($\frac{\partial Q}{\partial \mathbf{z}} = \mathbf{0}$), we get the linear system of equations that can be easily solved:

$$\mathbf{z} = (\mathbf{I} + \lambda \mathbf{D'D})^{-1} \mathbf{x} \tag{6}$$

Penalized least squares has several advantages when comparing with the commonly used Savitsky-Golay smoother: (1) Can be programmed in less than ten lines of C++; (2) Adapts to boundaries automatically; (3) Handles missing values, even in large stretches; (4) When sparse matrices are being used, it is very fast; (5) Control over smoothness with one parameter (Eilers 2003). So it is very suitable for smoothing the massive chromatograms in quality control of herbal medicine.

3.3 Baseline Correction

Baseline drift always blurs or even swamps signals and deteriorates analytical results, particularly in multivariate analysis. It is necessary to correct baseline drift to perform further data analysis. Adaptive iteratively reweighted penalized least squares has been proposed based on penalized least squares (Chen et al. 2010; Zhang et al. 2010a, b; Zhang and Liang 2012).

By introducing weights vector of fidelity, and set to an arbitrary value, say 0, to weights vector at position corresponding to peak segments of **x**. Fidelity of **z** to **x** is changed to

$$F = \sum_{i=1}^{m} w_i \left(x_i - z_i \right)^2 = \left(\mathbf{x} - \mathbf{z} \right)' \mathbf{W} \left(\mathbf{x} - \mathbf{z} \right) \tag{7}$$

W is a diagonal matrix with w_i on its diagonal.

Solve above linear equations, and the fitted baseline can be obtained easily:

$$\mathbf{z} = \left(\mathbf{W} + \lambda \mathbf{D}'\mathbf{D} \right)^{-1} \mathbf{W} \mathbf{x} \tag{8}$$

The adaptive iteratively reweight procedure is proposed to replace peak detection and special treatment steps:

$$Q^t = \sum_{i=1}^{m} w_i^t \mid x_i - z_i^t \mid^2 + \lambda \sum_{j=2}^{m} \mid z_j^t - z_{j-1}^t \mid^2 \tag{9}$$

In the starting steps, assigning $\mathbf{w} = \mathbf{1}$, otherwise, **w** can be obtained using following expressions adaptively:

$$w_i^t = \begin{cases} 0 & x_i \geq z_i^{t-1} \\ e^{\frac{t\left(x_i - z_i^{t-1}\right)}{\mid d^t \mid}} & x_i < z_i^{t-1} \end{cases} \tag{10}$$

The flow chart describing architecture of the proposed algorithm is shown in Fig. 3. One can see from this figure that air-PLS doesn't need the peak detection for fitting the baseline. After initialization, air-PLS enters the adaptive iteratively reweighted procedure to eliminate the influence of peaks when fitting the baseline.

The air-PLS provides a simple, flexible, valid and fast algorithm for estimating baseline for chromatographic fingerprints. There is one crucial but intuitional parameter λ to control smoothness of fitted baseline. It gives an extremely fast and accurate baseline corrected signals.

3.4 Peak Alignment

Peak shifts among fingerprints have a strong impact on the basic chemometric algorithms such as PCA and PLS. Peak alignment is also a crucial preprocess steps to reduce the variation in peak positions, which can improve useful information extraction using chemometrics and statistics. Many approaches has been proposed to align retention time shifts including dynamic time warping (DTW) (Athanassios et al. 1998), correlation optimized warping (COW) (Nielsen et al. 1998), parametric time warping (PTW) (Eilers 2004), recursive alignment by FFT (RAFFT) (Wong et al. 2005), recursive segment-wise peak alignment (RSPA) (Veselkov et al. 2009), icoshift, alignDE (Zhang et al. 2011), CAMS (Zheng et al. 2013) and MWFFT (Li et al. 2013). But currently, chromatogram often contains several of thousands

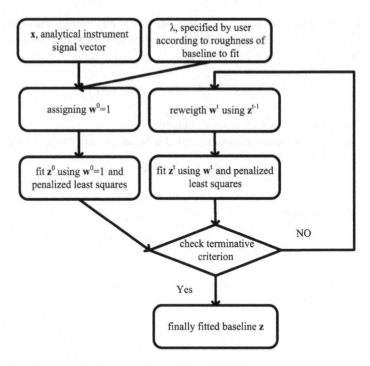

Fig. 3 Flow chart describing framework of airPLS algorithm

data points, original COW are not suitable for these signals due to large requirements in both execution time and memory, and DTW often "over-warps" signals
and introduces artifacts into the aligned profiles when signals were only recorded
using a mono-channel detector. RAFFT accelerates the aligning procedure by Fast
Fourier Transform (FFT) Cross Correlation, which is is amazingly fast. But RAFFT
moves segments by insertion and deletion of data points at the start and end of segments without considering peak information, which may change the shapes of peaks
by introducing artifacts and removing peak points.

In order to align the fingerprints accurately in acceptable time, Fast Fourier
Transform Cross-Correlation is adopted, which can determine lag between two fingerprints. Here is one simple example for candidate shifts detection of simulated
chromatograms. Consider two chromatograms (the reference one is denoted as r and
test one is s) that differ by an unknown shift along the retention time. One can rapidly calculate cross-correlation c between s and r using FFT cross correlation, and
the candidate shifts between s and r can be found at the local maximums of c.
Figure 4 depicts this procedure visually. The number 20 of candidate shifts in Fig. 4
means shift the test profile by 20 points and the maximum cross-correlation between
test and reference profile will be obtained.

FFT cross correlation can only estimate linear shift between signals, but retention time shifts are often nonlinear for chromatogram of real sample. To solve the
nonlinear shifts among fingerprints, we proposed a multi-scale peak alignment
(MSPA) approach (Zhang et al. 2012), which can align nonlinear shifts from large

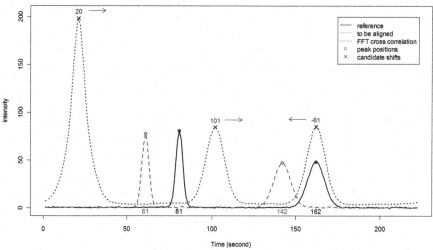

Fig. 4 Candidate shifts detection of simulated chromatograms by finding the local maximums in FFT cross-correlation

to small scale gradually. In MSPA method, chromatogram to be aligned will be iteratively divided into small segments and FFT cross correlation will be used to estimate candidate shifts for each segment and align peaks from large scale to small scale gradually. This strategy can solve the alignment of nonlinear retention time shifting problem by FFT cross correlation (Fig. 5).

The preprocess fingerprints of 38.

Aurantii Immaturus Fructus samples. are displayed in Fig. 6. The preprocess steps include denoising by whittaker smoother, baseline correction with air-PLS and peak alignment via MSPA.

3.5 Peak Detection

The peak height and area should be calculated for building calibration and classification model. So, the peak should be detected. The Haar Wavelet is applied to detect the peaks. Peak can be defined as a local maximum of N neighboring points, whose intensity is significantly larger than the noise level. The local maximums can be found from the derivative calculation via Haar CWT of the signal. Then, false positive peaks are eliminated from whose SNR is lower than a pre-specified threshold. Similar to finding of the peak position, the start and end points of each peak can also be found by this derivative calculation method. For each peak, its start and end points can be obtained by searching the nearest point from its peak position in the vector of detected peak position and peak width. Principles for peak detection and width estimation are concisely illustrated in Fig. 7. The middle part of the figure

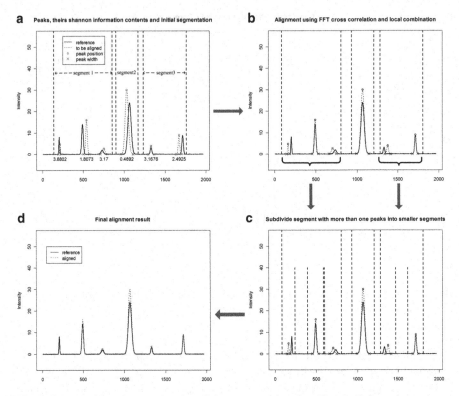

Fig. 5 Scheme of iterative segmentation of chromatogram based on Shannon information content to align nonlinear shift between signals

depicts derivative calculation via Haar CWT. The top and bottom parts of this figure describe peak detection and width estimation, respectively. During peak detection, Haar Wavelet has some advantages. The most obvious one is robust to noise. Haar Wavelet is much better than numeric differential, especially when noise is large (Zhang et al. 2012).

3.6 Multivariate Resolution

With the development of analytical instruments, especially with the development of the hyphenated chromatographic systems, such as GC-MS, HPLC-DAD, LC-MS and HPLC-NMR, the qualitative and quantitative ability has been enhanced significantly, since such instruments provide not only their separation ability but also their qualitative ability with spectroscopic profiles. Herbal medicine always contains a large number of chemical components. Even though the chromatographic conditions are optimized, it seems impossible to get a baseline separation with hundreds of analytes. In such a case, by direct similarity searches in MS database alone is hard to identify the compounds, which will even result in wrong conclusions.

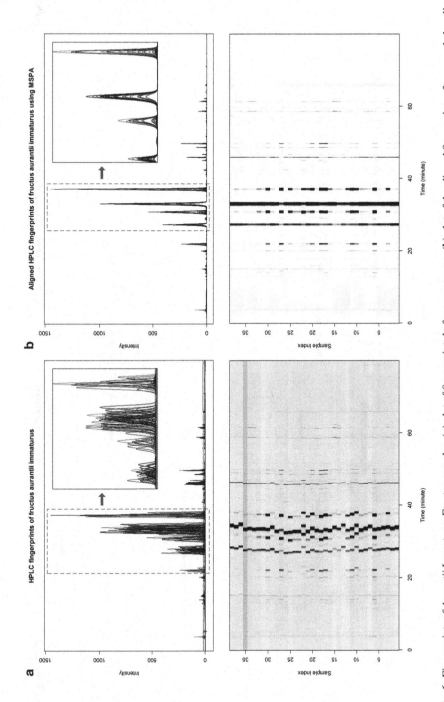

Fig. 6 Fingerprints of Aurantii Immaturus Fructus samples, (**a**) plot of fingerprints before preprocess, (**b**) plot of the aligned fingerprints after smooth, baseline correction and peak alignment

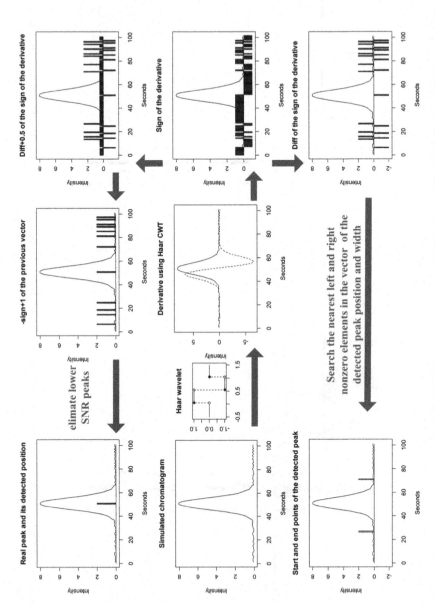

Fig. 7 Principles for peak detection and width estimation using derivative calculation based on Continuous Wavelet Transform with Haar wavelet as the mother wavelet

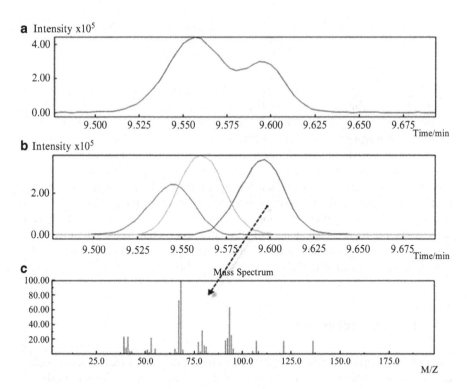

Fig. 8 Resolve overlap peaks using heuristic evolving latent projections method (**a**) overlap peaks before resolution; (**b**) pure chromatogram of each component; (**c**) pure mass spectrum

Fortunately, the chemometrics resolution methods provide powerful tools to resolve overlap peaks into pure chromatograms and/or spectra, which can improve the qualitative and quantitative results. Therefore, it is extremely necessary to resolve the overlapping peaks by means of chemometric techniques. One can observe the verlap peaks of total ion chromatogram in Fig. 8a. After resolving the overlap peaks using heuristic evolving latent projections method (Kvalheim and Liang 1992; Liang et al. 1992), one can obtain the pure chromatogram and mass spectrum of each component respectively. We have also evaluated the feasibility of sample classification of GC-ToF-MS dataset without the requirement for chromatographic deconvolution (Lu et al. 2011).

3.7   Similarity Analysis

The chromatographic fingerprints are constructed for the purpose of evaluating the quality of herbal medicines. One of the most common and easiest tools is similarity analysis based on the correlation coefficients. Correlation coefficients can take both the separation degrees and concentration distribution of components into consideration for evaluation the quality. The formula for correlation coefficient is:

$$r = \frac{\sum (x_i - \bar{x})(y_i - \bar{y})}{\sqrt{\sum (x_i - \bar{x})^2} \sqrt{\sum (y_i - \bar{y})^2}} \tag{11}$$

In Eq. 11, x_i and y_i is the i-th elements of fingerprints **x** and **y**. $\bar{x}$ and $\bar{y}$ are the means of fingerprints **x** and **y** respectively.

Similarity can be calculated based on entire fingerprint, peak area or peak height against the fingerprint of standard sample, mean or median of dataset. The similarity estimation based on correlation coefficient may be used as a standard even this is very simple. However, there are several disadvantages of the simple correlation coefficient: (1). the mean or median fingerprint as standard is influenced by the dataset; (2). how to determine the subjective threshold for quality control; (3). the major peaks have a high contribution to the similarity (Liang et al. 2004; Tistaert et al. 2011). For these disadvantages of correlation coefficient based similarity analysis, pattern recognition and machine learning are applied to build exploration, calibration and classification models to extract the quality information.

3.8 Pattern Recognition

Since the inherent "uncertainty" of secondary metabolic substances of herbal medicines, it seems subjective to define an absolute reference fingerprint for similarity analysis. The quality control based on certain biomarker compounds might not be reliable too. The concept of class of herbal medicines sounds more reasonable for the quality control purpose. Thus, the pattern recognition methods should be taken into consideration for reasonable definition of the class of the herbal medicine. Exploratory data analysis, cluster analysis and classification can be used to gain insight in the structure of the multivariate fingerprints and develope rules for the classification of new herbal medicine samples.

Exploratory data analysis can be used as an approach to summarize the main characteristics of chromatographic fingerprints in easy-to-understand form, often with visual graphs. Principal Component Analysis (PCA) (Wold et al. 1987), Projection Pursuit (PP) (Friedman and Tukey 1974) and Multidimensional scaling (MDS) (Kruskal 1964; Borg and Groenen 2005) are techniques often used in visualization for exploring similarities or dissimilarities in fingerprints. These techniques are based only on the fingerprints. Variables of fingerprints are transformed into two or three latent variables (LV), which can summarize the main patterns of variation between the samples. Then the latent variables can be drawn on the plots, which may reveal groups of observations, trends of the herbal medicine samples.

Cluster analysis is the task of assigning a set of fingerprints into groups so that the fingerprints in the same cluster are more similar to each other than to those in other groups. It is a common technique to define classes for herbal medicines. Cluster analysis techniques can be divided into two categories: hierarchical and non-hierarchical. Hierarchical clustering (Johnson 1967) falls into two types: agglomerative (bottom up approach) and divisive (top down approach). Hierarchical clustering has the distinct advantage that any valid measure of distance can be used. In fact, the observations themselves are not required: all that is used is a matrix of distances. Non-hierarchical clustering methods such as k-means (Hartigan and Wong 1979), fuzzy c-means (Bezdek and Ehrlich 1984) is often an iterative process based on the given parameters such as distance function, the number of expected clusters. It is necessary to modify preprocessing and parameters until achieving the desired clustering results.

Classification is an instance of supervised learning, where class (such as species, origins, parts of the plant or harvest times) of each fingerprint is available. Generally speaking, classification make use of a calibration set with information represents classes to build a model. The model is then validated by an independent test set and used to predict the classes of new samples. There are numerous classification techniques, the most popular techniques for building the classification model of herbal medicines including principal component analysis-mahalanobis distance (PCA-MD) (De Maesschalck et al. 2000), partial least squares-discriminant analysis (PLS-DA) (Matthew and William 2003), soft independent modeling of class analogy (SIMCA) (Wold and SjÖStrÖM 1977), linear discriminant analysis (LDA) (Fisher 1936), support vector machines (SVM) (Vapnik 1998), Random Forests (Breiman 2001) and etc. PCA-MD employs the mahalanobis distance in principal component space as numeric indices for assigning the class for unknown samples. Partial least squares was originally designed for solving the col-inearity problem in regression. After binary coding the groups of samples, PLS2 can be used as an approach for multi-category classification. One advantage of PLS-DA is that the scores and loadings can be used for a graphical presentation of the results and be helpful in the interpretation of the group characteristics. SIMCA is a supervised classification method, which is based on disjoint principal component models. The term soft means that the classifier can identify samples as belonging to multiple classes. In order to build the SIMCA classification model, the PCA models are built repeatedly for the samples belonging to each class, and only the significant principal components are retained. LDA is closely related to PCA in that they both look for linear combinations of variables which best explain the data. LDA explicitly attempts to model the difference between the classes of data. PCA-MD, PLS-DA, SIMCA and LDA are all linear classifiers. For some complex samples like herbal medicine, classes may not be separable by a linear boundary. SVM can efficiently perform non-linear classification via kernel trick, implicitly mapping their inputs into high-dimensional feature spaces. Random forests is an ensemble classifier that consists of many decision trees built by bagging idea and the random selection of features, which can also model the nonlinear relationships between variables. One can choose the pattern recognition methods according to the characteristic of datasets of herbal medicines.

From Fig. 9a, the correlation coefficients of 6, 17, 18 and 27 samples are small. The first two score of PCA are displayed in Fig. 9b, which have explained the 70 % variance (information) of the fingerprints. The 6, 17, 18 and 27 samples are far from the main group in the score plot. The dendrogram of HCA of 38 Aurantii Immaturus Fructus samples is shown in Fig. 9b. The 6, 17, 18 and 27 samples are also agglomerated into one group which is different from the main group. The results of similarity analysis, PCA and HCA can be used to verify each other. Figure 9d is the score plot of classification models built by PLS-DA.

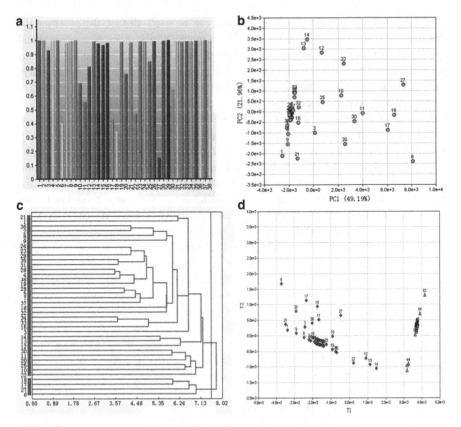

Fig. 9 Similarity analysis and pattern recongnition results of fingerprints of Aurantii Immaturus Fructus samples. (**a**) Results of similarity analysis; (**b**) exploratory data analysis using PCA; (**c**) Cluster analysis by HCA; (**d**) Classification models built by PLS-DA

4 Conclusion

It is not a simple task of applying modern technologies to quality control of the herbal medicines because of the complexity in chemical compounds. Chromatography with various detectors offers a powerful tool for separating the complex compounds to create a characteristic fingerprint. The use of chromatographic fingerprints of herbal medicines for quality control of herbal medicines is definitely a progress. Advantages and disadvantages of different chromatographic techniques for the quality control herbal medicines are discussed, such as gas chromatography for volatile components, liquid chromatography and hyphenation chromatographic system.

The quality information of herbal medicines should be mined from fingerprints, which are certainly a large dataset. They should be processed sufficiently and systematically through chemometrics methods. Therefore, we have devoted to the use of preprocess and pattern recognition for fingerprints of herbal medicines. Firstly, the Shannon information content is introduced to optimize experimental parameters. Then the features of the preprocess methods such as smoothing, baseline correction, peak alignment and peak detection are discussed to improve the quality of the generated fingerprints. Furthermore, characteristics of pattern recognition methods such as similarity analysis, exploratory data analysis, cluster analysis and classification for extracting the quality information are also elucidated.

The researchers can generate proper fingerprints for herbal medicines with chromatographic fingerprinting and preprocess, analyze, interpret and extract useful information from these datasets within an acceptable time using chemometric techniques. Chromatographic fingerprint analysis can ensure the maintenance of the consistent quality of samples for biological and pharmacological research.

References

A.J. Alpert, Hydrophilic-interaction chromatography for the separation of peptides, nucleic acids and other polar compounds. J. Chromatogr. **499**, 177–196 (1990)

K. Athanassios, F.M. John, A.T. Paul, Synchronization of batch trajectories using dynamic time warping. AIChE J. **44**, 864–875 (1998)

J.C. Bezdek, R. Ehrlich, FCM: the fuzzy c-means clustering algorithm. Comput. Geosci. **10**, 191–203 (1984)

I. Borg, P.J.F. Groenen, *Modern Multidimensional Scaling: Theory and Applications* (Springer, New york, 2005)

L. Breiman, Random forests. Mach. Learn. **45**, 5–32 (2001)

M.M. Bushey, J.W. Jorgenson, Automated instrumentation for comprehensive two-dimensional high-performance liquid chromatography of proteins. Anal. Chem. **62**, 161–167 (1990)

S. Chen, X.N. Li, Y.Z. Liang, Z.M. Zhang, Z.X. Liu, Q.M. Zhang et al., Raman spectroscopy fluorescence background correction and its application in clustering analysis of medicines. Spectrosc. Spect. Anal. **30**, 2157–2160 (2010)

L. Ciesla, M. Waksmundzka-Hajnos, Two-dimensional thin-layer chromatography in the analysis of secondary plant metabolites. J. Chromatogr. A **1216**, 1035–1052 (2009)

R. De Maesschalck, D. Jouan-Rimbaud, D. Massart, The mahalanobis distance. Chemometr. Intell. Lab. Syst. **50**, 1–18 (2000)

P. Drasar, J. Moravcova, Recent advances in analysis of Chinese medical plants and traditional medicines. J. Chromatogr. B-Anal. Technol. Biomed. Life Sci. **812**, 3–21 (2004)

G. Du, H.Y. Zhao, Q.W. Zhang, G.H. Li, F.Q. Yang, Y. Wang et al., A rapid method for simultaneous determination of 14 phenolic compounds in Radix Puerariae using microwave-assisted extraction and ultra high performance liquid chromatography coupled with diode array detection and time-of-flight mass spectrometry. J. Chromatogr. A **1217**, 705–714 (2010)

P.H.C. Eilers, A perfect smoother. Anal. Chem. **75**, 3631–3636 (2003)

P.H.C. Eilers, Parametric time warping. Anal. Chem. **76**, 404–411 (2004)

R.A. Fisher, The use of multiple measurements in taxonomic problems. Ann. Hum. Genet. **7**, 179–188 (1936)

J.H. Friedman, J.W. Tukey, A projection pursuit algorithm for exploratory data analysis. IEEE Trans. Comput. **100**, 881–890 (1974)

N. Fuzzati, Analysis methods of ginsenosides. J. Chromatogr. B-Anal. Technol. Biomed. Life Sci. **812**, 119–133 (2004)

F. Gong, Y.Z. Liang, P.S. Xie, F.T. Chau, Information theory applied to chromatographic fingerprint of herbal medicine for quality control. J. Chromatogr. A **1002**, 25–40 (2003)

J.A. Hartigan, M.A. Wong, Algorithm AS 136: a k-means clustering algorithm. J. Roy. Stat. Soc. Ser. C Appl. Stat. **28**, 100–108 (1979)

J. Heaton, L. Whiley, Y. Hong, C.M. Sebastian, N.W. Smith, C. Legido-Quigley, Evaluation of Chinese medicinal herbs fingerprinting by HPLC-DAD for the detection of toxic aristolochic acids. J. Sep. Sci. **34**, 1111–1115 (2011)

P. Hemstrom, K. Irgum, Hydrophilic interaction chromatography. J. Sep. Sci. **29**, 1784–1821 (2006)

Y. Hu, Y.Z. Liang, B.Y. Li, X.N. Li, Y.P. Du, Multicomponent spectral correlative chromatography applied to complex herbal medicines. J. Agric. Food Chem. **52**, 7771–7776 (2004)

S.C. Johnson, Hierarchical clustering schemes. Psychometrika **32**, 241–254 (1967)

M.J. Kim, H.A. Ki, W.Y. Kim, S. Pal, B.K. Kim, W.S. Kang et al., Development of radiation indicators to distinguish between irradiated and non-irradiated herbal medicines using HPLC and GC-MS. Anal. Bioanal. Chem. **398**, 943–953 (2010)

H.L. Koh, A.J. Lau, E.C.Y. Chan, Hydrophilic interaction liquid chromatography with tandem mass spectrometry for the determination of underivatized dencichine (beta-N-oxalyl-L-alpha, beta-diaminopropionic acid) in Panax medicinal plant species. Rapid Commun. Mass Spectrom. **19**, 1237–1244 (2005)

J.B. Kruskal, Multidimensional scaling by optimizing goodness of fit to a nonmetric hypothesis. Psychometrika **29**, 1–27 (1964)

O.M. Kvalheim, Y.Z. Liang, Heuristic evolving latent projections: resolving two-way multicomponent data. 1. Selectivity, latent-projective graph, datascope, local rank, and unique resolution. Anal. Chem. **64**, 936–946 (1992)

B.Y. Li, Y. Hu, Y.Z. Liang, L.F. Huang, C.J. Xu, P.S. Xie, Spectral correlative chromatography and its application to analysis of chromatographic fingerprints of herbal medicines. J. Sep. Sci. **27**, 581–588 (2004)

S.L. Li, P. Li, L.H. Sheng, R.Y. Li, L.W. Qi, L.Y. Zhang, Live cell extraction and HPLC-MS analysis for predicting bioactive components of traditional Chinese medicines. J. Pharm. Biomed. Anal. **41**, 576–581 (2006)

X.-R. Li, Y.-Z. Liang, T. Zhou, L.-X. Zhang, C.-D. Hu, Comparative analysis of volatile constituents between recipe jingfangsan and its single herbs by GC-MS combined with alternative moving window factor analysis method. J. Sep. Sci. **32**, 258–266 (2009)

S.-L. Li, H. Shen, L.-Y. Zhu, J. Xu, X.-B. Jia, H.-M. Zhang et al., Ultra-high-performance liquid chromatography-quadrupole/time of flight mass spectrometry based chemical profiling approach to rapidly reveal chemical transformation of sulfur-fumigated medicinal herbs, a case study on white ginseng. J. Chromatogr. A **1231**, 31–45 (2012)

Z. Li, J.J. Wang, J. Huang, Z.M. Zhang, H.M. Lu, Y.B. Zheng et al., Nonlinear alignment of chromatograms by means of moving window fast Fourier transfrom cross-correlation. J. Sep. Sci. **36**, 1677–1684 (2013)

Y.Z. Liang, O.M. Kvalheim, H.R. Keller, D.L. Massart, P. Kiechle, F. Erni, Heuristic evolving latent projections: resolving two-way multicomponent data. 2. Detection and resolution of minor constituents. Anal. Chem. **64**, 946–953 (1992)

Y.Z. Liang, P.S. Xie, K. Chan, Quality control of herbal medicines. J. Chromatogr. B **812**, 53–70 (2004)

Y. Liang, P. Xie, F. Chau, Chromatographic fingerprinting and related chemometric techniques for quality control of traditional Chinese medicines. J. Sep. Sci. **33**, 410–421 (2010)

H. Lu, D. Gan, Z. Zhang, Y. Liang, Sample classification of GC-ToF-MS metabolomics data without the requirement for chromatographic deconvolution. Metabolomics **7**, 191–205 (2011)

B. Matthew, R. William, Partial least squares for discrimination. J. Chemometr. **17**, 166–173 (2003)

N.-P.V. Nielsen, J.M. Carstensen, J. Smedsgaard, Aligning of single and multiple wavelength chromatographic profiles for chemometric data analysis using correlation optimised warping. J. Chromatogr. A **805**, 17–35 (1998)

A. Savitzky, M.J.E. Golay, Smoothing and differentiation of data by simplified least squares procedures. Anal. Chem. **36**, 1627–1639 (1964)

C.E. Shannon, A mathematical theory of communication. ACM SIGMOBILE Mobile Comput. Commun. Rev. **5**, 3–55 (2001)

C. Tistaert, B. Dejaegher, Y. Vander Heyden, Chromatographic separation techniques and data handling methods for herbal fingerprints: a review. Anal. Chim. Acta **690**, 148–161 (2011)

M.C. Tseng, M.J. Tsai, J.H. Lin, K.C. Wen, GC/MS analysis on anorectics adulterated in traditional Chinese medicines. J. Food Drug Anal. **8**, 315–330 (2000)

V.N. Vapnik, *Statistical Learning Theory*, vol. 2 (Wiley, New York, 1998)

K.A. Veselkov, J.C. Lindon, T.M.D. Ebbels, D. Crockford, V.V. Volynkin, E. Holmes et al., Recursive segment-wise peak alignment of biological H-1 NMR spectra for improved metabolic biomarker recovery. Anal. Chem. **81**, 56–66 (2009)

S. Wold, Pattern recognition by means of disjoint principal components models. Pattern Recognit. **8**, 127–139 (1976)

Wold S, SjÖStrÖM M (1977) SIMCA: a method for analyzing chemical data in terms of similarity and analogy. In *Chemometrics: Theory and Application*, vol. 52 (American Chemical Society), pp. 243–82, 1155 Sixteenth Street, NW, Washington, DC 20036 USA

S. Wold, K. Esbensen, P. Geladi, Principal component analysis. Chemometr. Intell. Lab. Syst. **2**, 37–52 (1987)

J.W.H. Wong, C. Durante, H.M. Cartwright, Application of Fast Fourier Transform crosscorrelation for the alignment of large chromatographic and spectral datasets. Anal. Chem. **77**, 5655–5661 (2005)

P.S. Xie, S.B. Chen, Y.Z. Liang, X.H. Wang, R.T. Tian, R. Upton, Chromatographic fingerprint analysis – a rational approach for quality assessment of traditional Chinese herbal medicine. J. Chromatogr. A **1112**, 171–180 (2006)

Y. Xie, Z.-H. Jiang, H. Zhou, X. Cai, Y.-F. Wong, Z.-Q. Liu et al., Combinative method using HPLC quantitative and qualitative analyses for quality consistency assessment of a herbal medicinal preparation. J. Pharm. Biomed. Anal. **43**, 204–212 (2007)

S.-Y. Xue, Z.-Y. Li, H.-J. Zhi, H.-F. Sun, L.-Z. Zhang, X.-Q. Guo et al., Metabolic fingerprinting investigation of Tussilago farfara L. by GC-MS and multivariate data analysis. Biochem. Syst. Ecol. **41**, 6–12 (2012)

Z.-D. Zeng, Y.-Z. Liang, Y.-L. Wang, X.-R. Li, L.-M. Liang, Q.-S. Xu et al., Alternative moving window factor analysis for comparison analysis between complex chromatographic data. J. Chromatogr. A **1107**, 273–285 (2006)

Z.-M. Zhang, Y.-Z. Liang, Comments on the baseline removal method based on quantile regression and comparison of several methods. Chromatographia **75**, 313–314 (2012)

Z.M. Zhang, S. Chen, Y.Z. Liang, Baseline correction using adaptive iteratively reweighted penalized least squares. Analyst **135**, 1138–1146 (2010a)

Z.M. Zhang, S. Chen, Y.Z. Liang, Z.X. Liu, Q.M. Zhang, L.X. Ding et al., An intelligent background-correction algorithm for highly fluorescent samples in Raman spectroscopy. J. Raman Spectrosc. **41**, 659–669 (2010b)

Z.-M. Zhang, S. Chen, Y.-Z. Liang, Peak alignment using wavelet pattern matching and differential evolution. Talanta **83**, 1108–1117 (2011)

Z.-M. Zhang, Y.-Z. Liang, H.-M. Lu, B.-B. Tan, X.-N. Xu, M. Ferro, Multiscale peak alignment for chromatographic datasets. J. Chromatogr. A **1223**, 93–106 (2012)

C. Zhao, Y. Zeng, M. Wan, R. Li, Y. Liang, C. Li et al., Comparative analysis of essential oils from eight herbal medicines with pungent flavor and cool nature by GC-MS and chemometric resolution methods. J. Sep. Sci. **32**, 660–670 (2009)

Y.B. Zheng, Z.M. Zhang, Y.Z. Liang, D.J. Zhan, J.H. Huang, Y.H. Yun et al., Application of fast Fourier transform cross-correlation and mass spectrometry data for accurate alignment of chromatograms. J. Chromatogr. A **1286**, 175–182 (2013)

H. Zhu, Y. Wang, H. Liang, Q. Chen, P. Zhao, J. Tao, Identification of Portulaca oleracea L. from different sources using GC MS and FT-IR spectroscopy. Talanta **81**, 129–135 (2010)

A New Methodology for Uncovering the Bioactive Fractions in Herbal Medicine Using the Approach of Quantitative Pattern-Activity Relationship

Foo-tim Chau, Qing-song Xu, Daniel Man-yuen Sze, Hoi-yan Chan,
Tsui-yan Lau, Da-lin Yuan, Michelle Chun-har Ng, Kei Fan,
and Daniel Kam-wah Mok, and Yi-zeng Liang

Abstract The Quantitative Pattern-Activity Relationship (QPAR) approach has been proposed recently by us and applied to the herbal medicine Radix *Puerariae Lobatae* and a related synthetic mixture system. Two different types of data from the chromatographic fingerprint and related bioactivity capacities of the samples were correlated quantitatively. The method thus developed provided a model for predicting total bioactivity from the chromatographic fingerprints and features in the chromatographic profiles responsible for the bioactivity. In this work, we propose a new methodology called QPAR-F here, to provide another piece of information: recommending the bioactive regions to facilitate bioassay-guided fractionation

F.-T. Chau (✉)
Department of Applied Biology and Chemical Technology, The Hong Kong
Polytechnic University, Hung Hom, Kowloon, SAR Hong Kong, People's Republic of China

State Key Laboratory of Chinese Medicine and Molecular Pharmacology,
Shenzhen, People's Republic of China
e-mail: bcftchau@polyu.edu.hk

Q.-S. Xu (✉)
School of Mathematics and Statistics, Central South University,
Changsha, People's Republic of China
e-mail: qsxu@csu.edu.cn

D.M.-Y. Sze • M.C.-H. Ng
Department of Health Technology and Informatics, The Hong Kong Polytechnic University,
Hung Hom, Kowloon, SAR Hong Kong, People's Republic of China

H.-Y. Chan • T.-Y. Lau • D.K.-W. Mok
Department of Applied Biology and Chemical Technology, The Hong Kong
Polytechnic University, Hung Hom, Kowloon, SAR Hong Kong, People's Republic of China

D.-L. Yuan • Y.-Z. Liang
College of Chemistry and Chemical Engineering, Research Center of Modernization
of Chinese Medicines, Central South University, Changsha, People's Republic of China

K. Fan
School of Information Technologies, University of Sydney, Sydney, Australia

J. Poon and S.K. Poon (eds.), *Data Analytics for Traditional Chinese Medicine Research*,
DOI 10.1007/978-3-319-03801-8_9, © Springer International Publishing Switzerland 2014

and related studies. QPAR-F makes use of chromatographic profiles instead of individual data points utilized in our previous work. The chromatograms of the system concerned are firstly divided into different regions or related fractions representing different groups of constituents. Then different combinations of these regions using the exhaustive searching strategy are processed by the partial least squares (PLS) methods to build models. The optimal models give smaller errors between the predicted and measured total bioactivity capacities. The performance of the proposed QPAR-F methodology is first evaluated by a known mixture system with combinations with active ingredients. The results confirmed that QPAR-F works very well in predicting the total antioxidant bioactivity capacities and the active regions could be correctly identified. These findings are very helpful in planning the bioassay-guided fractionation. For this data-mining process, only limited chemical and bioactivity information of the original samples or crude extracts are required. No prior knowledge of activities of the fractions under study is needed. The QPAR-F methodology was also applied to the herbal medicine, Radix *Puerariae Lobatae* and similar predicted models give smaller errors between the predicted and measured total antioxidant bioactivity capacities could be successfully built.

1 Introduction

There has been an upsurge of scientific research on the pharmacological activity of herbal medicine (HM) in recent years owing to the wide acceptance of taking HM as therapeutic agents. It is well known that natural sources including HM have not been very well explored like modern medicines, but it is thought that they will provide vast resources for drug development. Indeed, most of the drug substances nowadays originated from natural products or inspired by natural products (Harvey 2008).

Today, more emphasis has been put on the search of the novel compounds from HM. Yet, this is always challenging. Usually, the bioactivity of a HM, a complicated multi-component system, is screened first. On account of the limitation of the bioassay methods, very little and quite often even no information is available on individual HM ingredients that contribute to the bio-response. In recent studies, multiple chemical constituents in HM were tentatively identified by LC-MS and the HM bioactivities were investigated using selected in-vitro bioassay carried out in parallel (Bravo et al. 2007; de Mejía et al. 2010; Rauter et al. 2009).

Through the data acquired, investigation of the relationship between the HM chemical composition and bioactivity was attempted. The aim was to establish the active components that are responsible for related pharmacological activities. Furthermore, the discovery of these components is also very helpful in quality control. Mostly, the quality of HMs and dietary supplements is assessed through quantifying a few target compounds with some called markers. In many cases, this is not good enough because the biological activity is contributed by various components. For instance, Rijk et al. reported that the markers of steroids were not identified in the dietary supplements under study (Rijk et al. 2009). Yet, the biological screening test gave positive results. They attributed this to the presence of other steroids which were identified by the LC-MS/MS study. This showed the need to identify the bioactive candidates.

Different strategies have been mapped out to find bioactive candidates in complex systems like HMs. Bioassay-guided fractionation (BGF) is one of them (Ene et al. 2009; Han et al. 2009; Hostettmann et al. 2001; Othman et al. 2006; Pesin et al. 2010; Peters et al. 2010). The BGF process mainly involves confirming the HM extract to be bioactive first using one to several selected bioassays, then fractionating the active extract and testing the fractions obtained by the same screening methods. Fractionation will be repeated on the active fractions found and, ultimately, the target components within the active fractions will be isolated (Hostettmann et al. 2001; Shi et al. 2009). These bioactive candidates may be novel or known already. High speed countercurrent chromatography (HSCCC) and high-performance liquid chromatography (HPLC) on the preparative scale, supercritical fluid chromatography (SFC) and thin layer chromatography (TLC) are very often used in these investigations. As for characterization and structure elucidation of the target compounds, mass spectrometry (MS) and nuclear magnetic resonance (NMR) spectrometry are popular and powerful tools (Ene et al. 2009; Jerz et al. 2010; Othman et al. 2006; Peters et al. 2010; Wu et al. 2008).

Although BGF has its merits and is widely accepted by the industrial and academic sectors, it is time consuming and costly with repeated fractionation and bioassay measurements even with the help of automated devices. Also, at the very beginning, it is hard to identify the target compounds among many constituents in the sample for isolation and it is important to avoid selecting the wrong ones or known active compounds. Chemical characterization of the chemical constituents of the sample and crude extracts before or simultaneously with the BGF could assist to certain extent. Despite that, very little information about bioactive regions or HM constituents can be provided from BFG. It should be mentioned that BGF has also been applied to study compounds with other types of activity, such as those that are harmful and a risk to human health (Jhoo et al. 2006; Ratnayake and Lewandowski 2010; Uhlig et al. 2005).

In order to speed up the experimental work on determination of active compounds and structural identification using BGF, chemical analysis and bioassay study have been coupled together to facilitate online screening of bioactive ingredients without the need of isolation (Shi et al. 2009). Most of them have focused on the antioxidant assay and required special instrumental set-ups. Another strategy in detecting bioactive compounds is based on relating the chemical compositions and bioassays of the HM together through chemometric data processing techniques. In studying the Chinese medicine formula Qi-Xue-Bing-Zhi-Fang, this was found to be bioactive and fractionation was carried out on the crude extract to get six fractions (Wang et al. 2006; Xiao et al. 2006). Then these fractions with different contents were put together for further investigation. Based on the experimental data acquired, Cheng et al. established the quantitative composition-activity relationship (QCAR) between these fractions and their bioactivity levels. Through these relationships, the bioactive fractions were identified and confirmed by experimental findings. More than that, Cheng et al. attempted to find the optimal combination of the bioactive fractions from the established relationship. Later, these workers did another study (Wang et al. 2010). This time, they selected three known chemical components from the herbal formula shenmai that was reported to be bioactive. Then the related biological screening tests were carried out on different compositions of the three assigned contents according to the experimental design. After the results were obtained, the compositions of the three target compounds with optimal bioactivity were established.

Recently, our laboratory led by Chau et al. investigated the chemical composition and antioxidant activity of an HM, Radix *Puerariae Lobatae* (gegen, YG), a complicated mixture system. They developed models for the HM based on the quantitative pattern-activity relationship (QPAR) approach through these two types of data, chromatographic and bioactivity data, to come up with a model which predicts the level of bioactivity from the chromatographic fingerprint and reveals the features in the chromatographic profile for the bioactivity (Chau et al. 2009). The chemometric tool, target projection method and selectivity ratio, were utilized to scan the whole YG chromatograms to achieve the purpose. In this way, all the active and inactive components in the herbal medicine as detected by the separation instrument and the methods used were considered in assessing their bioactivity capacities. The outcomes were that more bioactivity information concerning the chemical composition of the HM was included compared to the conventional methods with just a few target compounds being considered.

In another work also by our laboratory, 60 synthetic mixtures with 12 chemical components of which 7 possessed antioxidant activity were created and investigated by the QPAR approach (Kvalheim et al. 2011). Excellent prediction performance of antioxidant strength from the bioactive signature was obtained. Moreover, the model established could even be able to rank 6 of the 7 bioactive strengths. The reason why one of the two least bioactive components was not found is that the ratios of bioactive capacity of the two most active components to the two least active ones were close to 100 to 1.

In this study, we propose a new methodology, QPAR-F, to tackle the problem of finding bioactive fractions in fractionation related studies such as BGF. Different regions within the chromatogram of the mixture system were input for data treatment so as to provide another piece of information: recommending the bioactive fractions to facilitate bioassay-guided fractionation and related works. Here, we considered that a fraction can be represented by the profile structures or partitioned regions in the chromatogram. The chromatogram from an analytical instrument, such as HPLC, may be exactly the same as that from the scaling-up process by, for example, preparative HPLC. Even if this is not so, the retention time and the spectral information acquired from the former can still help to identify the chemical components involved in the latter process.

In carrying out the QPAR-F computation, the chromatograms of the samples of the mixture system of interest are divided into several regions randomly or according to the actual information. These regions are combined together in different ways. Then data from the training set are utilized to establish models from various kinds of combinations using an exhaustive searching strategy and the partial least squares (PLS) method. As a result, the bioactivity capacities of the samples in the test set could be predicted. Here, we assume that the agreement between the predicted and observed values depended on whether the appropriate bioactive regions are included or not. Hence, the errors or differences are used to follow the bioactivity of the components in the regions involved.

In this work, the performance and the validity of the assumption of the proposed QPAR-F methodology are scrutinized by the synthetic mixture system which involves the preparation of mixtures with seven known antioxidants and five inactive compounds at different concentration levels through uniform design. Experiments are carried out to obtain their HPLC chromatograms and antioxidant activity data by the FRAP assay (Benzie and Strain 1996). Afterward, QPAR-F is applied to these data using three divided regions with prediction errors calculated.

From the result obtained, the assumption is found to be valid and the proposed QPAR-F algorithm works very well in identifying the bioactive regions correctly. In addition, the results obtained from different models are consistent and followed closely the assumption made. With the success of the QPAR-F methodology to the known mixture system, it is then applied to the herbal medicine, Radix *Puerariae Lobatae*. The three divided regions are also used for PLS modeling and the results obtained are compared with the experimental findings.

In the following, we will discuss in detail the QPAR-F methodology and the results obtained from the QPAR-F analyses on the synthetic mixture system and the herbal medicine, Radix *Puerariae Lobatae* (YG).

2 Theory

2.1 Prediction Model for Bioactivity by the PLS Model

Denoting the data matrix of the chromatograms of the crude extracts or samples, and the divided regions for setting up combinations as $\mathbf{X}$ and the vector of bioactivity as $\mathbf{y}$, the following formula relates these two types of data

$$\mathbf{y} = \mathbf{X}\mathbf{b} + \mathbf{e} \tag{1}$$

with b and e being the vector of regression coefficients and error vector respectively. Partial least squares (PLS) methodology (Wold et al. 1999, 2001) was applied here to estimate b and establish the model.

In the PLS algorithm, when k PLS components are used, the data matrix $\mathbf{X}$ is decomposed in a fashion similar to that of principal component analysis, generating a matrix of scores, $\mathbf{T}_k$ and loadings or factors, $\mathbf{P}_k$, with the residual matrix of $\mathbf{X}$

defined as $\mathbf{E}_k$. Similar analysis is applied to $\mathbf{y}$, producing a matrix of scores, $\mathbf{T}_k$, and loading vector, $\mathbf{q}_k$, with $\mathbf{f}_k$ being the error vector of $\mathbf{y}$ (Xu et al. 2001).

$$\mathbf{X} = \mathbf{T}_k\mathbf{P}_k^{\mathrm{T}} + \mathbf{E}_k \tag{2}$$

$$\mathbf{y} = \mathbf{T}_k\mathbf{q}_k + \mathbf{f}_k \tag{3}$$

$$\mathbf{T}_k = \mathbf{X}\mathbf{H}_k \tag{4}$$

Finally, the estimated vector of regression coefficients $\mathbf{b}$ is obtained as follows:

$$\hat{\mathbf{b}} = \mathbf{H}_k\left(\mathbf{T}_k^{T}\mathbf{T}_k\right)^{-1}\mathbf{H}_k\mathbf{X}^{T}\mathbf{y} \tag{5}$$

Through these equations, the estimated bioactivity can be computed:

$$\hat{\mathbf{y}} = \mathbf{X}\hat{\mathbf{b}} \tag{6}$$

For new objects, their predicted bioactivity can be obtained by:

$$\check{\mathbf{y}}_{new} = \mathbf{X}_{new}\check{\mathbf{b}} \tag{7}$$

The samples in the data set can be divided into two groups, a training set and a test set. The data of the training set is used to estimate the regression coefficients $\mathbf{b}$ and build the model. The number of PLS components used in the model can be determined by cross validation. The test set is used to assess the prediction ability of the model established. The performance of the model thus obtained is evaluated in this work by evaluating the root mean squared errors (RMSE) of training (RMSET) and RMSE of prediction (RMSEP).

2.2   The QPAR-F Methodology

In this study, we tried to discover the relationship between different profile regions within the chromatogram and measured total antioxidant capacity (TAC) of the sample. In doing so, the whole chromatogram was divided into several regions randomly according to the profile structures in the first stage. Then, the proposed QPAR models for predicting the related TACs were built by using different combinations of these regions through the algorithm mentioned in the above section.

Here we considered that the best combination was the one that resulted in the best agreement with the smallest error between the measured and the predicted TACs. Based on this, we applied the exhaustive searching strategy to find out the best combination from the combinations set. In this work, the total number of divided regions within a combination for modeling was varied and all possible combinations were generated and subjected to the PLS modeling. Variations of the outcomes from these models can provide valuable information about the bioactive regions hidden in the chromatograms of the mixture and HM studied. Furthermore, they can also help us to know better about the contributions of individual regions with active and/or inactive compounds to the total activity. In this manner, the results obtained through the proposed QPAR-F methodology are helpful to direct the bioassay-guided fractionation. Here we utilize the synthetic mixture system (MIX) as an example to illustrate how the QPAR-F methodology works.

Figure 1 shows the workflow chart of the QPAR-F procedure using the chromatogram of the mixture system MIX with three divided regions. In the first step, the whole MIX chromatogram is divided into three profile regions randomly or based on the information available. Then, all possible combinations of these regions are generated. For instance, Comb 1 only contains Region 1; Comb 4 consists of Region 1 and Region 2, while Comb 7 includes all the three regions representing the whole chromatogram. In the second step, PLS models are established based on all these combinations. The matrix $\mathbf{X}$ is used to store the data of the region(s) of a combination while the TAC values of all samples can be found in vector $\mathbf{y}$ as mentioned in Sect. 2. Through these two data sets, the model is constructed. For each combination, the number of PLS components in the model is determined using tenfold cross validation (Burman 1989). By comparing the outcomes from these PLS models, contributions of the selected regions to the TAC can be revealed under the assumption made. In addition, we can identify the bioactive regions and formulate a model with the right combination of these regions to give the best predictive ability for TAC.

3 Experimental Section

3.1 Sample Preparation

Fifty eight synthetic mixtures were prepared with the compositions with twelve compounds at different concentration levels according to the uniform design table. These chemicals were gallic acid (GA), hydroxybenzoic acid (HB), puerarin (PU), daidzin (DZ), coumaric acid (CMA), rutin (RT), quercetin dehydrate (QT), genistein (GS), kaempferol (KF), emodin (ED), betulinic acid (BA) and ursolic acid (UA). Details can be found in Reference (Kvalheim et al. 2011). With regard to Radix *Puerariae Lobatae*, all samples were extracted under the conditions as stated in our previous study (Chau et al. 2009).

3.2 Chromatographic Analyses

An Agilent 1100 series HPLC system with a diode-array-detector (DAD) was used to analyze MIX and YG. The reversed-phase, ODS hypersil column with the

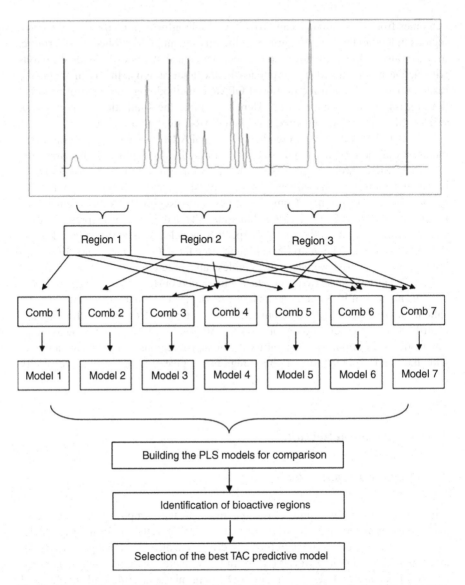

Fig. 1 The workflow chart of the QPAR-F methodology using the synthetic mixture system (MIX) as an example

dimension of the column being 250×4.6 mm and the particle size being 5 μm was used. For analyzing MIX, the mobile phase consisted of 0.1 % phosphoric acid in double deionized water (solvent A) and 0.1 % phosphoric acid in methanol (solvent B). The gradient elution program followed that of Kvalheim et al. (2011). As for analyzing YG extracts, acetonitrile (solvent A) and 0.3 % acetic acid in double deionized water (solvent B) were utilized with the gradient elution reported before (Chau et al. 2009).

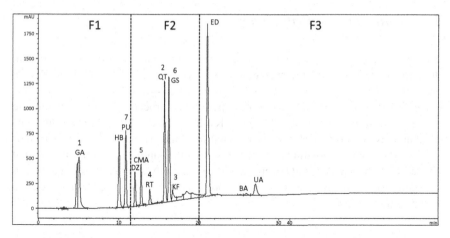

Fig. 2 The three divided regions in the chromogram of MIX44 with labels of peak number and the components involved (See Sect. 3.1)

3.3 Preparation of Fractions of MIX and YG

3.3.1 Preparation of the MIX Fractions

All the fractions of MIX F1, F2 and F3 were prepared by mixing the chemical compounds with the same concentration levels as those in MIX44 (see Fig. 2.). F1 was composed of GA, HB and PU. F2 contained DZ, CMA, RT, QT, GS and KF, while F3 was made up by ED, BA and UA.

3.3.2 Preparation of YG Fractions

The extract of the sample labeled as YG81 was fractionated into three fractions, F1, F2 and F3 by the Hewlett Packard 1100 preparative series HPLC instrument coupled with DAD and equipped with an ODS hypersil column of dimensions 250×21.2 mm and the particle size being 5 µm. The injection volume was 150 µl. The mobile phase flowed at 20 ml min^{-1} under the same elution profile used for analyzing YG extracts. F1, F2 and F3 were collected within 2 min to 11 min, 11 min to 18 min, and 18 min to 40 min respectively. All these fractions were collected by Foxy® Jr. fraction collector (ISCO, Inc., USA) and freeze dried after solvent removal using rotatory evaporation. The dried samples were used later for both antioxidant activity measurement and chromatographic characterization with the same chromatographic system used for the YG extracts.

3.4 Antioxidant Activity Assay

The antioxidant activities of all samples, fractions and the 12 compounds of MIX at different concentrations were measured by the FRAP method as proposed by Benzie and Strain (1996) with the use of a COBAS FARA II spectrofluorometric centrifugal analyzer (Roche). Details about the experimental procedure can be found in the published work of Chau et al. (2009) and Kvalheim et al. (2011). In brief, the antioxidant activity of the sample was evaluated from the change of the absorbance of the FRAP reagent at 593 nm after the addition of the sample for 4 min. It was then converted to the FRAP value to represent the total antioxidant capacity. A series of concentrations of ascorbic acid were also prepared for monitoring the performance of the instrument.

3.5 Data Analysis

All the data preprocessing and QPAR-F analyses were performed with the method proposed in the previous works (Eilers 2004; Tomasi et al. 2004) with Matlab R2007a software from the MathWorks.

4 Results and Discussion

The QPAR-F methodology proposed in this study was applied for identification of bioactive regions related to drug screening of two different mixture systems. The QPAR approach was adopted with the use of two different types of data obtained from the chemical fingerprints and total antioxidant activity measurements. In carrying out the QPAR-F calculation, the chromatograms of samples of the system were all divided in the same way into several regions. Then different combinations of these divided regions were designed and utilized for modeling so as to predict the total antioxidant capacities of the samples concerned through the proposed algorithm.

In the QPAR-F methodology, we assumed that the difference between the predicted and the measured TAC depended on which regions or regions were selected. The magnitude of the difference could provide valuable information about bioactivities of the components involved. In this way, models which included bioactive regions were expected to give more accurate prediction than those without. To investigate this, we started with the synthetic mixture system (Kvalheim et al. 2011), an idealized system with all the related properties known for methodology evaluation and assessment. Then, the assumption was applied to a real system, Radix *Puerariae Lobatae*, a herbal medicine, for further verification.

Fig. 3 The prediction errors
of PLS models based on
different combinations
of the three chromatographic
regions of MIX
(See Fig. 2 and Table 1)

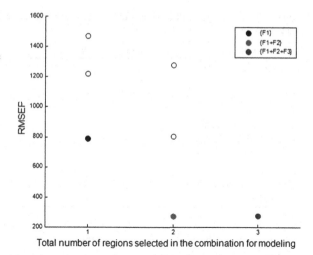

Total number of regions selected in the combination for modeling

4.1 The Synthetic Mixture System (MIX)

Fifty-eight synthetic mixtures with two outliers being removed, as in our previous study (Kvalheim et al. 2011) were used in this investigation. They were grouped randomly into a training set (38 samples) and a test set (20 samples). Then, the chromatogram of each one was divided into three regions, F1, F2 and F3, with different numbers of peaks and profile structures. Figure 2 shows these three divided regions in the chromatogram of the MIX44 sample as an example. In the chromatogram, all the peaks of the 12 compounds were labeled with their abbreviations (see Sect. 3.1). Also, some peaks were marked with numbers 1–7 according to the relative levels of the antioxidant activity of the related compounds, from high to low. Here, F1, F2 and F3 referred to the components eluted from 0 min to 12 min, 12 min to 20 min and 20 min to 33 min respectively.

It should be noted that these three regions represent the three different fractions when fractionations are carried out on the crude mixture sample. Even if there are changes in the order of the eluted components during large-scale fractionation, the chemical and spectral information obtained from the profiles of these regions can still be used for identification of the components obtained from the two processes. Once the divided regions were available, different combinations of these three regions of all the 38 samples in the training set were generated following the QPAR-F procedure described in Fig. 1. They together with the measured TACs with experimental errors less than 6 % were submitted to PLS modeling. Through the established models, fingerprints of samples from the test set were fed in and the TACs were predicted.

Figure 3 depicts the results obtained as given in Table 1 with the RMSEPs coming from the test set. It can be seen that the plot provides an overview about the performance of different models according to the prediction errors. It is obvious

Table 1 Summary of the PLS models established based on different combinations of the three divided regions of MIX (See Figs. 2 and 3)

Regions for modeling	Number of latent variables	RMSET	RMSEP
One-region (1:3) model			
F1	3	813	790
F2	2	1,028	1,218
F3	1	1,311	1,467
Two-region (2:3) model			
F1 + F2	7	197	271
F1 + F3	5	804	802
F2 + F3	7	1,079	1,276
Three-region (3:3) model			
F1 + F2 + F3	11	143	275

that, different combinations gave different errors even though the numbers of the regions selected are the same. For instance, among all the one-region (1:3) models with only one divided region being selected from all the three divided regions available, the combination {F1} occupied the lowest position in the plot (Fig. 3), while {F2} was situated in-between {F1}and {F3}. If the QPAR-F assumption works, the relative strength of antioxidant activity of these fractions in descending order was F1, F2 and F3. If this is true, one would expect that {F1 + F2} gave lower RMSEP than {F1} if the activity of F2 is not too low. In addition, {F2 + F3} should locate in a higher position than {F1 + F3} in the 2:3 model plots. In fact, these were observed in Fig. 3. The addition of F3 to {F1 + F2} did not improve the agreement between the predicted and the measured TAC.

All these observations supported the observation that the active fractions were F1 and F2. F3 had very low activity and it may even inactive. Table 1 gives more details about the prediction errors obtained from models with different combinations of the divided regions. When only one region was considered in modeling, the RMSEPs based on {F1}, {F2} and {F3} were 790, 1,218 and 1,467 respectively. With the consideration of the experimental errors and the assumption of QPAR-F, F1 was clearly more active than F2 as their RMSEPs differed significantly from each other. Also, F3 was the least active. When two regions were put together, surprisingly, {F1 + F2} gave an error of 271 (Table 1), much lower than that of {F1} alone.

The marked improvement in the predictive ability showed that, in this system, a single active region is not sufficient to account for the total activity. Both F1 and F2 contributed to the total bioactivity significantly even though they contributed to different extent individually. Furthermore, when F3 was added for modeling with the whole chromatogram being considered, there was no improvement in RMSEP (275). This strongly indicated that F3 played very little role to the bioactivity of the system. In other words, the ingredients within F3 were barely bioactive or even not active according to the assumption. This also explains why {F3} gave very high RMSEP in the 1:3 models. All these observations obtained from the QPAR-F 3-region modeling reveal that the magnitude of the RMSEP provides information consistently about how active a region or combination is. More than that, we can conclude that the activity strength of F1 is higher than that of F2, and in turn, higher than that of F3, when all the mixture samples in the training set are considered as a group in modeling.

In order to verify the conclusion drawn, separate experiments were carried out by testing newly prepared fractions related to F1, F2 and F3 for their TACs. Thus these fractions were prepared according to the chemical composition of the MIX44 sample and their TACs were measured. MIX 44 was selected because all the twelve components were present. The corresponding FRAPs thus obtained were 2,737, 2,085 and 74 respectively. It can be seen that these experimental findings supported the QPAR-F outcomes and also the assumption involved. In fact, when one looks closely into what components were present in the three fractions on preparing the mixtures, the most active antioxidant gallic acid (GA) was in F1 and the other less active ones were in F2 (see Fig. 2). There were no active ingredients in F3. This was also consistent with the RMSEP from {F1} being lower than that from {F2} in the 1:3 models and the {F1+F2} outperforming {F1+F3} in the 2:3 modeling as all active ingredients were included in QPAR-F computation.

In our previous work, we prepared the MIX samples with seven antioxidants having activity strengths of different extents (Kvalheim et al. 2011, article submitted for publication). At the highest concentration levels, GA, QT, KF, RT, CMA, GS and PU had FRAP values of 3,383, 2,250, 682, 476, 240, 30 and 26 respectively. Readings could be obtained for GS and PU at the concentration of 125 ppm or above. Hence, GA was the most active one. While QT and KF were the second and the third one from the FRAP assessment.

With the availability of these known properties, one can investigate the activity of the MIX fractions in more detail at the molecular level based on what components are present. As GA is present in F1 (Fig. 2), this explained why it was the most active fraction. The same argument can be applied to account for the activities of the other fractions. Thus, the results obtained from QPAR-F computation were further supported and confirmed by the known available information.

In summary, the QPAR-F methodology was proposed and an algorithm has been developed and applied to the synthetic mixture system MIX with known information. The chromatograms of the samples studied were divided into smaller regions first in order to carry out the QPAR-F algorithm. Then different combinations of these regions were utilized for PLS modeling.

The predicted total activity capacities from these models were compared with the experimental data. Here, we assumed that smaller differences between them come from the models using the combinations with appropriate bioactive regions included. From the results of MIX from QPAR-F analyses, one can clearly see that the assumption was valid and the proposed methodology preformed very well in identifying the active fractions. Experimental information available further supported this.

4.2 The Herbal Medicine YG

The 78 YG samples were grouped randomly into a training set (52 samples) and a test set (26 samples) for QPAR-F calculation. We took the same working procedure

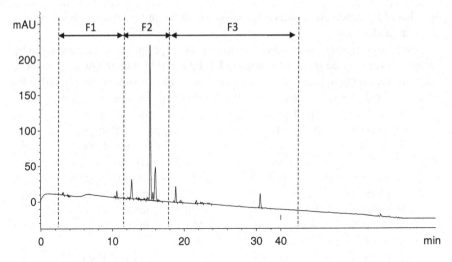

Fig. 4 The three divided regions in the YG chromatogram

Fig. 5 The prediction
errors of PLS models based
on different combinations
of the three divided regions
of YG (Fig. 5)

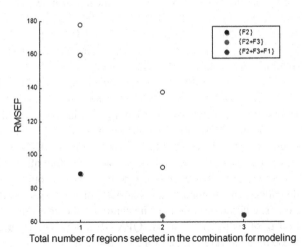

as that for MIX with the whole chromatogram being divided into three regions, F1,
F2 and F3 with elution times from 2 min to 11 min, 11 min to 18 min and 18 min to
40 min respectively (Fig. 4). The results obtained from different combinations of the
three divided regions were depicted in Fig. 5. Among all the 1:3 models, {F2} gave
the lowest RMSEP (89) while {F1} came up with the highest (178). With regard to
the 2:3 models, {F2 + F3} led to the lowest prediction errors. Addition of {F1} to
this combination with all the three regions involved did not reduce the RMSEP further. This indicated that F1 could not improve the predicted TAC, and it is relatively
not so active or even inactive compared to the other two. This observation is in line
with the outcome from the 1:3 modeling.

Table 2 Summary of results obtained results from models established based on different combinations of the three divided regions of YG (see Fig. 4)

Regions for modeling	Number of original variables	Number of latent variables	RMSET	RMSEP
One-region (1:3) model				
F1	1,460	5	124	178
F2	340	5	76	89
F3	668	4	151	160
Two-region (2:3) model				
F1 + F2	1,800	6	72	93
F1 + F3	2,128	7	97	138
F2 + F3	1,008	7	53	64
Three-region (3:3) model				
F1 + F2 + F3	2,468	5	55	64

Based on the experimental findings on the YG81 sample, the most antioxidant active fraction was F2 while the least one was F1 at the concentration of 1 mg/ml. The FRAP values of F2, F3 and F1 were 602, 136 and 83 respectively. The main reason why the YG81 sample was selected was that its FRAP value was close to the average of those from all the YG samples (Table 2).

5 Conclusions

Knowledge of active fractions can help to plan the bioassay-guided fractionation in drug screening more efficiently and effectively. These fractions may be represented by the regions as exhibited in the separation chromatogram of the system concerned. In this work, we propose a QPAR-F methodology based on approach of QPAR to establish the antioxidant active fractions from the chromatograms of a synthetic mixture system and the herbal medicine, Radix *Puerariae Locabae*. For the known mixture system, the active regions were identified successfully and their relative activity strength was also ranked. The results also confirmed the validity of the assumption that the predictive ability of the PLS model depended on the combination with appropriate bioactive regions being selected. When the QPAR-F was applied on the herbal medicine, the results obtained were consistent with those of the MIX system and they were also compared with the experimental findings.

Our work demonstrated that the proposed QPAR-F methodology is useful to help revealing information very efficiently which is important in the identification of bioactive fractions for drug development, discovering biomarkers and others. Unlike Cheng et al. (Wang et al. 2006; Xiao et al. 2006), no prior information about chemical and biological properties of the fractions or individual components are required in our study while establishing the QPAR relationship. Chemical and bioactivity information of the crude extract or the original sample are sufficient for the QPAR analysis.

Of course, chemical characterization on selected components of the crude extract might still be needed so as to reduce the chance of isolating known bioactive compounds. This novel QPAR-F approach can help to solve partly the technical problems encountered in the drug development of natural products (Li and Vederas 2009). It is worthwhile to mention that the new QPAR methodology is not only good for discovery of active chemical fractions of herbal medicines, it can also be applied to chromatograms of other complex mixtures, to find out biochemical active fractions.

In the past decade, chemical fingerprints obtained from separation instruments have been widely accepted by authorized agencies in the world as an alternative to monitor the quality of HM products (Chau et al. 2010; Zeng et al. 2008). Through these, all the active and inactive components as detected by the methods used are established, in contrast to the traditional procedures which utilize only a few markers that may be active or inactive compounds. It can be seen that through the proposed QPAR-F methodology, the chemical fingerprint can be transformed to the bioactivity fingerprint because the active regions with biomarkers present in the fingerprint are identified. It is much better to use this kind of fingerprint to assess a HM product as the functional activity is a key measure of the quality. In fact, other kinds of activity such as toxicity, smell, taste, etc. can also be considered as long as the relevant data are used for the QPAR-F modeling. With the availability of these activity fingerprints, the chemical composition of HMs can be standardized to much higher and accurate levels within the safety limits. Also, the composition of the compound HM formulation with more than one component herbs involved can be optimized to the desired level of bioactivity. Furthermore, personalized HM medicines can be prepared according to the required bioactivity level to meet the needs of individual patients.

Acknowledgments We would like to thank Professor Xie Pei-shan of Macau Institute for Applied Research in medicine and Health and Dr. Chen Si-bao of State Key Laboratory of Chinese Medicine and Molecular Pharmacology for herbal collection. Thanks are also due to the University Grant Committee (UGC) for financial support of the Area of Excellence (AoE) Project 'Chinese Medicine Research and further development" (AoE/B-10-01). Thanks are also to the Innovative Technology Research Syndicate (ITRS) (GHP/037/05) and the Taskforce on Development of Niche Area of the Hong Kong Polytechnic University, Hong Kong (BB8H and BB6R).

References

I.F.F. Benzie, J.J. Strain, The ferric reducing ability of plasma (FRAP) as a measure of "antioxidant power": The FRAP assay. Anal. Biochem. **239**, 70–76 (1996)

L. Bravo, L. Goya, E. Lecumberri, LC/MS characterization of phenolic constituents of mate (Ilex paraguariensis, St. Hil.) and its antioxidant activity compared to commonly consumed beverages. Food Res. Int. **40**, 393–405 (2007)

P. Burman, A comparative-study of ordinary cross-validation, v-fold cross validation and the repeated learning-testing methods. Biometrika **76**, 503–514 (1989)

F.T. Chau, H.Y. Chan, C.Y. Cheung, C.J. Xu, Y. Liang, O.M. Kvalheim, Recipe for uncovering the bioactive components in herbal medicine. Anal. Chem. **81**, 7217–7225 (2009)

F.T. Chau, K.P. Fung, C.M. Koon, K.M. Lau, S.Y. Wei, P.C. Leung, Bioactive Components in Herbal Medicines: Experimental Approach, in *Herbal Medicine: Biomolecular and Clinical Aspects* (Taylor Francis Group, LLC, Boca Ration, 2010)

E.G. de Mejía, Y.S. Song, C.I. Heck, M.V. Ramírez-Mares, Yerba mate tea (Ilex paraguariensis): phenolics, antioxidant capacity and in vitro inhibition of colon cancer cell proliferation. J. Funct. Foods **2**, 23–34 (2010)

P.H.C. Eilers, Parametric time warping. Anal. Chem. **76**, 404–411 (2004)

A.C. Ene, S.E. Atawodi, D.A. Ameh, G.I. Ndukwe, H.O. Kwanashie, Bioassay-guided fractionation and in vivo antiplasmodial effect of fractions of chloroform extract of Artemisia maciverae Linn. Acta Trop. **112**, 288–294 (2009)

Q.B. Han, Y. Zhou, C. Feng, G. Xu, S.X. Huang, S.L. Li, C.F. Qiao, J.Z. Song, D.C. Chang, K.Q. Luo, H.X. Xu, Bioassay guided discovery of apoptosis inducers from gamboge by high-speed counter-current chromatography and high-pressure liquid chromatography/electrospray ionization quadrupole time-of-flight mass spectrometry. J. Chromatogr. B **877**, 401–407 (2009)

A.L. Harvey, Natural products in drug discovery. Drug Discov. Today **13**, 894–901 (2008)

K. Hostettmann, J.L. Wolfender, C. Terreaux, Modern screening techniques for plant extracts. Pharm. Biol. **39**(Suppl), 18–32 (2001)

G. Jerz, S. Wybraniec, N. Gebers, P. Winterhalter, Target-guided separation of Bougainvillea glabra betacyanins by direct coupling of preparative ion-pair high-speed countercurrent chromatography and electrospray ionization mass spectrometry. J. Chromatogr. A **1217**, 4544–4554 (2010)

J.W. Jhoo, J.P. Freeman, T.M. Heinze, J.D. Moody, L.K. Schnackenberg, R.D. Beger, K. Dragull, C.S. Tang, C.Y.W. Ang, In Vitro cytotoxicity of nonpolar constituents from different parts of Kava plant (Piper methysticum). J. Agric. Food Chem. **54**, 3157–3162 (2006) http://www.ncbi.nlm.nih.gov/pubmed/16608246

O.M. Kvalheim, H. Chan, I.F.F. Benzie, Y.-t. Szeto, A.H.-c. Tzang, D.K. Mok, F.-t. Chau, Chromatographic profiling and multivariate analysis for screening and quantifying the contributions from individual components to the bioactive signature in natural products. Chemometr. Intell. Lab. Syst. **107**, 98–105 (2011)

J.W.H. Li, J.C. Vederas, Drug discovery and natural products: end of an era or an endless frontier? Science **325**, 161–165 (2009)

R. Othman, H. Ibrahim, M.A. Mohd, M.R. Mustafa, K. Awang, Biassay-guided isolation of a vasorelaxant active compound from Kaempferia galanga L. Phytomedicine **13**, 61–66 (2006)

I.S. Pesin, E.K. Akkol, F.N. Yalcin, U. Koca, H. Keles, E. Yesilada, Wound healing potential of Sambucus ebulus L. leaves and isolation of an active component, quercetin 3-0-glucoside. J. Ethnopharmacol. **129**, 106–114 (2010)

R.J.B. Peters, J.C.W. Rijk, T.F.H. Bovee, A.W.J.M. Nijrolder, A. Lommen, M.W.F. Nielen, Identification of anabolic steroids and derivatives using bioassay-guided fractionation, UHPLC/TOFMS analysis and accurate mass database searching. Anal. Chim. Acta **664**, 77–88 (2010)

S. Ratnayake, P. Lewandowski, Rapid bioassy-guided screening of toxic substances in vegetable oils that shorten the lide of SHRSP rats. Lipids Health Dis. **9**, 13–16 (2010)

A.P. Rauter, A. Martins, R. Lopes, J. Ferreira, L.M. Serralheiro, M.E. Araújo, C. Borges, J. Justino, F.V. Silva, M. Goulart, J.T. Oates, J.A. Rodrigues, E. Edwards, J.P. Noronha, P. Pinto, H.M. Filipe, Bioactivity studies and chemical profile of the antidiabetic plant Genista tenera. J. Ethnopharmacol. **122**, 384–393 (2009)

J.C.W. Rijk, T.F.H. Bovee, S. Wang, C.V. Poucke, C.V. Peteghem, M.W.F. Nielen, Detection of anabolic steroids in dietary supplements: the added value of an androgen yeast bioassay in parallel with a liquid chromatography–tandem mass spectrometry screening method. Anal. Chim. Acta **637**, 305–314 (2009)

S.Y. Shi, Y.P. Zhang, X.Y. Jiang, X.Q. Chen, K.L. Huang, H.H. Zhou, X.Y. Jiang, Coupling HPLC to on-line, post-column (bio)chemical assays for high–resolution screening of bioactive compounds from complex mixtures. TrAC Trends Anal. Chem. **28**, 865–877 (2009)

G. Tomasi, F. van den Berg, C. Andersson, Correlation optimized warping and dynamic time warping as preprocessing methods for chromatographic data. J. Chemom. **18**, 231–241 (2004)

S. Uhlig, A.C. Gutleb, U. Thrane, A. Flåøyen, Identification of cytotoxic principles from Fusarium avenaceum using bioassay–guided fractionation. Toxicon **46**, 150–159 (2005)

Y. Wang, X.W. Wang, Y.Y. Cheng, A computational approach to botanical drug design by modeling quantitative composition–activity relationship. Chem. Biol. Drug Des. **68**, 166–172 (2006)

Y. Wang, L.Y. Yu, L. Zhang, H.B. Qu, Y.Y. Cheng, A novel methodology for multicomponent drug design and its application in optimizing the combination of active components from Chinese medicinal formula Shenmai. Chem. Biol. Drug Des. **75**, 318–324 (2010)

S. Wold, M. Sjöström, L. Eriksson, in *The Encyclopedia of Computational Chemistry*, Partial Least Squares (PLS) in chemistry 2006–2020 (1999)

S. Wold, M. Sjostrom, L. Eriksson, PLS–regression: a basic tool of chemometrics. Chemometr. Intell. Lab. Syst. **58**, 109–130 (2001)

S.H. Wu, L. Yang, Y. Gao, X.Y. Liu, F.Y. Liu, Multi-channel counter-current chromatography for high-throughput fractionation of natural products for drug discovery. J. Chromatogr. A **1180**, 99–107 (2008)

X.F. Xiao, Y.Y. Cheng, L.Y. Zheng, C.L. Rui, Z.Q. Zhong, Multiple chromatographic fingerprinting and its application to the quality control of herbal medicines. Anal. Chim. Acta **555**, 217–224 (2006)

Q.S. Xu, Y.Z. Liang, H.L. Shen, Generalized PLS regression. J. Chemometr. **15**, 135–148 (2001)

Z.D. Zeng, F.T. Chau, H.Y. Chan, C.Y. Cheung, T.Y. Lau, S.Y. Wei, D.K.W. Mok, C.O. Chan, Y.Z. Liang, Recent advances in 'Compound-oriented' and 'Pattern-Oriented' quality control of herbal medicines. Chin. Med. **3**, 9 (2008) http://www.cmjournal.org/content/3/1/9

An Innovative and Comprehensive Approach in Studying the Complex Synergistic Interactions Among Herbs in Chinese Herbal Formulae

Chun-Hay Ko, Lily Chau, David Wing-Shing Cheung, Johnny Chi-Man Koon, Kwok-Pui Fung, Ping-Chung Leung, Simon K. Poon, and Clara Bik-San Lau

Abstract Traditional Chinese Medicine prescriptions depend not only on the individual herbs, but the interactions among herbs within an herbal formula. With examples, this chapter presents an innovative and comprehensive approach to studying the complex synergistic interactions among herbs in Chinese herbal formulae. In multi-targeted *in vitro* studies, we have integrated the use of the Combination Index and a statistical test of synergy to demonstrate not only the effectiveness of the combined use of herbs, but of the variation of their relationship on each mode of action. We report one of the first applications of statistical interpretations of combination effects of herbs in complex herbal formulae and the feasibility of applying this methodology in combinatory study of herbs.

C.-H. Ko • D.W.-S. Cheung • J.C.-M. Koon • P.-C. Leung • C.B.-S. Lau (✉)
Institute of Chinese Medicine, The Chinese University of Hong Kong,
E205, Science Centre East Block, Shatin, New Territories, Hong Kong

State Key Laboratory of Phytochemistry and Plant Resources in West China, The Chinese University of Hong Kong, Shatin, New Territories, Hong Kong
e-mail: gohey@cuhk.edu.hk; davidcheung@cuhk.edu.hk; johnnykoon@cuhk.edu.hk; pingcleung@cuhk.edu.hk; claralau@cuhk.edu.hk

L. Chau • S.K. Poon (✉)
School of Information Technologies, University of Sydney, Sydney, NSW 2006, Australia
e-mail: lily@it.usyd.edu.au; simon.poon@sydney.edu.au

K.-P. Fung
Institute of Chinese Medicine, The Chinese University of Hong Kong,
E205, Science Centre East Block, Shatin, New Territories, Hong Kong

State Key Laboratory of Phytochemistry and Plant Resources in West China, The Chinese University of Hong Kong, Shatin, New Territories, Hong Kong

School of Biomedical Sciences, The Chinese University of Hong Kong,
Shatin, New Territories, Hong Kong
e-mail: kpfung@cuhk.edu.hk

J. Poon and S.K. Poon (eds.), *Data Analytics for Traditional Chinese Medicine Research*, 173
DOI 10.1007/978-3-319-03801-8_10, © Springer International Publishing Switzerland 2014

1 Introduction

Traditional Chinese Medicine (TCM) is characterised by regulating the integrity of the human body and has accumulated over a few thousand years of experience in the use of herbal formulae for managing diseases. TCM has been widely used in ethnic communities for the treatment of a variety of diseases and is recognised as an attractive alternative to conventional medicine (Tang and Eisenbrand 1992; Chan 1995; Cheung et al. 2012). It is believed that within a herbal formula, the core herbs provides the main therapeutic actions, secondary herbs enhance or assist the effects of the principal herbs and the remaining herbs play modulatory roles such as treatment of accompanying symptoms, moderation of harshness and toxicity, enhancement of the delivery of herbal ingredients and harmonisation (Tang et al. 1998).

Formulating herbal combinations is a methodology used in herbal medicine that offers promising treatment over a single herb. TCM prescriptions depend not only on the individual herbs, but the interactions among herbs within an herbal formula. By combining herbs, it is possible to enhance superior medicinal properties while neutralising toxic effects. With examples, this chapter describes a novel methodology to statistically interpret the complex synergistic interactions among herbs in Chinese herbal formulae.

Previously, the study of the roles of each herb in a 2-herb formula and their synergistic interactions were investigated. The 2-herb formula NF3 (containing Astragali Radix (AR) and Rehmanniae Radix (RR) in the ratio of 2:1) was found to enhance diabetic wound healing in diabetic rats through the actions of angiogenesis, anti-inflammation and tissue regeneration (Tam et al. 2011). The diabetic wound healing effect was attributed to the synergistic interaction between its two component herbs, AR and RR. AR plays a preeminent role in the anti-inflammatory and fibroblast-proliferating activities of NF3. The inclusion of RR, however, is crucial for NF3 to exert its overall wound-healing as well as the underlying angiogenesis-promoting effects (Lau et al. 2012).

In recent years, there has been increasing concern about the application of bioinformatics and systems biology approaches for deciphering the scientific basis and the systematic features of TCM (Chen et al. 2009). Formal studies of chemical combinations began with agricultural poisons (Poch 1993; Bliss 1939), leading to broader pharmacological uses and drug developments (Araujo et al. 2005; Boik et al. 2008; Lee et al. 2007), particularly addressing life-threatening diseases such as cancer and HIV (Topaly et al. 2002). Herbal medicines have adopted these mathematical models in order to analyse their multi-targeted interactions (Cheung et al. 2012; Li and Zhang 2008).

Combination analysis typically utilises the classical isobolographic analysis introduced by Loewe and Muischnek in 1926, which have been extended by several formal methodologies to cater for variable potency ratio such as the Mixture (surface response) model (Tallarida 2001; White et al. 2003), the Combination index (CI) (Chou and Talalay 1983, 1984; Chou 2010), and the Bayesian model (Hennessey et al. 2010). The Combination Index is the most widely used numeric test in the field of pharmacology, with applications primarily used for *in vitro* anticancer drug testing such as cancer and HIV-1 (Tang et al. 1998; Pegram et al. 2004; Topaly et al. 2002). However, Greco describes the inherent nonlinear nature of the median-effect plot which therefore leads to incorrect calculations of the Combination Index for mutually non-exclusive combinations (Greco et al. 1995). The reproducibility of CI results are also poor as observed in a re-analysis of 136 data sets where only 28 % of results were in close agreement with the conclusions between the Chou–Talalay approach and a log-linear based regression approach (Fang et al. 2008; Gennings and Carter 1995). Tallarida's regression-based surface response methodology has found applications in toxicology, including food, drug and alcohol abuse (Lamarre et al. 2013; Lamarre and Tallarida 2008). However, Tallarida's methodology is limited to two herbal formulations.

This chapter will detail with examples, the innovative and comprehensive approach to studying complex synergistic interactions among herbs in Chinese herbal formulae. This methodology integrates the approaches from Chou's Combination Index and Tallarida's surface response for application to high dimensional modelling with statistical confidence.

2 Methodology

The innovative approach to studying complex synergistic interactions involves two primary steps. Step 1 involves understanding the role of each individual herb of an herbal formula in different mechanisms of action. This includes evaluating the potential synergistic, additive or antagonistic effects using Chou's Combination Index (CI). Step 2 involves analysing the degrees of herb-herb interaction using experimental designs of dose-ratio and verified by a test of significance.

2.1 Constant Fixed-Ratio Design

Experiments were designed where drugs were administered in a constant fixed ratio to simplify the analysis of synergy. Both the Danshen-Gegen (DG) combination and Epimedii Herba–Ligustri Lucidi Fructus–Psoraleae Fructus (ELP) combination were administered in amounts such that the proportion of each herb remained at a constant at 7:3 (according to traditional formula ratio) and 5:4:1 (according to our previous study (Siu et al. 2013)) ratio, respectively. This ratio design added to unity to allow an analysis of each constituent as a function of the proportions in the combination.

In this fixed-ratio design, the herbal constituents are administered in amounts that keep the dose proportions constant. According to Tallarida (2000), the benefit of fixed-ratio design can simplify the analysis of the data, and the results can be translated to production as manufactured combination product often has constant proportion of the ingredients.

Dose concentrations were organised such that doses were serially doubled on each increment. In regards to DG's effects, cells were treated with 5 increasing doses on nitric oxide (NO) production, 4 increasing doses on foam cell formation and 7 increasing doses on vSMC proliferation (Cheung et al. 2012). In regards to ELP's effects on osteoblast formation, rat bone mesenchymal stem cells were treated with 4 increasing doses of different combinations of herbal treatment. The bone formation marker, alkaline phosphatase activities (MSC-ALP) were determined at day 5. Details of the cell culture procedure, osteogenic differentiation and enzyme activities determination are described in our previous report (Siu et al. 2013).

2.2   Application of Chou's Combination Index

Dose-effect relationships were firstly analysed using the median-effect method described in (Chou and Talalay 1984; Chou 2010) as a preliminary numeric test. The Combination Index (CI) defines synergy as $CI < 1$ and antagonism as $CI > 1$ with respect to the additive effect ($CI = 1$). The CI was calculated using the 'CalcuSyn' software (Chou and Hayball 1996) according to the classic isobologram equation for n drugs described in Eq. 1

$$CI = \sum_{J=1}^{n} \frac{(D)_j}{(ED)_j} \tag{1}$$

In Eq. 1, the denominator is the sum of $(ED_{50})_1$, $(ED_{50})_2$, ... $(ED_{50})_n$, each of which represent the doses of constituent 1, constituent 2, ..., constituent n acting alone that is required to produce a chosen effect level (usually ED_{50}). The numerator is the sum of each constituent dose D_1, D_2, ... D_n as they act in combination to produce the same $x\%$ effect in the experiment where x is typically 50 %. The ED_{50} benchmark is typically used to ensure a half maximal effective dose for 50 % of the population. However, in herbal formulations, hebs have an inherent low-performing overall effect in the system in which they interact. This is because herbs do not have strong targeted effects, but moderately-strong multi-targeted effects. Consequently, for herbal formulations, ED_{25} is a more appropriate benchmark for herbal combinations. Chou's CI analysis is manipulated in this methodology as a means of eliminating combinations that displays strong antagonism, particularly if the herbal combination is high in dimension.

2.3   Extension of Tallarida's Regression

Following preliminary analysis with Chou's CI analysis, the synergistic effect can subsequently be tested for statistical significance by extending Tallarida's regression model as described in (Chau et al. 2013). Tallarida's methodology involves comparing the expected additive effect curve Z_{add} with that of the experimental combination curve Z_{mix} on an effect versus log(dose) curve. Z_{mix} can accordingly be tested against the reference curve in order to observe if the curve significantly falls above the additive line (synergistic), below the additive line (antagonistic) or close to the additive line (additive). This test can equivalently be expressed in Eqs. 2 and 3.

$$\text{synergism} : Z_{mix} < Z_{add} \tag{2}$$

$$\text{sub additive} : Z_{mix} > Z_{add} \tag{3}$$

To test if the interaction is statistically significant, a t-test based on the difference of two means is used, described in Eq. 4.

$$t' > |T| \tag{4}$$

where

$$t' = \frac{X - Y}{\sqrt{\left(SE_x\right)^2 + \left(SE_y\right)^2}}$$

$$T = \frac{t_{add}\left(SE_x\right)^2 - t_{mix}\left(SE_y\right)^2}{\left(SE_x\right)^2 + \left(SE_y\right)^2}$$

$$X = \log Z_{add} \quad Y = \log Z_{mix}$$

Following the determination of synergy, it is useful to explore the interactions of each combinatory subset to determine the optimal synergistic subset and thus infer the principal herb in the combination. The degree of interaction of each combination involves calculating the marginal contribution of each combination as defined in Eq. 5:

$$\left(a_1 a_2 \ldots a_n\right)_{marginal} = (-1)^n \left(n_1 a_1 + n_2 a_2 + \ldots + n_n a_n\right) - \left(a_1 a_2 \ldots a_n\right)_{mix}$$
$$+ \sum_{i=2}^{n-1} (-1)^{n+1-i} \left(i_{way}\right)_{mix} \tag{5}$$

where

$$i_{way_{mix}} = \prod_{i=1}^{n-i} s(i) \prod_{k=2}^{n-1} \prod_{j=i+1}^{k} s(j)$$

and
> n = number of drugs (or number of dimensions)
> $\underline{s}$ = set of drugs: $a_1, a_2, \ldots, a_n$ in the proportion $n_1 : n_2 : \ldots : n_n = 1$

$$n_1 + n_2 + \ldots + n_n = 1$$

This extension to Tallarida's methodology allows for the analysis of the degree of interaction within combinatory subsets of the herbal formulation as well as the statistical significance of the interaction. Overall, the higher dimensions model involves first utilising Chou's Combination Index to eliminate strong antagonistic combinations, followed by the extension of Tallarida's regression methodology to verify the type of interaction within combinatory subsets and testing for statistical significance.

3   Application of Methodology

Application of the higher dimensional model and test is described with two real-world dataset examples. The two-herb formula DG (Danshen and Gegen in the ratio of 7:3) and the 3-herb formula ELP (Epimedii Herba (E) and Ligustri Lucidi Fructus (L) and Psoraleae Fructus (P) in the ratio of 5:4:1) will be used to illustrate its application. From the analysis of the type and degree of interaction within combinatory subsets, it is possible to infer both the optimal synergistic subset and the principal herb responsible for effective treatment.

3.1   Descriptive Statistics

Prior to analysis, information can be inferred from descriptive statistics of the raw data. In reference to Cheung et al. 2012, the Danshen–Gegen (DG) combination was used to treat anti-inflammation, anti-foam cell formation and anti-vSMC proliferation. The dose response curve of DG is generally observed to be synergistic in the suppression of LPS-induced NO production as DG lies significantly above both the individual herbs D and G. Slight synergistic effects is observed for the inhibition of foam cell formation as the DG curve closely models the D curve, and only slightly outperforms D under ED_{90}. With respect to the inhibition of vSMC proliferation, antagonistic interaction is generally observed as DG underperforms herb D. It can therefore be generally concluded that the combination effects of DG in anti-inflammation, anti-foam cell formation and anti-vSMC proliferation were found to be synergistic, additive and antagonistic, respectively.

Similarly, descriptive statistics can be performed on ELP data. Data collected for ELP and their effects on osteoblast differentiation (MSC-ALP activity) can be summarised in Table 1. The effect at dose zero (control) was discounted from the remaining effects to ensure that any effects attributable from the background effects have been discounted.

Table 1 Dose-effect data averages for osteoblast differentiation (MSC-ALP activity)

Dose (µg/ml)	Effect						
	ELP	EL	EP	LP	E	L	P
100	57.9920	79.6640	18.2787	114.6415	39.5322	34.0054	1.7749
50	45.9803	58.1416	−3.0944	43.6250	32.6969	35.8403	−5.9106
25	32.5216	27.6973	2.0927	26.0187	8.0427	21.5528	−12.7936
12.5	2.4378	−2.1078	−5.2552	17.0867	−15.1272	12.8551	−6.8357
0	0.0000	0.0000	0.0000	0.0000	0.0000	0.0000	0.0000

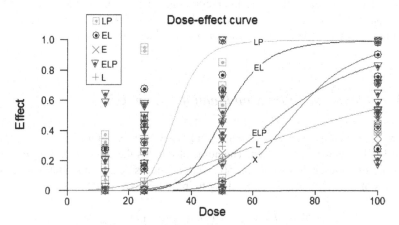

Fig. 1 Dose-effect curve for osteoblast formation (MSC-ALP activity) generated from CalcuSyn. *Effects ≤0 were reset to 1E-7 and effects >1 were reset to 0.9999999 due to the limitation of CalcuSyn in handling effect data that does not lie in between 0 and 1 exclusive. **Herb combination EP and herb P are not shown as they are slowly increasing curves that resemble a horizontally flat line at effect 0

Table 1 can be summarised in the dose-effect curve shown in Fig. 1. In Fig. 1, herb P and herb formulation EP are not shown as their performance are lower than the control scenario of no herbs. This horizontally flat curve will affect the standard deviation of herb combinations that consist of P or EP interactions. This is because Tallarida's regression depends on the prediction of dosage levels at a certain ED value. If the dose-effect curve is relatively flat, the predicted dosage at any ED value will be largely extrapolated and thus lack statistical confidence. Difficulties will therefore arise in concluding if synergistic interactions exist in larger combinations. For example, ELP may conclude to be synergistic from regression, however, a statistical test will reveal that herb P's presence will significantly affect the statistical significance of ELP usage. This may include the effect of falsely shifting down the ELP curve further than what is theoretically expected. Herb P is therefore more likely to create a false antagonistic effect due to the large amount of variance it carries. Further, from Table 1, it is indicative that herb P does not distinctly or directly affect osteoblast formation. Consequently, any statistical conclusion should be used with care as the statistical power will be considerably low. It is clear that a relatively flat dose-effect curve will hinder the statistical validity and conclusions of interacting components.

It is also observable from Fig. 1 that herb combination LP demonstrates a strong exponentially increasing relation to treating osteoblast differentiation, followed by herb combination EL. In terms of synergistic interaction, ELP is observed to outperform herb L at approximately ED_{25} and underperform herb E at approximately ED_{75}. An initial additive assumption is therefore assumed with the ELP herb combination in osteoblast differentiation. Nevertheless, regression analysis is performed on the data to reveal interesting interactions not dependent on the high standard variation of the herbs. However, further pharmacological tests and inferences are required to deterministically describe *in vitro* interactions.

3.2   Calculation of the Combination Index (CI)

In application of the herbal combination at ED_{50}, Chou's Combination Index is generated as below using CalcuSyn. The numerator holds the dosages of drug E, L and P acting in combination to inhibit 50 % effectiveness. The denominator holds the dosages of drug E, L and P acting along to inhibit 50 % effectiveness.

$$CI = \frac{\left(D_{50}\right)_{ELP(E)}}{\left(ED_{50}\right)_E} + \frac{\left(D_{50}\right)_{ELP(L)}}{\left(ED_{50}\right)_L} + \frac{\left(D_{50}\right)_{ELP(P)}}{\left(ED_{50}\right)_P}$$

Extending DG Combination Index analysis to include similar ED ranges, the results can be summarised in Table 2. Anti-inflammation demonstrates increasing synergy as the effect level increases, while anti-vSMC demonstrates increasing antagonism. Anti-foam cell formation however, demonstrates synergy when beyond ED_{50}. Though the Combination Index analysis lacks statistical validity, the calculated CI for the DG combination lies in the experimented dosage range. Thus, there is

Table 2 CI results for DG (Danshen–Gegen) in treating: anti-inflammation (Assay I), anti-foam cell formation (Assay II) and anti-vSMC proliferation (Assay III) (Cheung et al. 2012)

ED values	Assay I		Assay II		Assay III	
	CI	Dose	CI	Dose	CI	Dose
ED_{25}	0.9152	0.31	1.9430	0.29	3.7103	0.03
ED_{50}	0.7500	0.54	1.0300	0.34	2.0200	0.08
ED_{75}	0.6471	0.93	0.8529	0.41	4.3827	0.25

Table 3 Combination Index results based on data averages of osteoblast differentiation (MSC-ALP activity)

	ELP		EL		EP		LP	
ED values	CI	Dose (µg/ml)	CI	Dose (µg/ml)	CI	Dose (µg/ml)	CI	Dose (µg/ml)
ED_{25}	1.3578	34.70	1.9430	50.39	3.7103	218.30	0.5692	20.05
ED_{50}	1.1765	63.49	1.0490	58.06	4.0323	277.81	0.1294	23.10
ED_{75}	1.5247	116.16	0.8529	66.90	4.3827	353.54	0.0368	26.60

some confidence in the identified synergistic interactions, as opposed to extrapolated-based CI values.

The Combination Index results for the ELP combination can be summarised in Table 3. Due to the large variation in the raw data, especially with herb P's effects, data averages were used to calculate the CI as opposed to using the complete dataset.

From Table 3, several different types of interactions can be observed. In particular, it is observed that the ELP combination varied its direction around the additive-antagonistic line. This is justified from Fig. 1 where the interactions of ELP lied between herb L at lower effect levels, and herb E at higher effect levels. Combination EL generally observed synergistic effects beyond ED_{50} and continued to increase at higher effect levels. Combination EP however, demonstrated continued strong antagonism as the effect levels increased such that in order to reach ED_{25}, a large dose of 218.30 µg/ml is required, exceeding the dose regimen of the experiment. This out of range value is expected as EP demonstrated a relatively flat dose-response curve in Fig. 1. Finally, combination LP demonstrated significant synergistic effects, approaching the ideal zero CI value at a rapid rate.

3.3 Regression Analysis

In application of both DG and ELP formulations, each experimental combination was analysed via regression to estimate their ED_{50} doses and variance. Cheung et al. (2012) outlines the initial steps to determining G's dose at ED_{50}. As doses were doubled on each increment, a log transformation of base two was used to ensure the linearity of the data analysis, and thus maintaining the validity in extending upon Tallarida's methodology. With reference to the supplementary data presented in Cheung et al. (2012), a statistical test of significance can be performed on DG's suppression of NO production.

Table 4 Regression coefficients and ED$_{50}$ data for experimental osteoblast differentiation (MSC-ALP activity) results

	ELP	EL	LP	EP	E	L	P
Observation	48	32	32	32	16	16	16
s	32.220	42.089	42.368	34.845	9.536	13.062	12.452
α	−57.642	−100.998	−109.256	−30.643	−80.208	−13.389	−22.234
β	17.976	27.576	31.027	6.541	18.863	7.774	3.272
$\log_2(Herb)$	5.988	5.476	5.133	12.328	6.903	8.154	22.080
$Herb_{50}$	63.475	44.499	35.085	5,141.425	119.656	284.861	4.43E+06

$$Value\ of\ D\ at\ ED_{50} : Y = 52.5503 + 63.2619\,Log(dose)$$
$$\Rightarrow Log(ED_{50}) = -0.0403 \pm 0.1516$$
$$\Rightarrow D_{50} = 0.9114 \pm 0.3178$$

$$Value\ of\ G\ at\ ED_{50} : Y = 46.9808 + 51.5477\,Log(dose)$$
$$\Rightarrow Log(ED_{50}) = 0.0586 \pm 0.1336$$
$$\Rightarrow D_{50} = 1.1444 \pm 0.3515$$

$$Value\ of\ DG\ at\ ED_{50}\,(Z_{mix}) : Y = 71.3030 + 72.7996\,Log(dose)$$
$$\Rightarrow Log(Z_{mix}) = -0.2926 \pm 0.0529$$
$$\Rightarrow Z_{mix} = 0.5098 \pm 0.0620$$

$$Z_{add} = 0.9114 \times 0.7 + 1.1444 \times 0.3 = 0.9813 \pm 0.2462$$
$$t' = 7.5179, T = 2.0508$$

Since Z_{mix} (0.5098) <Z_{add} (0.9813), this indicates the DG combination is synergistic. Further, the t-test criterion is satisfied $|t'|$ (7.5179) >T (2.0508), indicating the DG synergistic interaction is statistically significant. Applying this high dimensional regression model on the ELP combination, the regression coefficients on the effect versus log(dose) curve can be summarised in Table 4. Regression at dose zero is ignored as there are no observed effects (NOEL) at any biologically significant endpoint.

Continuing with the ELP example, the regression equation can be expressed as $Y = -57.642 + 17.9\log_2(dose_{ELP})$. Solving for $dose_{ELP}$ (or Z_{mix}) gives a dose of 63.475 at ED$_{50}$. The standard error corresponding to the dose is 47.329, calculated using

$$SE_{ED} = 2.3 \cdot Herb_{ED} \sqrt{\frac{s^2}{\beta^2}\left[\frac{1}{N} + \frac{\left(Herb - \overline{\log dose}\right)^2}{S_{xx}}\right]}$$

where N represents that number of observations and $\overline{\log dose}$ is the mean of dosage data that have utilised the log transformation.

With the experimental values calculated, the additive reference curve can be computed by weighting the individual herbs in a 5:4:1 ratio, $Z_{add}=0.5E+0.4L+0.1P$ where E, L and P are the doses derived from regression analysis at ED_{50}. At ED_{50}, $Z_{add}=4.43E5\pm1.47E7$ where the standard deviation $SE(Z_{add})$ was calculated by weighting the standard error of the participating herbs, variance $V(Z_{add})=0.5^2SE_E+0.4^2SE_L+0.1^2SE_P$.

Testing for synergy, it is observed that $Z_{mix}<Z_{add}$ and thus, ELP is synergistic at ED_{50}. To test the statistical significance of this synergy, the t-test described in Eq. 4 is applied

$$t' \left(\frac{\log(4.43E5)-\log(63.475)}{\sqrt{\left(\frac{1.47E7}{2.3*4.43E5}\right)^2+\left(\frac{47.429}{2.3*63.475}\right)^2}} \right)$$
$$> \left| T\left(\frac{t_{16+16+16-3-1}(1-\alpha)\cdot(14.44)^2-t_{32-2}(1-\alpha)\cdot(0.324)^2}{(1.44.44)^2+(0.324)^2} \right) \right|$$

where α is the significance level used to compute the confidence level of $(1-\alpha)\%$. In this example, $\alpha=5\%$ is used.

Note the denominator on the LHS has terms $\log(SE(Z_{add}))$ and $\log(SE(Z_{mix}))$ where the latter is equivalent to dividing the $SE(Z_{mix})$ term by 2.3 and the Z_{mix} term at the desired ED value.

Evaluating the t-test, $t'(0.8841)<|T(2.0154)|$, indicating that the ELP interaction is not statistically significant at ED_{50}. This indicates the ELP ratio combination has a sub-additive effect on osteoblast differentiation. The regression methodology of calculating doses at ED_{50}, identifying synergy and testing for significance can be repeated for several ED values, summarised in Table 5.

From Table 5, it is observed that synergy is present at ED_{25}, ED_{50} and ED_{75} for all combinations of ELP, EL, EP and LP. However, this synergy is only statistically significant for EL combinations. Comparatively, Chou's CI from Table 3 indicates synergy with ELP, EL and LP for ED_{50} and ED_{75} levels. The test of statistical significance from regression analysis highlights the importance of a statistical test in analysing significance. Otherwise, Chou's CI results will produce two false synergistic interactions (ELP and LP). In addition, LP showed synergy at ED_{25}. Though LP demonstrated clear synergy in Fig. 1, herb P and its large standard error impacted on the statistical significance of LP, thus attributing a large variance in LP's Z_{add} value. A summary of the interacting herbs and its statistical significance is shown in Fig. 2.

Table 5 Determination of interaction and testing for significance for osteoblast differentiation (MSC-ALP activity)

Mix	ED$_\%$	Z$_{mix}$	Z$_{add}$	t-test
ELP	ED$_{25}$	24.2073 ± 16.0326	$2{,}255.72 \pm 4.07 \times 10^4$	$t'(0.8339) < |T(2.0154)|$
	ED$_{50}$	63.4753 ± 47.3287	$4.43 \times 10^5 \pm 1.47 \times 10^4$	$t'(0.8841) < |T(2.0154)|$
	ED$_{75}$	166.443 ± 221.37	$8.85 \times 10^7 \pm 4.26 \times 10^9$	$t'(0.9080) < |T(2.0154)|$
EL	ED$_{25}$	23.7380 ± 16.5637	40.1535 ± 15.7349	$t'(2.1794) > |T(2.0423)|$
	ED$_{50}$	44.4993 ± 28.8061	193.080 ± 351.170	$t'(2.5099) > |T(2.0423)|$
	ED$_{75}$	83.4186 ± 77.2535	$1{,}342.93 \pm 6{,}432.15$	$t'(1.8901) < |T(2.0423)|$
EP	ED$_{25}$	$363.594 \pm 2{,}495.70$	$3{,}739.10 \pm 6.78 \times 10^4$	$t'(0.3989) < |T(2.0423)|$
	ED$_{50}$	$5{,}141.42 \pm 7.24 \times 10^4$	$7.39 \times 10^5 \pm 2.45 \times 10^7$	$t'(0.4568) < |T(2.0423)|$
	ED$_{75}$	$7.27 \times 10^4 \pm 1.56 \times 10^6$	$1.48 \times 10^8 \pm 7.11 \times 10^9$	$t'(0.4794) < |T(2.4486)|$
LP	ED$_{25}$	20.0712 ± 13.8007	$4{,}463.70 \pm 8.13 \times 10^4$	$t'(0.9833) < |T(2.4486)|$
	ED$_{50}$	35.0855 ± 19.4806	$8.87 \times 10^5 \pm 2.95 \times 10^7$	$t'(1.2174) < |T(2.4486)|$
	ED$_{75}$	61.3313 ± 41.7771	$1.77 \times 10^8 \pm 8.53 \times 10^9$	$t'(1.0248) < |T(2.4486)|$

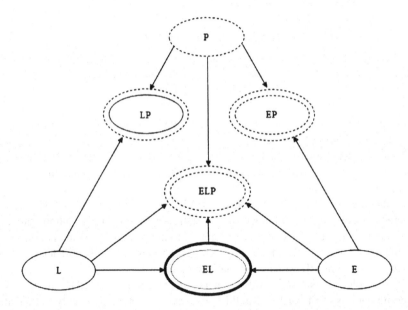

Fig. 2 A summary of the interacting combinatory subsets within ELP and its effect on osteoblast differentiation (MSC-ALP activity). For combinatory sets, the *inner line* represents the type of interaction: synergism (*solid line*) or antagonism (*dashed line*); and the *outer line* represents the statistical significance: not significant (*dashed line*) or statistically significant (*thick solid line*). For single components, a *dashed line* indicates the component performed worse than the control and a *solid line* indicates the component performed better than the control

As a post-processing step, the marginal contribution for each combinatory subset can be calculated to describe the role of interacting herbs. The marginal contribution for the ELP formulation is summarised in Table 6. It is observed that all pairwise interactions are synergistic while the three-way interaction is antagonistic. As both

Table 6 Marginal contribution of ELP combinatory subset for osteoblast differentiation (MSC-ALP activity)

	Marginal	Interaction	Rank
LP	8.87E5	Synergistic	1
EP	7.34E5	Synergistic	2
EL	1.49E2	Synergistic	3
ELP	−1.18E6	Antagonistic	4

Tables 4 and 5 agree in the antagonistic interaction of ELP, this implies that the interaction on the third dimension is predominately derived from the three-way interaction, over-riding any synergistic interacting pairwise combinations. As the marginal interaction calculation extends upon regression analysis, herb P's large standard error will further affect the magnitude of the marginal interaction. In particular, combinations involving herb P will always have a large magnitude and rank, and thus lack in statistical confidence. It is only combination EL that has some statistical confidence in its synergistic interaction. As a consequence, the large synergistic pairwise contribution combined with the dominant three-way antagonistic effect gave an overall antagonistic ELP interaction. Similarly, as EP is demonstrated to be antagonistic from both CI and regression analysis, but synergistic in marginal contribution, this indicates that EP is dominated by the individual effects of herbs E and P. The interaction between EP, though synergistic, is not large enough compared to the individual interaction. Thus, ELP has an overall antagonistic effect.

Observing the magnitude or rank of the pairwise synergy within ELP from Table 6, this suggests that the optimal synergy lies in the two dimensional LP combination. Further analysing the rank of the pairwise interaction, herb P appears in both the first and second rank. This suggests that herb P may be the principal interacting drug in the combination. This is against preconception as herb P demonstrated a relatively flat dose-response curve in Fig. 1. Referring back to Fig. 1 and analysing the individual herbs at ED_{50}, herb L is a more consistent performer than P, responsible for the overall synergy of LP and EL.

By combining Chou's Combination Index and the extended Tallarida's methodology, it was possible to identify the type of interaction and test for statistical significance. Application to the DG and ELP combinations demonstrated the feasibility of applying this high dimensional model and test to describing the effects between interacting components. Post-processing interacting combinatory subsets further illuminated the mechanisms and roles each herb plays in a specific combination.

4 Discussion

Application of the higher dimensional model has some inherent limitations, particularly as it was designed primarily for pharmacological use in drug development. Issues may also arise with application to combining herbs and their inherent low-performing nature. Nevertheless, the combined framework of Chou's CI and extended Tallarida's test aids in the understanding and difference between effectiveness and marginal contribution.

4.1 Pharmacological Usage

The integrated Chou and Tallarida model was designed for pharmacological use and may therefore experience issues with accuracy and validity on application to more complex systems. Though an herb may be underperforming or vary in performance and reliability does not necessitate the removal of that herb. As the body is a complex system, an herb combination with an outlier herb that may not be core in one treatment, may be core in another treatment. This is the whole basis of herbal treatment, affecting multiple areas of its environment. As the body is a multi-targeted and multi-outcome environment, herb combinations may be helpful in affecting other interacting components of the environment. As highlighted in Chau et al. (2013), the higher dimensional model is designed for pharmacological use, performing more accurately in *in vitro* studies for the purpose of drug development.

4.2 Low Performing Herbs

When analysing the ELP formulation, it was observed that herb P's low-performing effects affected the statistical validity of analysing any formulations consisting of herb P. Herb P and any other herb that underperforms compared to the control variable and demonstrates a relatively flat dose-response curve will always affect the standard error of any preceding results. If an herb has difficulty reaching the ED_{50} value, this means the derived calculations used in analysis will be a large extrapolated result with little confidence. One such consequence of an estimated result is that false synergistic interactions may be detected. As the regression analysis depends on both Z_{add} and Z_{mix} of which Z_{add} has been severely compromised in terms of statistical validity, regression calculations will always claim synergistic results. The criterion after all observes $Z_{mix} \ll Z_{add}$. However, it is not until the test of statistical significance that the false synergies are exposed. This test then concludes any false interactions as a questionable interaction termed "sub-additive"; not purely antagonistic, but at best, sub-additive. A low-performing herb therefore poses challenges in statistical validity, but when mixed with certain drugs, the reliability and standard error may become stable.

Due to the low-performing and off-target nature of herbs in contrast to western medicine, the notion of ED_{50} is not as important in analysis. Though combined interactions may enhance a beneficial effect, these off-target herbs may still never cumulate to effects as great as ED_{50}. Thus, when analysing herbal combinations, if ED_{50} is not statistically relevant, analysing between ranges $ED_{20} - ED_{30}$ may be more realistic. Herbs generally work as an overall well-being treatment and thus less restrictive ED ranges should be used for analysis.

4.3 Effectiveness Versus Marginal Contribution

Evaluating combinations at higher dimensions observed a difference between effectiveness and marginal contribution. In terms of effectiveness, formulations EL and LP demonstrated overall synergistic effects, though LP with a smaller level of confidence. In terms of marginal contributions, LP, EP and EL demonstrated synergistic pairwise effects. This difference aids in the understanding of higher order interactions. For example, a synergistic interaction may involve competing lower-order interactions, involving either synergistic or antagonistic interactions, with a dominant synergistic subset. An antagonistic interaction may also be made up of synergistic interacting pairs, but the dominant interaction is the individual herb. Where an antagonistic interaction is made up of synergistic interacting subsets, this can indicate that there exists a smaller and more effective subset involving fewer herbs that is more optimal in treatment. By analysing both effectiveness and marginal contribution, an indication of the core herbs can be deduced.

5 Conclusion

In the multi-targeted *in vitro* studies, we have integrated the use of the Combination Index and a statistical test to demonstrate not only the effectiveness of the combined use of herbs, but of the variation of their relationship on each mode of action. We report one of the first applications of statistical interpretations of combination effects of herbs in complex herbal formulae and the feasibility of applying this methodology in combinatory study of herbs. This study not only highlighted the potential herbal combinations of DG (Danshen and Gegen) and ELP (Epimedii Herba, Ligustri Lucidi Fructus and Psoraleae Fructus), but the design of future promising and low-cost means of novel drug discovery.

References

R.P. Araujo, E.F. Petricoin, L.A. Liotta, A mathematical model of combination therapy using the EGFR signaling network. Biosystems **80**(1), 57–69 (2005)

C.I. Bliss, The toxicity of poisons applied jointly. Ann. Appl. Biol. **26**(3), 585–615 (1939)

J.C. Boik, R.A. Newman, R.J. Boik, Quantifying synergism/antagonism using nonlinear mixed-effects modeling: A simulation study. Stat. Med. **27**(7), 1040–1061 (2008)

K. Chan, Progress in traditional Chinese medicine. Trends Pharmacol. Sci. **16**, 182–187 (1995)

L. Chau, S.K. Poon, J. Poon, Identifying high dimensional statistically significant synergistic interactions in dose response, in *34th Annual Conference of the International Society for Clinical Biostatistics*, Aug 25–19, Munich, (2013)

X. Chen, H. Zhou, Y. Liu, J. Wang, H. Li, C. Ung, L. Han, Z. Cao, Y. Chen, Database of traditional Chinese medicine and its application to studies of mechanism and to prescription validation. Br. J. Pharmacol. **149**(8), 1092–1103 (2009)

W.S. Cheung, C.M. Koon, C.F. Ng, P.C. Leung, K.P. Fung, S.K. Poon, C. Lau, The roots of Salvia miltiorrhiza (Danshen) and Pueraria lobata (Gegen) inhibit atherogenic events: A study of the combination effects of the 2-herb formula. J. Ethnopharmacol. **143**(3), 859–866 (2012)

T. Chou, Drug combination studies and their synergy quantification using the Chou-Talalay method. Cancer Res. **70**(2), 440–446 (2010)

T. Chou, M. Hayball, *CalcuSyn Windows Software for Dose Effect Analysis* (Biosoft, Cambridge, 1996)

T.C. Chou, P. Talalay, Analysis of combined drug effects: a new look at a very old problem. Pharmacol. Sci. **4**, 450–454 (1983)

T. Chou, P. Talalay, Quantitative analysis of dose-effect relationships: the combined effects of multiple drugs or enzyme inhibitors. Adv. Enzyme Regul. **22**(0065–2571), 27–55 (1984)

H.B. Fang, D.D. Ross, E. Sausville, M. Tan, Experimental design and interaction analysis of combination studies of drugs with log-linear dose responses. Stat. Med. **27**(16), 3071–3083 (2008)

C. Gennings, J.W.H. Carter, Utilizing concentration–response data from individual components to detect statistically significant departures from additivity in chemical mixtures. Biometrics **51**(4), 1264–1277 (1995)

W.R. Greco, G. Bravo, J.C. Parsons, The search for synergy: a critical review from a response surface perspective. Pharmacol. Rev. **47**(2), 331–385 (1995)

V.G. Hennessey, G.L. Rosner, R.C. Bast, M.-Y. Chen, A Bayesian approach to dose-response assessment and synergy and its application to in vitro dose-response studies. Biometrics **66**(4), 1275–1283 (2010)

N. Lamarre, R. Tallarida, A quantitative study to assess synergistic interactions between urotensin II and angiotensin II. Eur. J. Pharamacol. **586**(1–3), 350–351 (2008)

N. Lamarre, R. Raffab, R. Tallarida, Cocaine synergism with alpha agonists in rat aorta: computational analysis reveals an action beyond reuptake inhibition. Drug and Alcohol Depend. **129**(3), 226–231 (2013)

K.M. Lau, K.K. Lai, C.L. Liu, J.C.W. Tam, M.H. To, H.F. Kwok, C.P. Lau, C.H. Ko, P.C. Leung, K.P. Fung, S.K. Poon, C.B.S. Lau, Synergistic interaction between Astragali Radix and Rehmanniae Radix in a Chinese herbal formula to promote diabetic wound healing. J. Ethnopharmacol. **141**, 250–256 (2012)

J.J. Lee, M. Kong, G.D. Ayers, R. Lotan, Interaction index and different methods for determining drug interaction in combination therapy. J. Biopharm. Stat. **17**(3), 461–480 (2007)

X.J. Li, H.Y. Zhang, Synergy in natural medicines: Implications for drug discovery. Trends Pharmacol. Sci. **29**(7), 331–332 (2008)

M. Pegram, G. Konecny, C. O'Callaghan, M. Beryt, R. Pietras, D. Slamon, Rational combinations of trastuzumab with chemotherapeutic drugs used in the treatment of breast cancer. J. Natl. Cancer Inst. **96**(10), 739–749 (2004)

G. Poch, *Combined Effects of Drugs and Toxic Agents* (Springer, New York, 1993)

W.S. Siu, H.L. Wong, C.P. Lau, W.T. Shum, C.W. Wong, S. Gao, K.P. Fung, C.B.S. Lau, L.K. Hung, C.H. Ko, P.C. Leung, The effects of an antiosteoporosis herbal formula containing epimedii herba, ligustri lucidi fructus and psoraleae fructus on density and structure of rat long bones under tail-suspension, and its mechanisms of action. Phytother. Res. **27**, 484–492 (2013)

R.J. Tallarida, *Drug synergism and Dose-Effect Data Analysis* (Chapman and Hall/CRC, Boca Raton, 2000)

R.J. Tallarida, Drug synergism: Its detection and applications. J Pharmacol. Exp. Ther. **298**(3), 865–872 (2001)

W.X. Tang, G. Eisenbrand, *Chinese Drugs of Plant Origin: Chemistry, Pharmacology and Use in Traditional and Modern Medicine* (Springer, Berlin, 1992)

W.-X. Tang, P.-Y. Cheng, Y.-P. Luo, R.-X. Wang, Interaction between cisplatin, 5-fluorouracil and vincristine on human hepatoma cell line (7721). World J. Gastroenterol. **4**(5), 418–420 (1998)

J.C.W. Tam, K.M. Lau, C.L. Liu, M.H. To, H.F. Kwok, K.K. Lai, C.P. Lau, C.H. Ko, P.C. Leung, K.P. Fung, C.B.S. Lau. The *in vivo* and *in vitro* diabetic wound healing effects of a 2-herb formula and its mechanisms of action. *J. Ethnopharmacol.* **134**, 831–838 (2011)

J. Topaly, S. Fruehauf, A. Ho, W. Zeller, Rationale for combination therapy of chronic myelogenous leukaemia with imatinib and irradiation or alkylating agents: Implications for pretransplant conditioning. Br. J. Cancer **86**(9), 1487–1493 (2002)

D.B. White, H.K. Slocum, Y. Brun, C. Wrzosek, W.R. Greco, A new nonlinear mixture response surface paradigm for the study of synergism: A three drug example. Curr. Drug Metab. **4**(5), 399–409 (2003)

Data Mining in Real-World Traditional Chinese Medicine Clinical Data Warehouse

Xuezhong Zhou, Baoyan Liu, Xiaoping Zhang, Qi Xie, Runshun Zhang, Yinghui Wang, and Yonghong Peng

Abstract Real-world clinical setting is the major arena of traditional Chinese medicine (TCM) as it has experienced long-term practical clinical activities, and developed established theoretical knowledge and clinical solutions suitable for personalized treatment. Clinical phenotypes have been the most important features captured by TCM for diagnoses and treatment, which are diverse and dynamically changeable in real-world clinical settings. Together with clinical prescription with multiple herbal ingredients for treatment, TCM clinical activities embody immense valuable data with high dimensionalities for knowledge distilling and hypothesis generation. In China, with the curation of large-scale real-world clinical data from regular clinical activities, transforming the data to clinical insightful knowledge has increasingly been a hot topic in TCM field. This chapter introduces the application of data warehouse techniques and data mining approaches for utilizing real-world TCM clinical data, which is mainly from electronic medical records. The main framework of clinical data mining applications in TCM field is also introduced with

X. Zhou (✉)
School of Computer and Information Technology, Beijing Jiaotong University,
Beijing 100044, China
e-mail: xzzhou@bjtu.edu.cn

B. Liu • X. Zhang • Q. Xie
China Academy of Chinese Medical Sciences,
Beijing 100700, China

R. Zhang • Y. Wang
Guanganmen Hospital, China Academy of Chinese Medical Sciences,
Beijing 100053, China

Y. Peng
School of Computing, Informatics and Media,
University of Bradford, BD7 1DP, UK

J. Poon and S.K. Poon (eds.), *Data Analytics for Traditional Chinese Medicine Research*,
DOI 10.1007/978-3-319-03801-8_11, © Springer International Publishing Switzerland 2014

emphasizing on related work in this field. The key points and issues to improve the research quality are discussed and future directions are proposed.

1 Introduction

As a system of healing and treatment, Traditional Chinese Medicine (TCM) has a long history in Chinese society (Anonymous et al. 2003). The philosophy of TCM very much reflects the classical Chinese belief that the life and activity of individual human beings has an intimate relationship with the environment. In TCM, the general principle of health and the ultimate goal of treatment are to maintain the balance of yin and yang (WHO Regional Office for the Western Pacific 2007) inside the human body. TCM defines a different methodology and approach for disease diagnosis and treatment, which has been widely accepted in China (Robinson 2006; Stone 2008; Tang et al. 2008a). The reported data of the National Bureau of Statistics of China in 2007 (The National Social Statistical Data of China 2007) shows that there are 2,720 TCM hospitals and 123,760 TCM clinicians (including physicians and apothecaries) in China. In 2007, the number of inpatients in TCM hospitals reached 6,930,000 and the number of visits to outpatients and emergency cases is about 2,210 million. Even the doctors trained in modern western medical programs in China consider that Chinese herbal medicine is safe and would like to use them to supplement western medicine in treating patients with chronic or intractable illness (Harmsworth and Lewith 2001).

In the past decades, TCM has been increasingly adopted as a complementary medical therapy around the world (Barnes et al. 2004; National Center for Complementary and Alternative Medicine 2008). Actually, TCM has been successfully applied to the treatment of various complex diseases (Flaws and Sionneau 2005), such as cancer (Konkimalla and Efferth 2008), rheumatoid arthritis (Rao et al. 1999), promyelocytic leukemia (Wang and Chen 2008; Wang et al. 2008), migraine (Diener et al. 2006; Bensoussan et al. 1998), and irritable bowel syndrome (Tsang 2007), and its effectiveness has been validated in modern clinical or laboratory studies. However, establishing a practical and rational efficacy assessment system is a vital issue if TCM is to be widely accepted and used (Xie and Gao 1994).

It is widely accepted in China that TCM and modern biomedicine are mutually beneficial and complementary in generating an understanding of the body and of disease phenomena (Chen et al. 2006). It is hoped that the integration of TCM and modern medical therapies will provide great possibilities for developing novel methods of disease treatment (Tu et al. 2008; Liu et al. 2004). One example is the integrated use of TCM and modern medicine in the treatment of SARS, which has proved to be more effective than the use of modern therapies alone (World Health Organization 2004).

Since 2003, there developed several basic TCM databases, such TCM bibliographic literature database, herbal medicine database, disease database and ancient literature database, for literature search and data sharing (Zhou et al. 2010a). Various computing and statistical methods have been used in TCM clinical studies, clinical decision support, and TCM knowledge discovery using these available data sources (Lukman et al. 2007).

Recently, evidence-based discovery using electronic medical records or electronic health records has been increasingly recognized as a necessary approach to explore the complicated regularities of disease phenomenon and the corresponding therapies. However, as a most important component of TCM data, due to the difficulty of data curation, large-scale clinical data (mainly from electronic medical records) has not been recognized and explored as important data mining data source until in recent years. Therefore, developing a TCM clinical data warehouse platform would be the essential task for large-scale TCM clinical data management and analysis.

Data warehouse (Inmon 2002) is a technical solution for immense data storage, management and processing. The increased demands on financial analysis (Silver et al. 2001), disease control (Wisniewski et al. 2003), clinical decision process (Banek et al. 2006), adverse drug events control (Einbinder and Scully 2002), laboratory test data analysis (Allard et al. 2003), information feedback for hospital practice management (Granta et al. 2006), large-scale radiologic and pathologic data management (Rubin and Desser 2008) and clinical data mining (DM) (Lyman et al. 2008) in healthcare have given rise to the research and development of clinical data warehouse (CDW). Clinical data warehousing is a difficult systematic task with many particular complicated issues, such as many-to-many relationships, entity-attribute-value (EAV) data structure and bi-temporal data (Pedersen et al. 1998). In this chapter, we intend to introduce the clinical data warehouse platform to integrate the clinical data from disparate data sources in different hospitals. The real-world data mining issues in clinical data warehouse are discussed and the related work using real-world clinical data are introduced. Due to the task disparity and heavy burden of practitioners in clinical environments, data quality would be one of the major issues to use data directly generated from clinical settings. Furthermore, data directly from real-world patients incorporates rich clinical phenotypic features at the individual level. Therefore, TCM clinical data would contain important phenotypic features to be used for phenotype-genotype association research.

2   TCM Clinical Data Warehouse: Platform and the Related Key Components

Data integration of medical data storage is challenging, hence the data warehouse architectures (Sahama et al. 2007) were studied to propose practical solutions to tackle data integration issues. Based on the TCM clinical reference information model (RIM), we introduce a data warehouse solution to process and analyze the large-scale TCM clinical data sources (Zhou et al. 2010b).

Compared with the clinical data of modern medicine, TCM clinical data have the distinct and significant information contents, such as symptom and sign, syndrome, formula and herb, as the core components. Moreover, the symptom and sign information with systematic description is the foundational information for syndrome diagnosis. Therefore, the medical record containing symptom and sign should be structured and relationally stored. However, the structured data entry of electronic medical record (EMR) is still a research issue that needs to be further explored (Los et al. 2004), and the manual structured medical record data entry is a labor-intensive task. Hence, although the free text in EMR data need further information extraction are in huge scale, the collected structured EMR (SEMR) data in medical domain are still very rare.

In 2002, we have developed a TCM SEMR system (Li et al. 2005a), which stores the SEMR data (e.g. the clinical events and entities contained in the chief complaint, histories and progress notes) in relational database. Using the SEMR system, we have manually collected about 50,000 inpatients data of diabetes, coronary heart disease (CHD), stroke and hepatitis from TCM hospitals or TCM wards. In addition, over 50,000 outpatient data cases, which record the outpatient clinical encounters of 48 highly experienced TCM physicians were collected. Furthermore, we have a systematic study on the TCM clinical terminology and nomenclature (Guo et al. 2007) to facilitate the data entry and standardized representation of structured information elements. To utilize and analyze the TCM clinical data for research purposes, we have developed a clinical data warehouse (CDW) system to support medical knowledge discovery and clinical decision making. By comprehensive analysis of the characteristics of TCM clinical data structure and the subjects of TCM clinical research topics, we have designed the RIM, the physical data model and the multidimensional data model for CDW. Meanwhile, we have developed an extraction-transformation-loading (ETL) tool, called medical integrator (MI), to take the tasks of clinical data integration, data cleaning and preprocessing. We have also integrated the DM systems, namely Oracle data miner (ODMiner) (Oracle data miner) and Weka (Witten and Frank 2005), and the business intelligence system (BusinessObjects) (BusinessObjects) to implement a TCM clinical intelligence analysis platform with data mining and online analytical processing (OLAP) abilities. Moreover, we have studied on the complex network phenomena of TCM clinical data (Zhou et al. 2007), and found that it will be a promising approach to analyze the TCM clinical data from complex network perspective. Currently, we have developed a complex network analysis (CNA) system, called *Liquorice* (previous named TCMNetBench), to automatically construct the corresponding network models and directly analyze the data from the CDW. In this section, we would introduce the key components of the TCM CDW (Fig. 1 depicts these key components).

2.1 Data Model of CDW

Information model design is the vital step of TCM CDW development. Medical information model like HL7 RIM (HL7 reference information model) is a complicated system with various classes and relationships to support general medical operational processes. The semantic network of unified medical language system (UMLS)

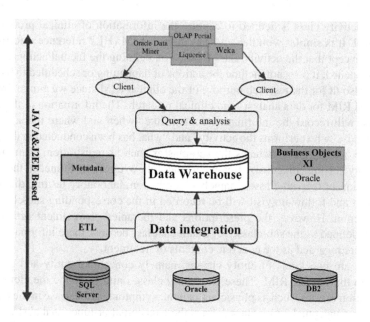

Fig. 1 The technique infrastructure of TCM clinical data warehouse

(Lindberg et al. 1993) is considered as the distinguished medical ontology in modern biomedical science, whose semantic types and structures proposed a global conceptual view of the medical terminologies. The main aim of UMLS is to bridge the gaps between different terminological systems used in the medical literature.

To help store the data elements for TCM clinical research using EMR data, we designed an information reference model to incorporate main information categories and the related elements with regard to clinical events and activities, and the related entities like patients, herbs and clinical terminologies as well. We consider that the main objective of TCM clinical research is to investigate on the relationships between different entities in each event and the relationships between different events. Therefore, we regard the clinical information as various kinds of events (phenomenon and activity), and in each event there have several conceptual entities and physical entities participated at a specific time point or in a time interval. More detailed description could refer to the published article (Zhou et al. 2010b).

Due to the variable and various kinds of manifestation information in clinical data, the EAV data model is preferred in the health-care information system. We also have implemented the TCM SEMR system based on EAV data model. In the EAV data model, each row of a table corresponds to an EAV triple: an entity, an attribute, and the attribute value. For example, the entity "patient" can have the attribute "postprandial blood sugar", a laboratory test result with a float value of 13.5. The EAV model facilitates the regular operations in health-care information system. In addition, it is flexible to be used in the data analysis applications. Hence, we also use EAV model to materialize all the phenomenon classes in physical data tables.

The activity class is defined to capture the information of clinical process and treatment. It is similar with the act class in HL7 RIM (HL7 reference information model) except that the activity class focuses on defining the factual actions, which have happened, it does not include the actions of happening or scheduled to happen. This is also fit for the research purpose of the clinical RIM since we aim to propose a general RIM for data analysis and clinical research. The information of the activity class will record the information content like "when and where the activity is performed", "who performs the activity" and "what has been conducted in the activity". The activity class includes the sub-classes such as registration, examination, laboratory testing, diagnosis, treatment and follow-up visit. Some of the result information of the sub-classes, namely examination, laboratory testing, diagnosis, treatment and follow-up visit will be recorded in the corresponding sub-classes of phenomenon. However, the prescriptions and therapies of treatment activity are directly defined as the sub-classes of treatment class because these information categories are regarded as the concrete contents of treatment.

There are two kinds of entity classes, namely conceptual entity and physical entity, in the clinical RIM. These two entity classes aim to define the elementary information classes, such as physician, patient, symptom, and disease in the clinical data. The conceptual entity class defines the conceptual or functional abstract entities, and the physical entity class represents the substantial and physical objects in the clinical data. The conceptual entity class gets the standardized terminology support from the existed clinical terminology systems such as UTCMLS (Zhou et al. 2004), TCM clinical terminology and nomenclature (Guo et al. 2007) and ICD-10 (it is inherited from the SEMR system). Because of the mixture of TCM and modern medical concepts and methods in current TCM clinical processes, some sub-classes of conceptual entity class like disease are also the mixture of TCM and modern medical classes. For example, we have defined two distinct disease classes, namely TCM disease and modern disease, in the model. The former represents the disease concept in TCM, while the latter is the modern medical concept. It is worth mentioning that the conceptual entity classes would be materialized as dictionary tables in the physical data model in data warehouse. The physical entity class defines the physical and substantial objects involved in the clinical practices. The sub-classes like patient, physician and medication are the core entities. The medication class includes the herb, Chinese traditional patent medicine and drug sub-classes. These sub-classes would be materialized to dictionary tables, in which some of the fields get the standardized terminology support from the conceptual entity class, such as herb effect and herb nature. Therefore, we construct the TCM RIM with an abstract level and granularity fitting for the TCM theoretical research purpose. The information classes like roles of HL7 RIM, which are mainly to support the clinical operation management, are not considered. We have the more detailed description of the RIM in the work (Zhou et al. 2007). Based on the defined information model, we have designed the physical data model to manage the detailed TCM clinical data from the heterogeneous operational data sources. The physical data model has 18 core physical data tables such as patient, clinical registration, diagnosis, clinical finding, laboratory test, order, clinical formula, drug, herb, progress notes and scale.

These core tables provide the storage schema for the detailed clinical data. Furthermore, to support the multidimensional analysis tasks such as OLAP, we have designed several core relational multidimensional data models as the basis of data marts. There are several significant subject analysis applications for TCM clinical research purpose, which have the corresponding relational multidimensional data models such as clinical formula, clinical diagnosis and clinical finding. For example, the clinical formula relational multidimensional data model is defined in snowflake schema, which has a clinical formula fact table with several related dimensional tables like patient, physician, time, diagnosis, herb and therapeutic method. The herb dimension is further normalized into multiple related tables such as herb nature and flavor table, herb efficacy table and herb channel entry table. The formula data model is used for the clinical formula prescription data analysis. The frequent formulae, herbs (also the herb properties) and therapeutic methods for a specific disease could be explored based on the clinical formula data model. The practical results showed that the RIM and multidimensional data model could support well for the clinical analysis applications (Bi et al. 2012).

2.2 Extraction-Transformation-Loading Tool

The ETL is the core component of a successful data warehouse system. Due to the requirement of complex clinical data structure transformation, flexible data checking, heterogeneous data sources integration and terminological standardization processing, even the commercial ETL systems can not fit well for the tasks. Using Java and Eclipse Rich Client Platform technique, we develop an ETL tool, medical integrator (MI), to implement the required functions. It has the key components such as data connection configuration, data checking, data integration (e.g. operational data source consolidation, data transformation and loading), data cleaning, data standardization and data transformation interface. Due to the distributed SEMR data collecting in different hospitals and wards, the data integration component has been developed to integrate the multiple operational data sources (e.g. inpatient and outpatient SEMR data) to one unified data structure, and load the transformed data into the TCM CDW. Recently, we have partitioned the CDW data storage to three distinct data schemas, namely, operational data stores, detailed data warehouse and multidimensional data marts and developed corresponding ETL components to perform data loading, data transformation and standardization tasks (Pan et al. 2012).

Because the EAV data structure is used in the SEMR system and strict data entry control is not applicable in the clinical practice, we should check each value of the original data to avoid loading the invalid data into the data warehouse. Furthermore, MI has focused on the particular functions like data standardization and data analysis interface. Data standardization process mainly concerns the standardization of the terminological data like clinical finding, diagnosis and treatment (e.g. herb name and description phrase of the therapeutic methods). The data analysis interface implements the functions of preparing the data for OLAP analysis and DM. It includes the components of data transformation of detailed physical data to multidimensional data, the transformation of EAV data to conventional data and the data exporting for statistical software. MI performs significant tasks to integrate and preprocess the heterogeneous TCM clinical data.

2.3   Online Analytical Processing and Data Analysis Components

Based on the multidimensional data model and ETL preprocessing, we have prepared the clinical data for OLAP analysis and data mining tasks. We develop the OLAP analysis applications (Bi et al. 2012) based on BO platform. To make the report-designing task available for clinical experts, we designed several semantic layers to map the physical data structures to domain knowledge categories by using BO Designer. Based on the semantic layers, even clinical experts can design their own reports according to their personal requirements. In addition, have developed a complex network analysis system, called *Liquorice*, for TCM clinical data. The complex network analysis system filters the data set directly from the data warehouse, and automatically constructs several interesting TCM clinical networks, such as herb combination network, symptom co-occurrence network and complication disease network. The constructed networks could be displayed and analyzed with manually tuned parameters. We implement the network visualization and analysis functions using JUNG graph package (http://jung.sourceforge.net/index.html). Using *Liquorice*, the clinical researchers could filter the data set from the huge CDW by the expected combinatorial conditions, such as inpatient of type 2 diabetes with thirst symptom and the outpatient data of a specific TCM physician with *Xiao Chaihu decoction* (XCD) treatment. Then the objective networks would be automatically constructed and stored based on the filtered data set. The metadata of the constructed network is also recorded in a table. Finally, the stored network data could be explored and visualized by searching the metadata table. Several properties like node size, node shape, node color, edge style, layout and scale of the visualized network can be configured and changed. The core sub-networks could be filtered and clustered by the ranking methods (e.g. degree and betweenness) and community identification algorithms respectively. To address community discovery from the dense networks, we have implemented a novel algorithm to extract the core hierarchical sub-networks from the constructed large-scale networks (Zhou et al. 2008).

3   Real-World Data Mining Issues in TCM Clinical Data Warehouse

There are common challenges of the medical data mining applications, such as, high dimensions with sparse values, multi-relational data schema and privacy-reserved data mining requirements. The main components of the TCM clinical data form a typical kind of the multi-relational data structure (Fig. 2). The TCM clinical

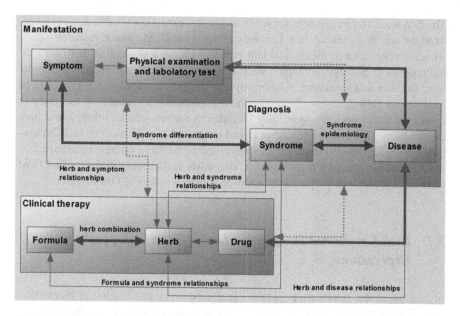

Fig. 2 The main topics of TCM clinical data mining. The *red thick lines* show the current TCM research topics. The *green thick lines* show the clinical data mining topics of modern biomedicine. The *grey thin lines* and *yellow thin lines* indicate the promising topics that should be further explored (Color figure online)

data are generated from a holistic information system with patient, manifestation, diagnosis, prescription and physician as the core components. Meanwhile, because there are no popular adopted clinical guidelines for clinical operations, the TCM theories and empirical knowledge that are charged by the individual TCM physician will be one of the main constraints of the clinical information. This means that besides the diagnosis and prescription, the manifestation will also be influenced by the different TCM physicians. Meanwhile, as time and space are the common features that will be considered in clinical operations, the diagnosis and prescription for the same patient (with identified manifestation) in the different time conditions (e.g. season and weather) may be diverse. Due to the hidden factors of TCM theories, empirical knowledge and environments, it is widely recognized that TCM has the individualized diagnosis and treatment mode in clinical practices. To get the reliable knowledge discovery results, it is necessary to analyze the TCM clinical data by keeping the different components of TCM clinical data as a whole. However, it will become a real challenge for data mining methods. Although has the problems of missing values, possible error information inputs and variable expressions, real-world TCM clinical data directly from EMR sources keeps individualized phenotype features, which has high value for evidence-based personalized medicine research. Therefore, inductive analysis of this kind of real-world empirical data from clinical practice is a key step for TCM clinical research. Moreover, study on the relationships between primary conceptual medical elements like disease, syndrome, symptom, herb and formula is the central topic of TCM clinical research.

The DM would be an efficient approach to get the related knowledge and evidences from the practical clinical data. Corresponding to the TCM clinical research topics, we have a depiction of the clinical DM topics in Fig. 2. It shows that there are various types of knowledge and topics, such as syndrome differentiation, herb combination, formula and syndrome relationships, and syndrome epidemiology, could be explored by DM methods. Currently, the related research focuses on the study of syndrome differentiation (generally includes syndrome epidemiology) and herb combination. However, due to the practical integrated clinical practice in TCM hospitals, there are various interesting topics could be further explored and studied on the relationships among manifestation, diagnosis and clinical therapy. The TCM CDW provides a well-prepared information source for clinical DM research.

3.1 Rich Structured Data with Flexible Terminological Expressions

In contrast to the quantitative variables (e.g. laboratory test results) of biomedical clinical data, the main contents (e.g. main complaints, histories and diagnoses) of TCM clinical data are originally expressed as natural language. Moreover, different from modern clinical medicine, TCM diagnosis and prescription is mainly based on the utilizing of the symptom information. Therefore, the structured EMR system should struggle to record the rich structured information expressed by natural language. Also TCM physicians prefer to use the idioms in clinical practice. Meanwhile, based on the TCM theories, TCM has a very elaborate differentiation of the manifestations of patient to make diagnosis and prescription. Hence, although the TCM clinical data will often be manually transformed as structured data, the incomplete information (the structured data will have inevitable loss of some information in the original natural language data) and the flexible terminological expressions will be popular. For example, TCM physician will often differentiate principal symptoms and secondary symptoms in the main complaints to make the accurate diagnosis and prescription. However, the differentiated information can not easily be recorded in the structured data. Furthermore, the synonymous and polysemous terms are difficult to be distinguished in the structured schema. Hence, the TCM clinical data with multi-dimensions and hierarchical information structures propose a real obstacle for CDM research.

3.2 Data Preprocessing

The poor data quality, inconsistent representation, and the requirement of transformation from EAV schema to flatten tables and the complicated domain knowledge make data preparation of CDM a labor intensive and error prone task. Moreover, TCM clinical data mainly consist of the medical terminologies, which have rich domain knowledge support, such as the clinical terminology systems. There are multi-granular and heterogeneous variables in the clinical data. The standardization of the symptom representation, and the feature reduction of symptom variables are the core problems in TCM clinical data preprocessing, because the symptom terms are various and diverse in different clinical cases. Unify the symptom terms to the distinct concepts will be the key problem to generate the standard variables. For example, the symptoms like fatigue and lower limbs fatigue will be recorded in the different clinical cases. It should unify the two terms at a common knowledge level. Otherwise, the two different granular terms with conceptual relationships will influence the analysis effect.

Usually there will be thousands of symptoms in a middle-scale TCM clinical data set, and also there are various locally dependent variables. It is a both necessary and effective step to reduce the dimensions and integrate the related variables for data mining tasks. For example, the symptom variables like fatigue, nightly cough, insomnia, dark purple tongue and deep pulse, may be related to each other. Hence, the feature extraction method (e.g. factor analysis) or the attribute interaction method (Jakulin and Bratko 2004) could be used to promote the data mining performance in the context of the local correlation between variables.

3.3 Post-Processing and Interpretation of the Data Mining Results

TCM has rich theoretical knowledge and the ability to deduce new concrete knowledge from the general principles. There are plenty of classical literatures to present the commonsensible knowledge. It is only the elaborate data mining results with both commonsense convincing and newly information that would be clinical useful and accepted by the TCM clinicians. The detailed level commonsense knowledge with high frequency in the clinical data is often not useful for TCM clinicians. However, the rare patterns with high interestingness may provide valuable information for researchers. For example, association rule mining is the preferred method to analyze the combination knowledge of herbs in the formulae. However, if the method only generates the high support association rules, it will often get no novel knowledge but common sense in TCM field. Whereas, the low support herb combinations with high lift values may provide useful information. Therefore, the discussion with domain experts will be a significant step to perform the analysis and elucidate the results. Often the results should be post-processed to visualize in a natural way by integrating more background knowledge. Usually the analysis procedure must be repeated many times to change the measures or algorithms to get the clinically meaningful results. Another important issue of data interpretation is the understanding of the TCM problem through data mining perspectives. There exist inaccurate interpretations of the data mining results in the previous related researchers, such as the variable clustering for syndrome epidemiology analysis that is discussed in (Zhang et al. 2007b).

4   Related Work on Real-World Clinical Data Mining

As a DM domain with high rewards and uniqueness (Cios and Moore 2002; Prather et al. 1997), medical DM has been a hot research topic in recent years. Mining over medical, health or clinical data is considered as the most difficult domain for DM (Roddick et al. 2003). There is plenty of related research in clinical DM (McSherry 1999; Harrison 2008; Bellazzi and Zupan 2008) of modern biomedicine. The study on the methods and data analysis of laboratory test results, medical images and demographics to make diagnosis or prognosis prediction are the main research topics (Tan et al. 2003; Kurgan et al. 2001; Richards et al. 2001). Compared with the clinical DM research in modern biomedicine, TCM clinical DM only becomes the hot topics in recent years. The related work of TCM knowledge discovery has been reviewed by Feng et al. (2006) and Lukman et al. (2007). Recently, Zha et al. (2007) used neural network to predict the role of diagnostic information in treatment efficacy of rheumatoid arthritis. Chen et al. (2008) had a comparative study on the five classification methods (e.g. SVM, neural network and decision tree) for syndrome differentiation of CHD using 1,069 clinical epidemiology survey cases. The result shows that SVM performs best in the prediction task. Tang et al. (2008b) have worked on the mining of the elder TCM masters' knowledge to visualize their thoughts and facilitate the knowledge transfer. To illuminate the statistical foundation and objective diagnosis standards of syndrome differentiation, Zhang et al. (2008a, b) proposed the latent tree model to learn the diagnosis structures from the TCM clinical data sets with symptom variables in an unsupervised way. The study showed that there exist natural clusters in the data sets, such as the data set of kidney deficiency syndrome with 2,600 cases, which correspond well to the syndrome types.

Besides using of the outpatient cases of highly experienced physicians, most of the previous work on TCM clinical data mining utilizes of observational clinical data of case report form, whose feature set is limited to predesigned medical elements. Not reflecting the individualized phenotypes of patients is one of the most recognized shortcomings of this kind of clinical data.

4.1   General Data Mining Methods for TCM Diagnosis and Treatment

We have successfully conducted several preliminary TCM clinical data analysis studies like acupuncture prescription knowledge discovery (Zhang et al. 2007a), the relationship between formula (herbs) and syndrome of T2DM affiliated metabolic syndrome (DAMS) (Ni et al. 2006), herb treatment for T2DM (Jian et al. 2007), cluster analysis on the syndrome types in patients with acute myocardial infarction (Gao et al. 2007), and the GPBT syndrome differentiation (Zhang et al. 2008). All the previous work has gotten the clinical useful results.

Here we give one example on finding the phenotype features of TCM diagnosis (i.e. syndrome differentiation) by using classification methods. We have conducted

Table 1 The experimental results of classification methods. The chief symptoms are ordered by attribute weight, prediction weight in SVM and ADTree respectively. The chief symptoms of Bayesian network are ranked by the ratio of the probability distribution of symptom on QIS syndrome and non- QIS syndrome

Classification method	Test mode	Prediction accuracy	The five suggested chief symptoms
SVM	Evaluate on training data	0.864	Costal pain (1.7166), back pain (1.1961), chest pain and oppression (1.0361), breathlessness (0.7063) and gastric pain (0.6704)
	10 cross-evaluation	0.812	Costal pain (1.7041), back pain (1.1745), chest pain and oppression (0.9662), breathlessness (0.7833) and gastric pain (0.6959)
ADTree	Evaluate on training data	0.841	Chest pain and oppression (0.732), gastric pain (0.592), dyspnea (0.402) and slow pulse (0.383)
	10 cross-evaluation	0.814	Chest pain and oppression (0.732), gastric pain (0.592), dyspnea (0.402) and slow pulse (0.383)
Bayesian network	Evaluate on training data	0.845	Costal pain (0.042/0.006), back pain (0.030/0.006), chest pain and oppression (0.042/0.011), gastric pain (0.077/0.023) and breathlessness (0.053/0.021)
	10 cross-evaluation	0.806	Costal pain (0.042/0.006), back pain (0.030/0.006), chest pain and oppression (0.042/0.011), gastric pain (0.077/0.023) and breathlessness (0.053/0.021)

the classification study on QIS syndrome differentiation of a high-experienced TCM physician to validate the possibility of inducing the common rules from clinical data by machine learning methods. We get 484 first encounter outpatient cases of the physician from the CDW. The data set has 102 standard symptom variables. It is a binary classification into QIS syndrome and non-QIS syndrome. The number of outpatient cases with QIS syndrome is 83. We use three classification methods, namely SVM, ADTree (Freund and Mason et al. 1999) and Bayesian network, in Weka 3.4.6 to learn the syndrome differentiation models. The prediction accuracy and the suggested chief symptoms are listed in Table 1. All the results are got with the default parameters. The results showed that the three methods have the acceptable prediction accuracies. In addition, there are common chief symptoms, such as costal pain, chest pain and oppression, and gastric pain, suggested by the three methods. The prediction accuracy of the SVM learned model is high over 86.4 % while in "evaluate on training data" test mode. The related variables with large positive weight are the variables of costal pain (1.7166), back pain (1.1961), chest pain and oppression (1.0361) and breathlessness (0.7063), gastric pain etc. These variables with positive values are considered as the chief symptoms of QIS syndrome. The discovered chief symptoms of QIS match well with the widely accepted clinical guidance in TCM practice. Hence, it indicates that the machine learning and DM methods could be a helpful approach for syndrome differentiation and syndrome epidemiology studies. It shows that SVM could be used for TCM clinical diagnosis study with high dimensions. Although Bayesian network has the visualization results that will facilitate the interpretation, the interpretation of the result with high dimensions is rather difficult. Hence, the dimension reduction issue should be further addressed in the large-scale TCM clinical DM research.

The herbs in the same formula are organized according to the principle of formula theories such as the monarch, minister, assistant and guide theory, to make a prescription with systematic efficacy. Herb combination and the basic formula with common herb combinations play a key role in the efficient clinical prescriptions. Hence, discovery of the common herb combinations from large-scale clinical formulae has been a significant research topic in TCM DM. Frequent itemset and association rule have been used as the general DM methods to find the interesting herb combinations. We have conducted several studies using association rule mining method, such as acupuncture prescription knowledge discovery (Zhang et al. 2007a). The work focuses on the empirical clinical acupuncture prescription of a doctor in acupuncture department of Guanganmen hospital, Beijing, China. Using the association rule mining method (Apriori) in Weka, we got 18 common acupuncture formulae from the 1,697 clinical prescriptions. The doctor indicates that one of the 18 acupuncture formulae is not a fixed prescription in his clinical practice. Therefore, finally, we get 17 useful acupuncture formulae (with name, acupuncture point composition, modifications, main efficacy, etc.) for different disease conditions, which reflect the empirical knowledge of the doctor. However, association rule mining has the shortcoming that it often generates large amount of rules due to the limited number of herbs (not over 1,000 herbs in clinical use) and acupuncture points (not over 400 points in the clinical use), and the almost unlimited clinical prescriptions. Furthermore, the rules generated by association rule method are often in low granularity, thus association rule method cannot capture the skeleton herb combination knowledge in the large-scale prescriptions.

In conclusion, the DM applications based on the TCM CDW get the promising results to help the knowledge distilling and discovery from large-scale clinical data. The results could be a good reference for clinical operations and Chinese patent medicine development. Based on the prepared clinical data from TCM CDW, we will conduct further studies on the various clinical DM topics as indicated in Fig. 2.

4.2 Complex Network Approaches for Clinical Herbal Combination Knowledge Discovery

We have implemented the hierarchical core sub-network structure discovery algorithm (Zhou et al. 2008) in the CNA system. The method constructs herb combination network from the complete connected sub-networks with the element herb as node of one formula, and then extracts the hierarchical core herb combinations from the constructed herb combination network. We have applied the method to several specific TCM prescription data sets extracted from the CDW, and got the clinical meaningful common herb combination patterns. We take the data analysis results from two data sets, namely the herb prescriptions of DAMS and the herb prescriptions of GPBT syndrome, to demonstrate the interesting analysis results.

Metabolic syndrome[1] is one of the significant complications of T2DM, which may have the symptoms and features of high blood pressure, central obesity, and fasting hyperglycemia. Distilling the common herb combination knowledge from the large numbers of clinical prescriptions for DAMS will help guide the efficient herb treatment. There are 188 inpatient cases of DAMS that have been treated with herb prescriptions, are filtered from the 5,000 over diabetes inpatient data according to the WHO standard. The data set has totally 752 herb treatment prescribed in the different encounters. The herb prescriptions have 320 different herbs and the constructed weighted herb combination network has 9,541 edges (two-item herb relationships). The extracted core herb combinations and main herb modifications of DAMS prescriptions are displayed in the right part of Fig. 3. The core herb combinations contain the herbs, such as *Chinese angelica, dwarf lilyturf tuber, milkvetch root, Chinese magnoliavine fruit* and *figwort root*. According to the efficacies of these five herbs, it shows that the organization principle of core herb prescription for DAMS is to *replenish qi and nourish yin* (one type of the TCM therapeutic methods). This reflects the basic pathogenesis of DAMS indicated in the previous research (Ni et al. 2006). Also, the main herb modifications for DAMS are the herb pairs like *gordon euryale seed* and *cherokee rose fruit, red poeny root* and *white peony root, indian bread* and *largehead atractylodes rhizome, danshen root* and *fresh rehmannia*, etc. These herb pairs are mainly prescribed to treat the accompanying syndromes, such as nephrosis and numbness of extremities, of the DAMS patients.

GPBT syndrome is a rather general syndrome in the patients with the diseases such as chronic gastritis, fatty liver, female infertility, liver cirrhosis and polycystic ovary syndrome. The pathogeneses and manifestations of GPBT syndrome are various. Hence, the herb prescriptions for the patients with GPBT syndrome are also various and individualized. The discovery of the common herb combination knowledge will be helpful to grasp the central rules of the prescriptions for GPBT syndrome. We get 1,287 clinical herb prescriptions of GPBT syndrome from the outpatient data of 21 high-experienced TCM physicians in the CDW. There are 367 distinct herbs in the data set, and the result weighted herb combination network has 13,428 edges, which is dense and hard to be directly understood. However, it is interesting that the extracted core herb combinations form a high-experienced classical formula, called *Xiaoyao San*. Although *Xiaoyao San* has been accepted as one of the classical formulae (e.g. *Xiao Jianzhong decoction, Chaihu Shugan San* and *Sijunzi decoction*) for GPBT syndrome treatment, it has not been suggested as the basic formula for GPBT syndrome treatment yet. Our result proposes a hypothesis that *Xiaoyao San* could be considered as the fundamental formula to treat the patient with GPBT syndrome. Also, the core herb combinations and the discovered main herb modifications (in the below left part of Fig. 3) provide the individualized therapies for reference in the clinical herb prescriptions for GPBT syndrome. For example, the herb pair of *danshen root* and *red pony root* would mainly be prescribed to patients with additional blood stasis syndrome. Based on the analysis result, we

---

[1] http://en.wikipedia.org/wiki/Metabolic_syndrome (Accessed: 2013 June 30th).

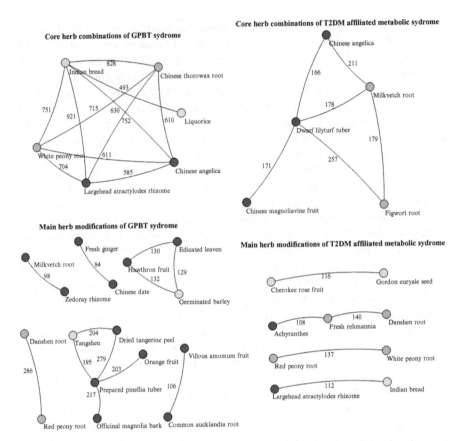

Fig. 3 The extracted core herb combinations and main herb modifications of GPBT syndrome and DAMS. The number labeled at the edge represents the co-occurrence of herb nodes. The color of nodes is defined according to the flavor and property of herbs (*red*: warm or hot herb property, *green*: cold or cool herb property, *yellow*: other herb property) (Color figure online)

have summarized several useful empirical formulae with herb constituents and dosages for the different types of patients with GPBT syndrome (Zhang et al. 2008).

4.3 Topic Models for Detection of Patient Groups and the Related Herb Prescriptions

Topic model, such as latent Dirichlet allocation (LDA) (Blei et al. 2003; Steyvers et al. 2007) is a widely-used statistical probability model that could find the latent topic in documents. While we consider patients with symptom and sign features as documents, we could apply topic model to analyze the clinical phenotypic topic structure of patients. Besides of symptoms and signs, other medical entities, such as herb prescriptions, diseases, are involved in TCM EMR data as well, therefore, multi-relational knowledge (like depicted in Fig. 2) that is meaningful for clinical tasks should be detected by topic model. Zhang et al. proposed several multi-relational topic models (Zhang et al. 2011) by extending the author-topic model to incorporate multiple relationships between symptoms, herb prescriptions and diagnoses. The proposed models were useful to extract the underlying common symptom groups of one specific general disease classification, like diabetes, stroke and heart disease. Furthermore, the herb constitutes of clinical prescriptions were also generated. To help generate more reliable multi-relational topics from real-world TCM clinical data, Jiang et al. (2012) applied LinkedLDA to symptom-herb topic detection.

4.4 Effectiveness Driven Clinical Knowledge Discovery by Using Markov Decision Model

Finding clinical regularities of diagnosis and treatment with good outcome is important in promoting the development of sustainable clinical solutions. Currently, information on effectiveness of treatment is often absent in most real-world TCM clinical data. Therefore, most related TCM clinical data mining tasks only generate empirical regularities with no constraints on clinical effectiveness. This means that it is difficult to judge which discovered regularities are effective for disease treatment. For example, association rule mining on herb combinations would generate rules like: if *herb A* is used, then *herb B* will be used with a probability of 100 %. However, the rule does not provide predictive information on the outcome of patients who have taken both *herb A* and *herb B*. Therefore, it is significant to explore clinical knowledge or hypothesis in the context of clinical effectiveness. Furthermore, because TCM theories are rather abstract and only provide the general principle for clinical operations, effective clinical treatment will largely depend on the empirical knowledge of TCM physicians. Therefore, it is promising to discover TCM clinical knowledge by integrating the clinical effectiveness analysis. For example, finding the effective herb–herb interactions from clinical prescriptions for specific disease conditions (Li et al. 2005a) would be useful to propose regularities for practical clinical treatment. In particular, real-world TCM clinical cases include individualised sequential treatment decision policies. If we can infer optimal or hypo-optimal sequential solutions with effectiveness from the clinical data, it will be a great help for TCM clinical trials and practical clinical treatments. Markovian decision processes (MDPs) and partially observable MDPs (Li et al. 2005b) are powerful mathematical frameworks for sequential planning under uncertainty and are potential methods to help plan the sequential treatment for specific diseases (Mackay and Taylor 2007). Feng et al. (Hripcsak et al. 2003) proposed an initial study on using MDP to model traditional Chinese medicine therapy planning to find the optimal sequential clinical treatment options for inpatients with type 2 diabetes. It inferred the model parameters (e.g. states, actions, rewards and transition functions) from clinical data set and used value iteration algorithm (Prather et al. 1997) to solve the MDP problem. The study shows that MDP model can be used to help identify useful clinical prescriptions from data and help to generate sequential TCM clinical guidelines for type 2 diabetes treatments.

5 Future Directions

In recent years, meaningful use and data mining from real-world EMR data has been recognized as an extremely important research task in medical field (Denny 2012; Roden et al. 2012). Integration of the clinical phenotype data with genotype data on individual patients would generate high valuable data sources for disease pathology and clinical solution research. Therefore, it is an essential step for translational medicine research, which aims to correlate basic discovery from bench to practical clinical solutions at bedside. Due to the rich phenotype information like symptoms and signs, behavior, and environmental factors, captured in TCM regular clinical settings, we consider real-world TCM clinical data a classical clinical phenotype data sources related to disease diagnosis and treatment. Therefore, integration of clinical phenotype and genotype information for biomedical knowledge discovery and hypothesis generation would be a potential direction of real-world TCM clinical data mining. Furthermore, as a well-developed clinical practice schema integrating with personalized treatment by multi-ingredients prescriptions, TCM contains high volume of clinical data that need perform clinical effectiveness evaluation to detect novel effective therapies for disease treatment. Thus, it is a high opportunity to develop new data mining methods in the constraint of effectiveness to find effective therapeutic knowledge. However, due to various complicated clinical tasks involved and diverse information incorporated, data quality will become a major obstacle for real-world TCM clinical data mining. Therefore, how to evaluate, monitor and improve the data quality of TCM clinical data during the data capture, integration and preprocessing stages, would be vital task to assure getting reliable knowledge discovery results. Hence, we consider three main directions that need be further addressed to meet the major challenges in real-world TCM clinical data mining.

5.1 Translational Biomedical Informatics for Clinical Phenotype and Genotype Association Discovery

To accelerate the translation of bench biological discovery to practical clinical solutions, translational medicine has been proposed as new promising discipline to integrate basic biology science with clinical medicine (Lean et al. 2008). Several translational medicine projects like eMERGE and I2B2 showed that current EMRs used for routine clinical care could be used to identify phenotypes for genetic studies (Kho et al. 2011). Real-world TCM clinical data includes rich disease phenotypes, and disease related environmental factors and behavior features. Most of these phenotype information relate to macro-level functional health status of human body, which is directly observable for patients and clinical practitioners. In one hand, like modern biomedical EMR, TCM clinical data could help generate clinical useful knowledge to improve the practical health solutions. In the other hand, while integrated with the available genomics data banks, it could also be used to accelerate the understanding of disease molecular pathologies and etiological mechanism by exploring the correlation between phenotypes and genotypes (Maricel 2009; Kohane 2011; Butte 2009). However, one obstacle of the utilizing of free text TCM EMR data is that the phenotype information is subjectively described in high-level knowledge representation approaches like natural languages and has semantic diversity in different clinical data sources. Therefore, with large-scale EMR data (in free text) available, two important steps should be conducted to make this kind of data usable for improving clinical solution development and disease genomics exploration. One essential step is automatic or semi-automatic extraction of medical named entities (mainly clinical phenotype entities) and their relationships from these data (Cohen and Hunter 2013). Another step is biomedical data integration (Payne 2012) to integrate both TCM clinical data and modern biomedical data by using TCM and medical terminology systems into a unified semantic medical knowledgebase. Furthermore, as a complex intervention method, TCM herbal prescriptions (acupuncture therapy as well) have a complicated molecular pharmacological effects and mechanisms. Real-world TCM clinical data would provide as a high valuable data sources for pharmacogenomics research (Wilke et al. 2011).

5.2 Effectiveness Driven Data Mining for Comparative Effectiveness Research

Managing and defeating diseases in real-world clinical setting is the final objectives of medical research and clinical studies. Real-world TCM clinical practice is practical clinical schema for personalized treatment and management of patients, in which new prescriptions with herbal combinations were introduced to treat individual patients. Each new proposed herb prescriptions were not evaluated by experimental results but were directly prescribed for patients. This means that TCM clinical practice is also a kind of real-world clinical study aiming to manage the patients by optimal therapies generated by TCM practitioners. This, in the other fold, would generate large-scale real-world clinical solutions that need be assessed to obtain the optimal ones. Therefore, comparative effectiveness research (CER) (Luce et al. 2009) using real-world clinical data from routine clinical care would be an extremely promising research direction in TCM field. Different from CER research in conventional medical field (Bayley et al. 2013), getting better effective therapies would be the major research task for TCM because too many personalized therapies were used in TCM clinical settings. From these immense personalized therapies, which consist of multiple herbal ingredients, we can get better clinical care solutions while using the outcome information for comparisons (Yan et al. 2013).

To meet these requirements, the new data mining methods or statistical models to find the structured relations between intervention constitutes and clinical phenotypes with the constraints of outcomes would be a inherent pursuit for TCM research. Probabilistic graphical model like Bayesian network (Pearl 2000) and probabilistic relational model (Friedman et al. 1999) would be one of the potential approaches to discover the significant phenotype-intervention correlation structures.

5.3 Data Quality Monitoring Methods to Prepare High Quality Clinical Data Sources

Data quality is a fundamental issue in secondary data analysis and comparative effectiveness research using EMR data (Sandra 2007). The real-world TCM clinical data is recorded for clinical operation purpose. It contains the necessary information (e.g. symptom, diagnosis, prescription and laboratory test result) that is relevant to the diagnosis and treatment of diseases. Other than the data used in secondary data analysis in modern medicine, the TCM clinical data includes most clinical variables and clinical information contents to support various clinical questions.

However, the primary issue in use of TCM clinical data for analysis is the existence of missing values and heterogeneous data representations. In general, the real-world clinical data would usually only record the abnormal values of the medical variables of patients. The negative variables are only recorded in the conditions of diagnosis differentiation purpose. Thus, most of the missing values could be considered as negative values. However, due to the personalized views of TCM physicians, some abnormal values would not be recorded in the clinical data if they were considered having no value for diagnosis and treatment. Therefore, the mixing conditions of missing values propose challenges for reliable data analysis.

Furthermore, heterogeneous data sources and rich classical references result in the various terminologies and phrases used in the clinical data. The same concepts may be represented by different synonymous terms. Also related but not identical phrases are frequently used in the data. Also data accuracy has become an important concept with the widespread use of computer-based systems for clinical and epidemiological research (Hogan and Wagner 1997).

Thus, with the structured clinical data prepared, there still needs a both reliable and efficient preprocessing step to filter the useful data set from the large-scale clinical data source, clean and integrate the data to provide high-quality data for further analysis.

Acknowledgements This work is partially supported by National 863 Program of China (2012AA02A609), NSFC Project (61105055, 81230086), China 973 Project (2014CB542900), National S&T Major Project of China (2009ZX09301-005-010, 2009ZX09502-031) and the Fundamental Research Funds for the Central Universities.

References

R.D. Allard, The clinical laboratory data warehouse. An overlooked diamond mine. Am. J. Clin. Pathol. **120**(6), 817–819 (2003)

Anonymous, *The Inner Canon of Emperor Huang*. (Chinese Medical Ancient Books Publishing House, Beijing, 2003)

M. Banek, A.M. Tjoa, N. Stolba, Integrating different grain levels in a medical data warehouse federation. in *Proceedings of the 8th International Conference of Data Warehousing and Knowledge Discovery*, ed by AM Tjoa, J Trujillo, Krakow, Poland, LNCS, vol. 4081 (Springer-Verlag, Heidelberg, 2006), pp. 185–194

P.M. Barnes, E. Powell-Griner, K. McFann, R.L. Nahin, Complementary and alternative medicine use among adults: United States, 2002. Adv. Data **343**, 1–19 (2004)

K.B. Bayley, T. Belnap, L. Savitz, A.L. Masica, N. Shah, N.S. Fleming, Challenges in using electronic health record data for CER: experience of 4 learning organizations and solutions applied. Med. Care. **51**(8 Suppl 3), S80-6 (2013)

R. Bellazzi, B. Zupan, Predictive data mining in clinical medicine: current issues and guidelines. Int. J. Med. Inform. **77**(2), 81–97 (2008)

A. Bensoussan, N.J. Talley, M. Hing, R. Menzies, A. Guo, M. Ngu, Treatment of irritable bowel syndrome with Chinese herbal medicine: a randomized controlled trial. JAMA **280**, 1585–1589 (1998)

Bi Lanxing, Zhou Xuezhong, Zhang Lei, Zhang Runshun, Multidimensional analysis for traditional Chinese medicine diagnosis and treatment on hepatitis diseases. IEEE HealthCom, Beijing, China, 2012, pp. 52–56

D. Blei, A. Ng, M. Jordan, Latent Dirichlet allocation. J. Mach. Learn. Res. **3**, 993–1022 (2003)

O. Brazhnik, J.F. Jones, Anatomy of data integration. J. Biomed. Inform. **40**(3), 252–269 (2007)

BusinessObjects, http://www.sap.com/solutions/sapbusinessobjects/index.epx. Accessed 18 Nov, 2013 (2013)

A.J. Butte, Translational bioinformatics applications in genome medicine. Genome Med. **1**(6), 64 (2009). doi:10.1186/gm64

K. Chen, A. Lu, S. Chen, B. Wei, W. Lu, D. Mu et al., Survey on the developing status of integrative Chinese and western medicine. Zhongguo zhong xi yi jie he za zhi **26**(6), 485–488 (2006) [in Chinese]

J. Chen, G. Xi, Y. Xing, J. Chen, J. Wang, Global comparison study of five data mining methods in predicting syndrome in coronary heart disease. J. Comput. Inf. Syst. **4**(1), 219–224 (2008)

K.J. Cios, G.W. Moore, Uniqueness of medical data mining. Artif. Intell. Med. **26**(1–2), 1–24 (2002)

K.B. Cohen, L.E. Hunter, Chapter 16: Text mining for translational bioinformatics. PLoS Comput. Biol. **9**(4), e1003044 (2013). doi:10.1371/journal.pcbi.1003044

J.C. Denny, Chapter 13: Mining electronic health records in the genomics era. PLoS Comput. Biol. **8**(12), e1002823 (2012)

A.M. Deshpande, C. Brandt, P.M. Nadkarni, Metadata-driven ad hoc query of patient data meeting the needs of clinical studies. J. Am. Med. Inform. Assoc. **9**(4), 369–382 (2002)

H.C. Diener, K. Kronfeld, G. Boewing, A. Molsberger, M. Tegenthoff, H.J. Trampisch et al., Efficacy of acupuncture for the prophylaxis of migraine: a multicenter randomised controlled clinical trial. Lancet Neurol. **5**, 310–316 (2006)

J.S. Einbinder, K. Scully, Using a clinical data repository to estimate the frequency and costs of adverse drug events. J. Am. Med. Inform. Assoc. **9**(6 Suppl 1), s34–s38 (2002)

Y. Feng, Z. Wu, X. Zhou, Z. Zhou, W. Fan, Knowledge discovery in traditional Chinese medicine: state of the art and perspectives. Artif. Intell. Med. **38**(3), 219–236 (2006)

B. Flaws, P. Sionneau, *The Treatment of Modern Western Medical Diseases with Chinese Medicine: A Textbook and Clinical Manual*, 2nd edn. (Blue Poppy Press, Boulder, 2005)

Y. Freund, L. Mason, The alternating decision tree learning algorithm, in *Proceeding of the 16th International Conference on Machine Learning*, ed. by I Bratko, S. Dzeroski, (Morgan Kaufmann, San Francisco, 1999), pp. 124–133

N. Friedman, L. Getoor, D. Koller, A Pfeffer, Learning probabilistic relational models, in *International Joint Conferences on Artificial Intelligence*, Stockholm, Sweden, 1999, pp. 1300–1309

Z. Gao, H. Xu, D. Shi, Z. Shi, X. Zhou, The cluster analysis on syndrome type of TCM in patients with acute myocardial infarction. J. Emerg. TCM **16**(4), 432–434 (2007) (in Chinese)

S.C. Garmon Bibb, Issues associated with secondary analysis of population health data. Appl. Nurs. Res. **20**, 94–99 (2007)

A. Granta, A. Moshyka, H. Diaba et al., Integrating feedback from a clinical data warehouse into practice organisation. Int. J. Med. Inform. **75**, 232–239 (2006)

Y. Guo, B. Liu, P. Li, X. Zhou, Ontology and standardization of the TCM terms. Chin. Arc. TCM **25**(7), 1368–1370 (2007) (in Chinese)

K. Harmsworth, G.T. Lewith, Attitudes to traditional Chinese medicine amongst western trained doctors in the People's Republic of China. Soc. Sci. Med. **52**(1), 149–153 (2001)

J.H. Harrison, Introduction to the mining of clinical data. Clin. Lab. Med. **28**(1), 1–7 (2008)

HL7 reference information model, http://www.hl7.org/Library/data-model/RIM/modelpage_mem. htm. Accessed 18 Nov, 2013 (2013)

W.R. Hogan, M.M. Wagner, Accuracy of data in computer-based patient records. JAMIA **4**, 342–355 (1997)

G. Hripcsak, S. Bakken, P.D. Stetson, V.L. Patel, Mining complex clinical data for patient safety research: a framework for event discovery. J Biomed. Inform. **36**(1–2), 120–130 (2003)

W.H. Inmon, *Building the Data Warehouse*, 3rd edn. (Wiley, Hoboken, 2002)

A. Jakulin, I. Bratko, Testing the significance of attribute interactions, in ICML (2004) Banff, Alberta, Canada pp. 409–416

Z. Jian, Q. Ni, X. Zhou, W. Xin, L. Lin, B. Liu, Study on treatment law of type 2 diabetes based on structural electronic medical record system. J. Shandong Univ. TCM **31**(3), 195–197 (2007) (in Chinese)

Z. Jiang, X. Zhou, J. Yu et al., Using link topic model to analyze traditional Chinese medicine clinical symptom-herb regularities. Healthcom, Beijing, China, 2012, pp. 15–18

M.G. Kann, Advances in translational bioinformatics: computational approaches for the hunting of disease genes. Brief. Bioinform. **11**(1), 96–110 (2009)

A.N. Kho et al., Electronic medical records for genetic research: results of the eMERGE consortium. Sci. Transl. Med. **3**, 79re1 (2011). doi:10.1126/scitranslmed. 3001807

I.S. Kohane, Using electronic health records to drive discovery in disease genomics. Nat. Rev. Genet. **12**(6), 417–428 (2011)

V.B. Konkimalla, T. Efferth, Evidence-based Chinese medicine for cancer therapy. J. Ethnopharmacol. **116**, 207–210 (2008)

L.A. Kurgan, K.J. Cios, R. Tadeusiewicz, M. Ogiela, L.S. Goodenday, Knowledge discovery approach to automated cardiac SPECT diagnosis. Artif. Intell. Med. **23**(2), 149–169 (2001)

M.E.J. Lean, J.I. Mann, J.A. Hoek, R.M. Elliot, G. Schofield, Translational research: from evidence-based medicine to sustainable solutions for public health problems. Br. Med. J. **337**, a863 (2008)

P. Li, B. Liu, T. Wen, Y. Wang, Y. Gao, H. Xu et al., Traditional Chinese medicine electronic medical record system and the reorganization of TCM theoretical knowledge (in Chinese). Chin. J. Inf. TCM **12**(4), 7–39 (2005a)

T. Li, G. Wang, L. Wang, B. Mao, Clinical trials of traditional Chinese medicine in China: status and evaluation. Chin. J. Evid-Based Med. **5**(6), 431–437 (2005b) [in Chinese]

J-H. Lin, P.J. Haug, Data preparation framework for preprocessing clinical data in data mining, in *AMIA Annual Symposium Proceedings*, 2006, pp. 489–493

D.A.B. Lindberg, B.L. Humphreys, A.T. McCray, The unified medical language system. Method Inf. Med. **32**, 281–291 (1993)

B. Liu, J. Hu, Y. Xie, W. Wen, R. Wang, Y. Zhang et al., Effects of integrative Chinese and western medicine on arterial saturation in patients with Severe Acute Respiratory Syndrome. Chin. J. Integr. Med. **10**(2), 117–122 (2004)

R.K. Los, A.M. Ginneken, M. Wilde, J. Lei, OpenSDE: row modeling applied to generic structured data entry. J. Am. Med. Inform. Assoc. **11**, 162–165 (2004)

B.R. Luce, J.M. Kramer, S.N. Goodman, J.T. Connor, S. Tunis, D. Whicher et al., Rethinking randomized clinical trials for comparative effectiveness research: the need for transformational change. Ann. Intern. Med. **151**, 206–209 (2009)

S. Lukman, Y. He, S.-C. Hui, Computational methods for traditional Chinese medicine: a survey. Comput. Methods Progr. Biomed. **88**, 283–294 (2007)

J.A. Lyman, K. Scully, J.H. Harrison Jr., The development of healthcare data warehouses to support data mining. Clin. Lab. Med. **28**(1), 55–71 (2008)

J. Mackay, A. Taylor, The use of routinely collected clinical data for large-scale pharmacogenetic studies. Int. J. Healthcare Technol. Manage. **8**(5), 492–502 (2007)

D. McSherry, Dynamic and static approaches to clinical data mining. Artif. Intell. Med. **16**(1), 97–115 (1999)

National Center for Complementary and Alternative Medicine, *The Use of Complementary and Alternative Medicine in the United States* (National Academies Press, 2008)

Q. Ni, S. Chen, X. Zhou, Z. Wei, Y. Gong, Y. Li et al., Study of relationship between formula (herbs) and syndrome about type 2 diabetes mellitus affiliated metabolic syndrome based on the scale-free network. Chin. J. Inf. TCM **13**(11), 19–22 (2006) (in Chinese)

Oracle data miner, http://www.oracle.com/technology/products/bi/odm/odminer.html. Accessed 2013 Nov 20 (2013)

J.A. Osheroff, J.M. Teich, B. Middleton, E.B. Steen, A. Wright, D.E. Detmer, A roadmap for national action on clinical decision support. J. Am. Med. Inform. Assoc. **14**(2), 141–145 (2007)

Pan Xishui, Zhou Xuezhong, Zhang Runshun, Song Hongmei, Enhanced data extraction, transforming and loading processing for traditional Chinese medicine clinical data warehouse. IEEE HealthCom, Beijing, China 2012, pp. 57–61

P.R. Payne, Chapter 1: biomedical knowledge integration. PLoS Comput. Biol. **8**(12), e1002826 (2012). doi:10.1371/journal.pcbi.1002826

J. Pearl, *Causality: Models, Reasoning, and Inference* (Cambridge University Press, Cambridge, 2000)

T.B. Pedersen, C.S. Jensen, Research Issues in clinical data warehousing, in *Proceedings of the 10th International Conference on Scientific and Statistical Database Management*, ed. by M. Rafanelli, M. Jarke, Italy, (IEEE Computer Society, Washington, DC, 1998), 1–3 Jul 1998, pp. 43–52

J.C. Prather, D.F. Lobach, L.K. Goodwin, J.W. Hales, M.L. Hage, W.E. Hammond. Medical data mining: knowledge discovery in a clinical data warehouse, in *Proceedings of the AMIA Annual Fall Symposium*, 1997, pp. 101–105

J.K. Rao, K. Mihaliak, K. Kroenke, J. Bradley, W.M. Tierney, M. Weinberger, Use of complementary therapies for arthritis among patients of rheumatologists. Ann. Intern. Med. **131**, 409–416 (1999)

G. Richards, V.J. Rayward-Smith, P.H. Sönksen, S. Carey, C. Weng, Data mining for indicators of early mortality in a database of clinical records. Artif. Intell. Med. **22**(3), 215–231 (2001)

N. Robinson, Integrated traditional Chinese medicine. Complement. Ther. Clin. Pract. **12**, 132–140 (2006)

J.F. Roddick, P. Fule, W.J. Graco, Exploratory medical knowledge discovery: experiences and issues. ACM SIGKDD Explor. Newsl. **5**(1), 94–99 (2003)

D.M. Roden, H. Xu, J.C. Denny, R.A. Wilke, Electronic medical records as a tool in clinical pharmacology: opportunities and challenges. Clin. Pharmacol. Ther. **91**(6), 1083–1086 (2012)

D.L. Rubin, T.S. Desser, A data warehouse for integrating radiologic and pathologic data. J. Am. Coll. Radiol. **5**, 210–217 (2008)

T.R. Sahama, P.R. Croll, A data warehouse architecture for clinical data warehousing, in *Proceedings of the 5th Australasian Symposium on ACSW Frontiers*, ed. by L. Brankovic, P. Coddington, J.F. Roddick, C. Steketee, J.R. Warren, A. Wendelborn, vol. 68 (Australian Computer Society, Darlinghurst, Australia, 2007), pp. 227–232

M. Silver, T. Sakata, H. Su et al., Case study: how to apply data mining techniques in a healthcare data warehouse. J. Healthc. Inf. Manag. **15**, 155–164 (2001)

M. Steyvers, T. Griffiths, Probabilistic topic models, in *The Handbook of Latent Semantic Analysis: A road to meaning* (Psychology Press, 2007), pp. 427–448

R. Stone, Chen Zhu interview: China's modern medical minister. Science **319**, 1748a–1749a (2008)

K.C. Tan, Q. Yu, C.M. Heng, T.H. Lee, Evolutionary computing for knowledge discovery in medical diagnosis. Artif. Intell. Med. **27**(2), 129–154 (2003)

J.-L. Tang, B. Liu, K.-W. Ma, Traditional Chinese medicine. Lancet **372**(9654), 1938–1940 (2008a)

X. Tang, N. Zhang, Z. Wang, Exploration of TCM masters knowledge mining. J. Syst. Sci. Comput. **21**(1), 34–45 (2008b)

The 2007 National Social Statistical Data of China. Available from: http://www.stats.gov.cn/tjsj/qtsj/shtjnj/2007/. Accessed 20 Oct 2009

The STRIDE clinical data warehouse. http://clinicalinformatics.stanford.edu/STRIDE/cdw.html. Accessed 8 July 2012 (2012)

I.K. Tsang, Establishing the efficacy of traditional Chinese medicine. Nat. Clin. Pract. Rheumatol. **3**, 60–61 (2007)

B. Tu, M.F. Johnston, K.K. Hui, Elderly patient refractory to multiple pain medications successfully treated with integrative East–West medicine. Int. J. Gen. Med. **1**, 3–6 (2008)

Z.-Y. Wang, Z. Chen, Acute promyelocytic leukemia: from highly fatal to highly curable. Blood **111**, 2505–2515 (2008)

L. Wang, G.-B. Zhou, P. Liu, J.-H. Song, Y. Liang, X.-J. Yan et al., Dissection of mechanisms of Chinese medicinal formula Realgar-Indigo naturalis as an effective treatment for promyelocytic leukemia. Proc. Natl. Acad. Sci. U. S. A. **105**, 4826–4831 (2008)

WHO Regional Office for the Western Pacific, *WHO International Standard Terminologies on Traditional Medicine in the Western Pacific Region*, Manila, Philippines (2007)

R.A. Wilke, H. Xu, J.C. Denny, D.M. Roden, R.M. Krauss, C.A. McCarty, R.L. Davis, T. Skaar, J. Lamba, G. Savova, The emerging role of electronic medical records in pharmacogenomics. Clin. Pharmacol. Ther. **89**(3), 379–386 (2011). doi:10.1038/clpt.2010.260

M.F. Wisniewski, P. Kieszkowski, B.M. Zagorski, W.E. Trick, M. Sommers, R.A. Weinstein, Development of a clinical data warehouse for hospital infection control. J. Am. Med. Inform. Assoc. **10**(5), 455–462 (2003)

I.H. Witten, E. Frank, *Data Mining: Practical Machine Learning Tools and Techniques*, 2nd edn. (Morgan Kaufmann, San Francisco, 2005)

World Health Organization, *SARS: Clinical Trials on Treatment Using a Combination of Traditional Chinese Medicine and Western Medicine*, Genevese, Switzerland (World Health Organization, 2004)

W. Xie, X. Gao, The idea and approach of the mutual complementarity and integration of TCM and western medicine. J. Chendu Coll. TCM **17**(2), 14–17 (1994) [in Chinese]

S. Yan, R. Zhang, X. Zhou, P. Li, L. He, B. Liu, Exploring effective core drug patterns in primary insomnia treatment with Chinese herbal medicine: study protocol for a randomized controlled trial. Trials **14**, 61 (2013). doi:10.1186/1745-6215-14-61

Q.L. Zha, Y.T. He, X.P. Yan, L. Su, Y.J. Song, S.P. Zeng et al., Predictive role of diagnostic information in treatment efficacy of rheumatoid arthritis based on neural network model analysis. Zhong Xi Yi Jie He Xue Bao **5**(1), 32–38 (2007) (in Chinese)

H. Zhang, C. Tian, B. Liu, X. Zhou, Y. Wang, Z. Liu. Study on the idea of clinical acupuncture point combination of TCM physician Tian. J. Clin. Acup. Mox. **23**(2), 36–38 (2007a) (in Chinese)

N.L. Zhang, X. Zhou, B. Liu et al., Interpreting results of variable clustering in TCM research. Chin. J. Inf. TCM **14**(7), 102–103 (2007b) (in Chinese)

R. Zhang, Clinical research on the syndrome structure and syndrome hierarchical differentiation of disharmony of liver and spleen syndrome. Ph.D thesis, Guanganmen hospital, China academy of Chinese medical sciences. 2008.5 (in Chinese)

N.L. Zhang, S. Yuan, T. Chen, Y. Wang, Latent tree models and diagnosis in traditional Chinese medicine. Artif. Intell. Med. **42**(3), 229–245 (2008a)

N.L. Zhang, S. Yuan, T. Chen, Y. Wang, Statistical validation of traditional Chinese medicine theories. J. Altern. Complement Med. **14**(5), 583–587 (2008b)

X. Zhang, X. Zhou, H. Huang et al., Topic model for Chinese medicine diagnosis and prescription regularities analysis: case on diabetes. Chin. J. Integr. Med. **17**(4), 307–313 (2011)

X. Zhou, Z. Wu, A. Yin, L. Wu, W. Fan, R. Zhang, Ontology development for unified traditional Chinese medical language system. Artif. Intell. Med. **32**(1), 15–27 (2004)

X. Zhou, The research on TCM clinical data warehousing and clinical data mining methods. Postdoctoral report, China academy of Chinese medical sciences, Beijing, 2007.3 (in Chinese)

X. Zhou, S. Chen, B. Liu, R. Zhang, Y. Wang, X. Zhang, Extraction of hierarchical core structures from traditional Chinese medicine herb combination network. in *Proceedings of 2008 International Conference on Advanced Intelligence*, ed. by Z. Shi, W. Horn, X. Wu (Posts & Telecom press, Beijing, 2008), pp. 262–267

X. Zhou, Y. Peng, B. Liu, Text mining for traditional Chinese medical knowledge discovery: a survey. J. Biomed. Inform. **43**, 650–660 (2010a)

X. Zhou, S. Chen, B. Liu, R. Zhang, Y. Wang, P. Li et al., Development of traditional Chinese medicine clinical data warehouse for medical knowledge discovery and decision support. Artif. Intell. Med. **48**(2–3), 139–152 (2010b)

TCM Data Mining and Quality Evaluation with SAPHRON™ System

Jing Yang, Hua Su, Guoshun Tang, Zihan Zheng, Yue Shen, Lei Zhang, Hongyan Wei, Songxia Yin, Lu Chen, Zirong Yang, and William Jia

Abstract Traditional Chinese Medicine (TCM) is an invaluable human heritage for its documented clinical experience of thousands of years. However, it remains problematic for how to make the best use of this treasure. A major concern of TCM modernization is the credibility of the information. A large number of these clinical records are scattered in various notes, books and research reports and there is absence of good tool to scientifically evaluate this tremendous amount of information. Our recent preliminary study has shown that the quality of TCM information is generally poor and unreliable. To provide a platform that provides TCM information with verified quality as a base for TCM-originated product development, we established a proprietary SAPHRON TCM data system to quantitatively evaluate the quality of TCM information, which ranks TCM prescriptions, herbs, active ingredients as well as potential lead compounds based on the reliability of available information for recommendation. Our results have showed that, scientific approaches with modern technology of informatics and statistics can be applied to TCM information in a high throughput fashion.

J. Yang • H. Su • G.S. Tang • Z.H. Zheng • Y. Shen • L. Zhang • H.Y. Wei • S.X. Yin • L. Chen • Z.R. Yang
Shanghai Innovative Research Centre of Traditional Chinese Medicine, Shanghai, China

W. Jia (✉)
Shanghai Innovative Research Centre of Traditional Chinese Medicine, Shanghai, China

Brain Research Centre and Department of Surgery, University of British Columbia, Vancouver, BC, Canada
e-mail: w.jia@ubc.ca

J. Poon and S.K. Poon (eds.), *Data Analytics for Traditional Chinese Medicine Research*, 215
DOI 10.1007/978-3-319-03801-8_12, © Springer International Publishing Switzerland 2014

1   Introduction

While herbal medicines have been used by all nations in the world for thousands of years, Traditional Chinese Medicine (TCM) is one of the most significant herbal medicines in human civilization. Over generations, TCM has been used to treat all clinical conditions and more importantly, the herb usage and clinical observations are recorded in numerous notes, books and research reports. Tremendous amount of written documents going back to 3,000 years ago have provided strong evidence of safety and effectiveness on Chinese herbs. Making good use of this treasure is an important task for TCM modernization.

On the other hand, quality of TCM information has always been questioned. Actually, much of the TCM information is either probably myths or based on anecdotal evidence. In addition, TCM theories, on which traditional herb usages in the clinic are based, are extremely diverse and often contradictory. This results in thousands of TCM prescriptions with completely different herb compositions for a very same clinical condition (Yan Liu et al. 2010; Zhiqiang Ouyang et al. 2007; Zhanpeng Tan et al. 2011). It is therefore very challenging to understand and select the best prescription and herb combination for further drug discovery with a logical and unbiased approach.

There are many TCM databases in China. However, the majority is encyclopedia-like, which have collected everything without further verification for quality of the information. Furthermore, those databases typically do not provide any tools for using the information to design new TCM products or to discover lead compounds for novel drugs. Realizing the above shortcomings of current TCM databases, we have established SAPHRON™ database at Shanghai Innovative Research Centre of Traditional Chinese Medicine after more than 10 years of efforts. SAPHRON database links diseases, prescriptions, herbs, active compounds and bioactivity of compounds together. Based on SAPHRON™ database, we developed a SIRC TCM Information Quality Evaluation System (STIQES) to address the quality issue of TCM information. The present article is to test the SAPHRON database and its use in early product development.

2   Assessment of Quality of Published TCM Clinical Trials

We have assessed 412 published clinical trials out of 5,559 searched publications that used TCM prescriptions to treat hyperlipidemia (Fig. 1). We then investigated the quality of each clinical trial with eight commonly used parameters for modern clinical studies and the results are shown in Fig. 1. Our results show that 7 % did not mention any specific criteria for efficacy evaluation; 26 % did not conduct any statistical analysis; 8 % did not use any objective measurements for efficacy; 59 % did not mention whether toxicity/side effects were observed; 28 % did not include a control group; 36 % were not randomized trials; 62 % involved less than 100

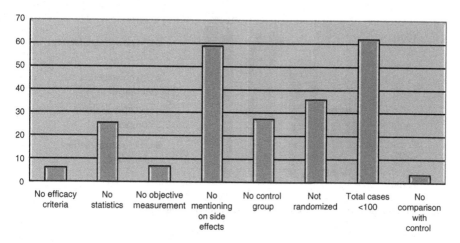

Fig. 1 Analysis of 412 clinical trials for hyperlipidemia

patients; even worse, 3 % trials included a control group but did not make any comparison with the TCM treated groups.

Taken together, only 55 trials in the 412 total reports did not have any of the eight deficiencies above.

3 Quality of Studies on TCM Formulated Products

Formulated TCM products have been widely used in clinic in China. For TCM usage, the formulated TCM products are supposed to be the best regulated as each product must go through clinical trials as regulatory procedures before being used in clinic. Unlike most TCM prescriptions that the decoctions are prepared by either patients themselves or TCM pharmacies using individual herbs, formulated TCM products are manufactured by TCM pharmaceutical companies with standardized GMP procedures. Therefore, it is expected that clinical data of those products may be more reliable. To test that, we have evaluated 115 reports of clinical studies on "Shenmai Injectable", a well-known TCM formulated product used as intravenously infusion for cancer management. This product has been granted the certificates of SFDA by seven manufacturers in China (Lixing Nie et al. 2011; Weirong Zhu et al. 2005; Weixin Guo et al. 2008; Minhua He et al. 2004; Yang Cao et al. 2006; Wei Hu et al. 2008; Li 2008).

As shown in Fig. 2, among the 115 studies, 51(45 %) did not mention the manufacturer of the product used in the clinical study. 90 reports (78 %) did not provide complete information about the herb composition of the product used for the study. 90 % of the studies did not give any information regarding SFDA registration number for the product used. Finally, none of the reports described how the product was extracted and formulated.

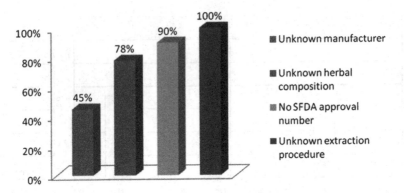

Fig. 2 Information from 115 references of "Shenmai Injectable"

While the above information may not be necessarily essential for a clinical report on western drugs, they are important for TCM clinical studies. This is because that there are seven pharmaceutical companies in China manufacturing the products that are all named "Shenmai Injectable". As the products are formulated extracts from the roots of *Ginseng Radix et Rhizoma* and *Ophiopogonis Radix* (Dwarf Lilyturf Tuber), it is necessary to identify the specific manufacturer for the product being trialed as each product may be manufactured by different procedures developed by each manufacture.

Furthermore, although all products in the 115 studies were called "Shenmai Injectable", some studies also contained *Schisandrae Chinensis Fructus* as a third herb component (Lu et al. 2004). In addition, only 18 studies disclosed some quantitative information of herb components and none of them mentioned any information about non-herb additives in the products used. Shi et al. have used peak-area ratios of characteristic components to compared four batches of "Shenmai Injectable" from the same manufacture (Shi et al. 2002). Their results showed that chemical ingredients can vary ±20 % from batch to batch. Another study (Xiaohui et al. 2006) has measured two principle components (PC1 and PC2) of "Shenmai Injectable" from three manufacturers and found the clusters of products from each manufacturer were completely non-overlapping when plotted in a PC1-PC2 plane. Given the fact that mechanism of action is unknown for most of TCM, variation in the concentrations of thousands of compounds may significantly affect the efficacy of the product. On the other hand, the SFDA certificate number is the identification for each drug in China that is not only the proof of approval for the product and also refers to specifics of the product for the approval. Without knowing the exact composition, the clinical data cannot be sensibly analyzed. Thus, owing to the lack of specifics and tremendous variation in chemical composition for the drugs used in each study, results of clinical studies on those products even under the same name are not comparable.

Taking together, the above analysis (Shi et al. 2002; Xiaohui et al. 2006) suggests that information quality of clinical trials on TCM is generally poor. This is partly attributed to substandard quality requirement for publication in TCM related journals, which may improve with time. However, the other problems (such as lacking information of herb or chemical composition in formulated TCM products) were inherited as the nature of this type of products due to industry trade secrets and government policies. In conclusion, while there is abundant clinical information for TCM, the above fatal flaws substantially reduced the credibility and value of such information.

The above preliminary analysis exemplified the variation in quality of TCM related information, which raised a serious question for product development from TCM herbs. Thus, a TCM database should not only serve as a knowledge resource but more importantly, should provide a function to evaluate and screen for the most creditable information that meets current standard of modern medical sciences. To this aim, we have established a novel approach using SAPHRON™ database developed by Shanghai Innovative Research Centre of Traditional Chinese Medicine. This platform takes approaches of statistics and informatics to evaluate the quality of TCM related literatures and to provide a screening system for TCM prescriptions, herbs and active compounds that can be used for product development.

4 SAPHRON™ TCM Information Platform

4.1 SAPHRON™ TCM Database

The SAPHRON™ TCM database was built in 2000 and it has been expended significantly since then after more than 12 years data construction. The database is constructed in an interactive framework that contains five independent sub-databases, namely TCM disease terminology, TCM prescriptions, TCM herbology, TCM phytochemistry and TCM pharmacology. The TCM disease terminology database collected 1,400 TCM disease terms that are all described in terms of both TCM and modern medicine. This database connects current disease terminology with TCM defined diseases, which are described in symptoms and syndromes. The TCM prescription database is a collection of more than 180,000 TCM formulas some of them were documented 3,000 years ago. While the database kept many original ancient TCM prescriptions, it collects and emphasizes more on TCM prescriptions that derived from ancient formulas and are currently used in clinic. The TCM herbology database has monographs of more than 9,000 TCM herbs with their full botanic definition as well as the process techniques used by TCM practitioners. The phytochemistry database contains more than 30,000 compound structures identified in TCM herbs with their full physical and chemical characteristics. Finally, the pharmacology database has more than 120,000 items of biological information for the compounds isolated from TCM herbs. Since the five sub-databases are built in an interactive manner, one can obtain a set of information for any TCM related questions from their clinical indications by both western and Chinese definition, formulas with various herb compositions, known compounds found in those herbs and their known biological and pharmacological activities.

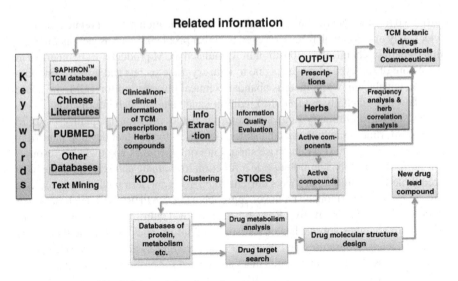

Fig. 3 SAPHRON™ TCM data mining & product design system

4.2 Outline SAPHRON™ TCM Information Platform

We have utilized the SAPHRON™ to establish a service platform as shown in Fig. 3 that can be used for screening TCM resources to provide information that are used to develop new products including novel TCM medicines, nutraceutical products, cosmetic products and lead compound discovery.

The first part of the system is data collection. Key words of both English and Chinese related to the topic of interest are generated. Using TEXT MINING technology, literatures potentially relating to the topic will retrieve from SAPHRON™ database as well as other public databases including VIP (http://www.cqvip.com/), PUBMED (http://www.ncbi.nlm.nih.gov/pubmed/) etc. Secondary, KNOWLEDGE DISCOVERY FROM DATABASE (KDD) techniques are applied to collect information from retrieved literatures and only those containing the information closely relating to the topic are selected. KDD is a process of knowledge creation from both structured (such as SAPHRON database) and unstructured (text, literature, etc.) sources. From those sources, KDD generate knowledge in a machine-readable format (Cunningham 2006). For instance, to obtain knowledge about a clinical trial literature, information such as numbers of recruited patients for the trial, dosage of treatment and rates of response, etc. are extracted from the related literature and organized into a form that can be stored in access format to facilitate further investigation. Thirdly, data collected from the KDD process are grouped with CLUSTER ANALYSIS to extract common features in each group. For the example of clinical trials, prescriptions utilized in the trials will be grouped according to the similarity of herb usage. Compounds contained in the herbs can be grouped based on the similarity in their scaffold structures. At the last stage of analysis, information of TCM

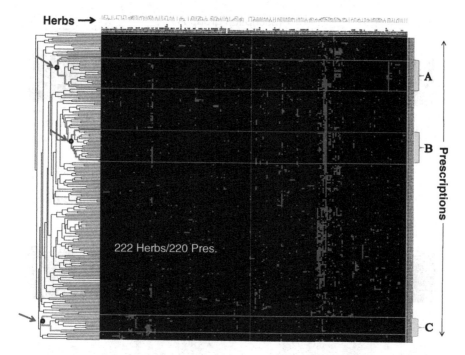

Fig. 4 Heat map of cluster analysis on 222 prescriptions and included 220 herbs

prescriptions, herbs of interest, and compound structures will be evaluated for their credibility and quality using SIRC TCM Information Quality Evaluation System (STIQES) (see below). Through STIQES, each prescription, herb or compounds with potential for treatment of a specific clinical indication will be scored and ranked according to their STIQES scores. The highest scored prescriptions, herbs, active fraction of herb extracts or compounds will be the recommended candidates for further development.

4.3 Cluster Analysis of Herb Usage in TCM Prescriptions

While individual TCM prescriptions vary significantly in herb usage and doses for treatment of the same clinical indication, most of the prescriptions can be grouped with a simple cluster analysis (Ye Liang et al. 2008; Gu 2010). Taking the same example for treating hyperlipidemia, 222 prescriptions were screened out of 412 clinic prescriptions on the basis of known specific herb composition and proportion, which is essential for prescription-herb cluster analysis. There are totally 220 herbs used for those prescriptions. Figure 4 shows the results as a heat map that provides a visible way to show frequencies of herb usage. When the prescriptions are clustered according to the similarity of their herb usage and weight of each herb in a prescription, groups are formed and showed in trees (left of the figure).

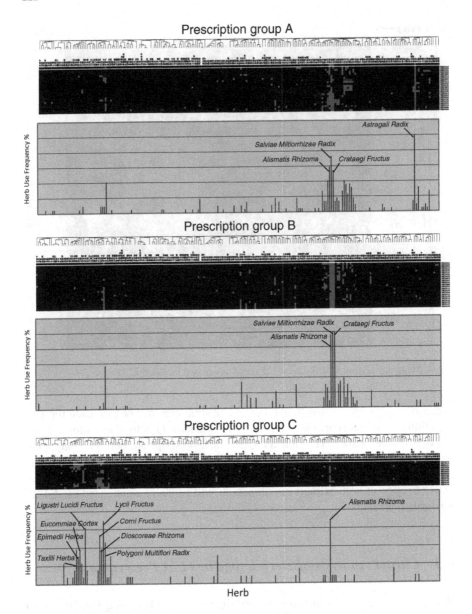

Fig. 5 Herb use frequency in prescription group A, B and C

Derived from cluster analysis, group A, B and C can be defined. In each prescription group, some of the herbs were commonly used, which are showed as regions with high density of red color in their heat maps. Details are showed in Fig. 5.

In group A, *Astragali Radix* is the principle component with a function of invigorating "qi". *Salviae Miltiorrhizae Radix et Rhizoma* and *Crataegi Fructus* are used as adjuvant ones to activate blood circulation. In addition, *Alismatis Rhizoma* is to promote urination and dispel dampness. Based on these herb compositions, it can be concluded that the prescriptions in this group are to treat hyperlipemia with a syndrome of "qi" deficiency caused "blood stasis" by TCM theory.

In group B, *Crataegi Fructus*, *Salviae Miltiorrhizae Radix* and *Alismatis Rhizoma* are the main components that activate blood circulation, remove blood stasis and to promote urination and dispel dampness. Since little *Astragali Radix* was used, the prescriptions in group B are mainly to treat hyperlipemia with blood stasis but not "qi" deficient.

In group C, *Ligustri Lucidi Fructus* is the principle component that is known for its function of reinforcing "liver" and "kidney", while *Lycii Fructus*, *Corni Fructus*, *Polygoni multiflori Radix*, *Dioscoreae Rhizoma*, *Taxilli Herba*, *Epimedii Folium* and *Eucommiae Cortex* are used as adjuvant ones. As mentioned above, *Alismatis Rhizoma* is to promote urination and dispel dampness. Thus, the prescriptions in group C are to treat hyperlipemia with "yin" deficiency of "liver" and "kidney".

It is worthwhile to point out that *Alismatis Rhizoma*, is commonly used for all the three groups. This herb is well known for the diuretics effect to eliminate dampness (Chinese Pharmacopoeia 2010; Chunping Yin and Jizhou Wu 2001; Wang et al. 2008), which is also consistent with the TCM theory that hyperlipemia is a disease closely related with increased "dampness". Modern pharmacology studies also support that *Alismatis Rhizoma* is useful for treating hyperlipemia (Hu et al. 2011; Shugang Yuan et al. 2011; Shuzi Li et al. 2008).

The results from the above statistical analysis reveal the most frequently used herbs for one indication such as *Alismatis Rhizoma*. Furthermore, grouping by cluster analysis provides an objective approach to distinct different treatments by TCM practitioners. These can be the difference based on individual patient's conditions (such as with or without "qi" deficiency) or based on specific TCM theories.

4.4 Frequency Analysis of Co-used Herbs to Reveal Possible Synergy Between Herbs

TCM herbs are typically used by decoctions of multiple herbs in clinic. Some rules are applied in TCM practice to allow certain herbs used together but others are exclusive to each other (Erxin Shang et al. 2010; Chen et al. 2012). While those rules are to be understood by modern pharmaceutical sciences for potential synergy or adverse interaction when herbs are co-decocted or co-administrated, we used clinical data to demonstrate how TCM herbs are combinedly used in prescriptions with creditable clinical evidence. Prescriptions for a given indication are first grouped by clustering to ensure that all the formulations are prescribed based on similar principles of TCM theories. Within a group, the most frequently used herbs are analyzed for the time it is used in combination with each of another herb used in all the prescriptions to treat the same indications. An example is shown in Table 1. In this case, *Puerariae Lobatae Radix* appeared with a 100 % frequency in a group

Table 1 Herb correlation analysis

	Herb name	Frequency of co-used herbs (No. of co-appearance/no. of total prescriptions)
Puerariae Lobatae Radix	*Astragali Radix*	1.000 (71/71)
	Rehmanniae Radix	0.859 (61/71)
	Dioscoreae Rhizoma	0.845 (60/71)
	Trichosanthis Radix	0.662 (47/71)
	Ophiopogonis Radix	0.592 (42/71)
	Schisandrae Chinensis Fructus	0.507 (36/71)

of 71 prescriptions for treating diabetes group. Some herbs in the group with high frequencies of co-use with *Puerariae Lobatae Radix* are listed in Table 1, which showed that, in this group of prescriptions for treating diabetes, *Puerariae Lobatae Radix* is always used with *Astragali Radix* and also co-used with *Rehmanniae Radix* and/or *Dioscoreae Rhizoma*.

4.5 STIQES (SIRC TCM Information Quality Evaluation System)

We have developed three STIQES systems for evaluate credibility and quality of information for prescriptions, herbs and potential lead compounds, respectively. STIQES is an itemized scoring system consentaneous with the principle of Evidence Based Medicine, which evaluates the above TCM related information from multiple aspects, including not only the evaluation of randomized trial with proper control group but also the availability of toxicity/side effect data and pharmacological study, quality of clinical studies, costs and environmental impact of each TCM product. The total STIQES score of each TCM related information determines the final list of prescriptions, herbs or compounds that are recommended for further verification.

5 General Discussion

SAPHRON™ TCM database has been established since 2000. During the past 13 years, we have vigorously verified the information contained in the database to ensure the accuracy and correctness of each piece of data. SAPHRON™ TCM Data Mining & Product Design System is a platform for drug discovery and product development using TCM information. While this system has been used successfully to identify TCM prescriptions, herbs and potential lead compounds for early stage development of TCM related products, it is still rather primitive and needs further development. Most TCM literatures are published in Chinese and so it shut out a large number of international researchers. On the other hand, there is lack of powerful software to extract information from Chinese literatures. A lot of work are still checked manually. The technology of bioinformatics for data mining and information extraction needs to be improved to increase the efficiency of data management. Also, information of TCM remedies are always more or less subjective and arbitrary. Modern statistical methods provide good tools to analyze those information. However, statistical tools utilized in the analysis of TCM data require optimization. For example, we still look for a good statistical tool to reasonably express the antagonistic relationship of herb usages. At the same time, statistical methods used in other fields can be expanded to researches of TCM prescription to find the possible laws of TCM treatment. Cluster analysis is widely used in biological studies to help the research on DNA or proteins by grouping. When this method used for TCM prescriptions, the distribution of herb usages for one indication can be visually presented. In our system, TCM prescriptions, herbs and lead compounds can be quantitatively evaluated from various angles of interest. Given the inherent nature of this type of information, any quantitative scoring has to be arbitrary. Therefore, interpretation of the final ranks for recommendation shall be dealt in caution. Furthermore, it needs to point out that any recommendations by the SAPHRON database services merely indicates the quality of information supporting the claims by literature but not to compare the effectiveness of the recommended TCM prescriptions, herbs or lead compounds. The purpose of SAPHRON TCM information services can only be seen as to provide a group of candidates that may have the best quality of supporting evidence for their claimed efficacy while one cannot rule out the possibility that others without strong evidence may be more effective. Therefore, with the improvements of publication of experimental approaches both in animals and in well-designed clinical trials, more effective researches can be traced by further studies.

References

S. Chen, Y. Tang, X. Liang, The simple discussion of evil compatibility in traditional Chinese medicine. J. Liaoning Univ. TCM **14**(2), 105–106 (2012)

Chinese pharmacopoeia, **1**, 212–213 (2010)

Chunping Yin, Jizhou Wu, Advances in studies on immunoregulation of Alism aorientalis and its active constituents. Chin. Trad. Herb. Drugs **32**(12), 1132–1133 (2001)

H. Cunningham, Information extraction, automatic, in *Encyclopedia of Language & Linguistics*, vol. 5, 2nd edn. Oxford: Elsevier, pp. 665–677 (2006)

Erxin Shang, Xinsheng Fan, Jinao Duan, Liang Ye, Data mining study on incompatibility characters of Chinese herbal medicine in accordance with association rules. J. Nanjing TCM Univ. **26**(6), 421–424 (2010)

Z. Gu, Research on prescription classification using text classification technology. J. Liaoning Univ. TCM **12**(2), 45–46 (2010)

X. Hu, Z. Cheng, S. Wang, N. Fang, S. Yu, Effects of Rhizoma Alismatis decoction on levels of blood lipids in rat. Lishizhen Med. Meteria Medica Res. **22**(9), 2073–2074 (2011)

D. Li, Study on the bacterial endotoxins test of Shenmai injection. Strait Pharm. J. **20**(3), 59–61 (2008)

Lixing Nie, Yan Liu, Gangli Wang, Hongyu Jin, Ruichao Lin, Direct determination of 26 elements in traditional Chinese medicine injection. Chin. Pharm. J. **46**(11), 866–868 (2011)

H. Lu, R. Chen, M. Wu, Evaluation of high-dose Senmai in treating patients with advanced cancer. Chin. Trad. Pat. Med. **26**(9), 729–731 (2004)

Minhua He, Jianxin Wu, Ping Zhou, Rongxiang Niu, Kunlun Tian, The protection effect of shenmai injection on rabbits with renal ischernic/reperfusion injurn. J. Chin. Clin. Med. **5**(6), 5–6 (2004)

X. Shi, J. Yang, C. Zhao, J. Xiong, G. Xu, Application of fingerprint chromatogram in quality control of Shen-Mai injection. Chin. J. Chromatogr. **20**(4), 299–303 (2002)

Shugang Yuan, Yingjie Zhang, Shaodan Ma, Guihua Su, Shibao Ruan, The optimal dose ratio experimental study of Zexie Tiaozhi granule on adjust lipids of hyperlipidemic rats. Clin. J. Chin. Med. **3**(16), 5–6 (2011)

Shuzi Li, Zaijiu Jin, Shanyu Zhang, The effects of alisma orientalis's extracts on blood lipid and antioxidation of experimental hyperlipidemia mice. China Pract. Med. **3**(32), 7–9 (2008)

L. Wang, Q. Wu, Q. Zhang, G. Peng, A. Ding, Basic study of diuretic active compounds in Rhizoma Alismatis. West China J. Pharm. Sci. **23**(6), 670–672 (2008)

Wei Hu, Junying Ding, Shixiang Jia, Zhongsi Lin, ShenMai injection combined with chemotherapy in the treatment of advanced lung cancer. J. Liaoning Univ. TCM **10**(11), 108–109 (2008)

Weirong Zhu, Lan Zheng, Yuanbiao Guo, Jianming Yuan, Xiaoheng Shen, Clinical research of intraperitoneal chemotherapy plus Shenmai injection in treating advanced colorectal cancer. J. Chin. Integr. Med. **3**(4), 266–269 (2005)

Weixin Guo, Qidong Yang, Xiaoyun Xie, Wang Miao, Effects of Shenmai injection on number and activity of endothelial progenitor cells from human peripheral blood. Stroke Nerv. Dis. **15**(1), 37–40 (2008)

F. Xiaohui, W. Yi, C. Yiyu, LC/MS fingerprinting of Shenmai injection: A novel approach to quality control of herbal medicines. J. Pharm. Biomed. Anal. **40**, 591–597 (2006)

Yan Liu, Xin Fan, Kang Li, Application of association rules on selecting the prescription from classics of traditional Chinese medicine. Chin. J. Hosp. Stat. **17**(4), 294–297 (2010)

Yang Cao, Peng Li, Kaiji Tan, Ruishen Chen, Clinical observation on Shenmai injection in preventing and treating adverse reaction of chemotherapy on advanced non-small cell lung cancer. Chin. J. Integr. Trad. West. Med. **26**(6), 550–552 (2006)

Ye Liang, Xinsheng Fan, Chongjun Wang, Erxin Shang, Fengying Zhao, Huan Zhang, Discussion data mining technology applying on prescription. Med. Inf. **21**(10), 1734–1737 (2008)

Zhanpeng Tan, Yi Luo, Jiqiang Li, The data mining analysis of the Chinese medicine principle and ZHENG-oriented effects of 43 medical records on dysentery by the contemporary famous veteran Chinese medical doctors. Clin. Med. Eng. **18**(3), 412–414 (2011)

Zhiqiang Ouyang, Lisheng Jiang, Ruyi Wang, Seqi Lin, Qiming Zhang, Qinglin Zha, Aiping Lv, The regularity of the compatibility and corresponding prescriptions with syndrome of treating toothache with TCM in 63 case of famous practitioner of Chinese medicine about toothache on publication. J. Jiangxi Univ. TCM **19**(5), 88–90 (2007)

An Overview on Evidence-Based Medicine and Medical Informatics in Traditional Chinese Medicine Practice

Kelvin Chan, Josiah Poon, Simon K. Poon, Miao Jiang, and Aiping Lu

Abstract This chapter describes how best to look at the evidence-base of the rich experience-based disciplines of traditional Chinese medicine in this era of highly advance of biomedicine, science-orientated development and information technology. It is emphasized that there is a need in using modified modalities that can focus on the inclusion of holistic TCM diagnosis and treatment outcomes of individual patients in randomized clinical trial for TCM products studies and that in practice individual patients' reported outcomes linked with biomedical parameters may provide evidence-base treatment efficacy. Using TCM formulae for treatment of female infertility as an example for IT contribution to data analysis, it is suggested that continuing feedback between practitioners in each field will help refining IT analysis of TCM informatics in general.

K. Chan (✉)
Faculty of Pharmacy, The University of Sydney,
Rm N502B, Building A15, Science Road, Sydney, NSW 2006, Australia

National Institute of Complementary Medicine, University of Western Sydney,
Richmond, NSW 2560, Australia
e-mail: kelvin.chan@sydney.edu.au

J. Poon • S.K. Poon
School of Information Technologies, The University of Sydney,
Sydney, NSW 2006, Australia
e-mail: josiah.poon@sydney.edu.au; simon.poon@sydney.edu.au

M. Jiang • A. Lu
Institute of Basic Research in Clinical Medicine, China Academy of Chinese Medical
Sciences, Dongzhimennei Nanxiaojie 16#, Beijing 100700, China

J. Poon and S.K. Poon (eds.), *Data Analytics for Traditional Chinese Medicine Research*,
DOI 10.1007/978-3-319-03801-8_13, © Springer International Publishing Switzerland 2014

1 Introduction

Traditional Chinese medicine (TCM) is a holistic medical practice that alleviates disease related syndromes and maintains good health by balancing the body, mind, and spirit into harmony (Jiang et al. 2012b). Currently, TCM has been increasingly accepted world-wide. The widespread use of TCM in the treatment of chronic diseases that conventional western medicine fails and the investigation of mechanisms of actions for Chinese herbal medicines and acupuncture treatment have produced massive publications in both basic and clinical literature (Jiang et al. 2012c).

Following the principle of evidence-based medicine, concrete evidence is needed to evaluate the efficacy of TCM (Lu and Chen 2009). Accordingly, in the past decade, since the first systematic review of TCM clinical research was published in 2002 (Nestler 2002), more clinical trials have also been published internationally, and, which has consequently increased the number of systematic reviews (SRs) and meta-analysis of TCM clinical trials (Jiang et al. 2012b), TCM has a long history but its efficacy is not as well-documented as one would hope. Proof of efficacy has to come from empirical researches, i.e. clinical trials, prospective experiments assessing the effects of medical interventions. Randomized Controlled Trials (RCTs) are regarded as golden clinical trial design. Since 2002, more and well-designed RCTs have been conducted worldwide to evaluate the efficacy of TCM.

2 Effectiveness Evaluation of TCM

More TCM clinical studies were reported in the past three decades (Fig. 1), and majority are observational ones since it is still difficult to conduct RCTs for TCM with its unique diagnostic and treatment approach. The observational clinical studies on TCM do show the efficacy for chronic diseases. For TCM treatment of chronic disease processes, individually prescribed, bulk-dispensed, water-based decoctions are the professional standard of care in China (Flaws 2005). This implies that decoctions have their own particular indications and uses in a large outpatient population. Usually nonrandomized controlled clinical trials and observational studies report indicated that decoctions' efficacy. Ideally, the efficacy of decoctions should be rigorously tested by RCTs. It is also difficult to include placebo herbal mixtures in the double-blind design.

Only recently, RCTs have been conducted in China to evaluate the effectiveness of proprietary traditional Chinese medicines (PTCMs) generated from well-known Chinese medicine formula and from currently effective practice formula in treatment of various diseases. Some studies have shown good effectiveness in not only the treatment of certain chronic diseases, such as hypertension (Liu et al. 2006a), gastroenteritis (Yu et al. 2007), diabetes mellitus (Tong et al. 2009), rheumatoid arthritis (Guo et al. 2008), cerebrovascular disease (Zhou et al. 2010a), intervertebral disc disorders (Qin et al. 2007), chronic obstructive pulmonary disease (COPD)

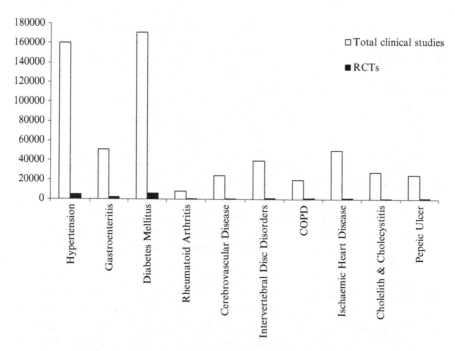

Fig. 1 The number of papers on total TCM clinical studies and RCTs published in China from 1979 to 2009 in Chinese BioMedical Literature Database (CBM) [http://sinomed.imicams.ac.cn/index.jsp]

(Xu et al. 2010c), ischaemic heart disease (Qing et al. 2009), cholelith & cholecystitis (Liu et al. 2005), and peptic ulcer (Gong et al. 2012; Wei Jinqi and Weining 1994); but also in the treatment of some virus infective disease including H1N1 influenza (Wang et al. 2011, 2012) and hand-foot-mouth disease (Li et al. 2013). However, the situation on the efficacy evaluation focus on PTCM is not enough since the clinical trials are difficult to evaluate the individually-prescribed decoctions. In fact, the bulk of current RCTs were assessing the efficacy of one TCM product or formula on a specific chronic disease diagnosed with western medicine (biomedicine) approach and aimed to prove the "one size fits all" hypothesis, while TCM practice is more personalized and the herbal combination is prescribed individually on the basis of each person's particular disease Pattern (ZHENG, syndrome).

As the evidence gathering tools both systematic reviews (SRs) and meta-analysis provide synthesis of published research papers. The number of SRs and meta-analysis on TCM is increasing rapidly after the evidence-based medicine (EBM) was introduced and practiced in China. The following accounts are recently published findings of SRs that explores a range of evidence on TCM for chronic diseases.

Using Chinese medicines for treatment of irritable bowel syndrome (Liu et al. 2006b) in 75 randomized trials 7,957 participants were included in the studies.

Some TCM formulae showed significant improvement of the global symptoms. Twenty-two TCM medicines demonstrated a statistically significant benefit for symptom improvement. Six tested PTCM showed additional benefit from the combination therapy compared with conventional mono therapy. Some Chinese medicines deserve further examination in high-quality trials.

In reviewing TCM treatments for type 2 diabetes mellitus (Liu et al. 2004), 66 randomized trials, involving 8,302 participants had been reported. Methodological quality was generally low. Some PTCM showed hypoglycemic effects in type 2 diabetes. Some PTCM deserved further examination in high-quality trials.

Danshen and related PTCM were introduced into clinical practice for treatment of ischaemic stroke in 1970 in China. Six trials involving 494 patients were reported (Wu et al. 2007). These Danshen products were associated with a significant increase in the number of patients with the positive outcomes. No deaths were reported within the first 2 weeks of treatment or during the whole follow-up period. The authors called for further high-quality randomized controlled trials should be performed.

Generally speaking in large TCM clinical practices where most extensive observational studies and substantial number available of RCTs and SRs have shown that efficacy of TCM was reflected in some advances in treatment of various diseases. Though the efficacy in some evaluated TCM treatments remains uncertain with RCTs and SRs, it should be carefully interpreted due to issues of methodology. On the other hand, most TCM clinical trials have been published in Chinese language and are inaccessible to scholars outside China for further analysis. To substantiate observations on positive findings, some PTCM and related composite formulae deserve further examination in high-quality trials based on TCM pattern differentiation. We expect that improvement on reporting more TCM clinical studies in high level international journals in the near future.

3   Safety Evaluation of TCM

TCM treatment using Chinese materia medica (CMM) or PTCM is regarded as a safe and effective system of medicine because TCM practice has served the community in China through several thousands of years with cumulative practice experience. TCM has also provided personalized therapy by using multi-component prescriptions that act with concerted actions derived from multi-target pharmacological actions (Chan 2005). Records of safety issues can be reviewed as follows.

Literatures on TCM safety and ADRs from 1978 to October of 2010 in the Sinomed database (http://sinomed.imicams.ac.cn/) were searched and there are altogether 30,631 related papers on this topic. The increasing literature number on ADRs after the year 2005 indicated the close attention to the safety issue of TCM in China. Table 1 showed the summary of adverse events for chronic diseases reported in SRs (TCM vs. Pharmaceuticals) focusing on the common chronic diseases in China. The conclusion exhibited a desirable safety profile of TCM comparing to pharmaceuticals.

Table 1 Summary of adverse events for chronic diseases reported in SRs (TCM vs. Pharmaceuticals)

Disease	Intervention	Year published	Journal	Authors' conclusions
Hypertension	Pharmaceuticals	2008	Chinese journal of evidence-based medicine	The incidence of adverse reaction is 9.66 % (Yi et al. 2008)
	TCM	2008	Liaoning journal of traditional Chinese medicine	The adverse effect is diarrhea, incidence rate is about 2.56 % (Wang et al. 2008)
Intervertebral disc disorders	Pharmaceuticals	2007	None	Many adverse events were reported, more details in the article (Vipond 2007)
	TCM	2009	Chinese journal of evidence-based medicine	No adverse events reported in included studies (Wang et al. 2009)
COPD	Pharmaceuticals	2005	The Cochrane library	There was an increased risk of adverse effects, including increased blood glucose, adrenal suppression and reduced serum osteocalcin (Walters et al. 2005)
	TCM	2009	Chinese journal of evidence-based medicine	Gastrointestinal adverse events reported in three RCTs. No serious adverse events from the herbal medicines were reported (Zhou et al. 2009)
Ischaemic heart disease	Pharmaceuticals	2010	Lancet	Serious drug-related adverse events were not significantly increased by fibrates (17,413 participants, 225 events), although increases in serum creatinine concentrations were common (1.99, 1.46–2.70; p<0.0001) (Jun et al. 2010)
	TCM	2008	Journal of the Fourth Military Medical University	No adverse events reported in included studies (Wang et al. 2009)

TCM prescriptions or PTCMs are prescribed to patients according to the principles of diagnosis and treatment in TCM practice, which is considered as safe through experience of test of time. Various studies have been reported outcomes of good safety and quality of TCM decoctions in treatment of some chronic diseases (Geng et al. 2010; Hsieh et al. 2010; Sze et al. 2011; Zhou et al. 2010b; Zhu et al. 2010). Majority of PTCMs have been reported to be safe (Deng et al. 2010; Fan et al. 2010; Jia et al. 2010; Wang et al. 2010; Xie et al. 2009; Xu et al. 2010a; Xu et al. 2010b; Zhao et al. 2010), yet it had been observed that the toxicity was augmented in PTCM comparing to TCM decoction due to the unsupervised long-period usage of PTCM and the improved surveillance effort recently introduced by national authority. To evaluate the safety of TCM is complicated by using conventional methodological approaches since TCM products are complex in composition, as in prescriptions containing multiple CMM, the lack of known synergetic active ingredients, the risk of contaminants such as pesticides, heavy metals and addition of other ingredients (sometimes pharmaceuticals), deterioration and variation in composition (Chan 2005). Furthermore, the interactions between TCM and pharmaceutical drugs might be another issues related to safety of TCM. All these issues should be addressed accordingly (Chan and Cheung 2000).

TCM safety profile is essential for TCM application in clinical practice, especially in patients with chronic diseases since they often need long term taking of those TCM products. Through clinical application based on TCM theory and strict quality control we can improve safer application of TCM. Nevertheless, TCM safety has not been fully determined and further studies are needed to explore the mechanisms of TCM products in order to decipher the toxic activities of TCM products.

4   General Issues in Evidence-Based Study of TCM

TCM has been involving the healthcare system in China for thousands of years, and supplies about one fourth medical services nowadays in China. More importantly, TCM takes an active role in prevention of diseases and rehabilitation after recovery from severe illnesses in China. To provide efficacy evidence, the design and reporting of clinical trials of TCM should follow the same guidelines as those for any other such research. However, there are some specific features and general issues in TCM practice that the design for clinical studies require modification from conventional approach because of both diagnosis and treatment paradigms are different from orthodox medical practice.

4.1   TCM Pattern Classification

Utilizing diagnostic principles in TCM practice, pattern classification is applied to stratify the patients and provide more suitable indications for inclusion criteria in RCT. However, the key problem which undermined the acceptance of RCTs in

TCM is the absence of standard TCM diagnosis criteria for patient recruitment into the RCTs.

In some RCTs design, patients with the same disease were recruited and received TCM or conventional treatment respectively but the information for TCM pattern classification was ignored. Thus in these clinical studies, conventional treatment tends to produce a better curative effect than TCM treatment, the RCT failed to evaluate the real efficacy of TCM.

In studies where the patients were given individual TCM prescription treatments according to their TCM pattern diagnosis the results may show efficacy, but to generalize the success of treatment efficacy is difficult unless the trial is sufficiently large to allow subgroup analyses. On the other hand, if patients with the same TCM pattern diagnosis can be recruited from those with a particular disease in conventional medicine in a trial, the same TCM treatment can be evaluated, and generalization about the therapy would be valid, but eligible patients available for such study could be small in number and difficult to recruit.

Increasing numbers of medical researchers recognized that the combination of disease diagnosis in biomedicine and pattern classification in TCM is essential for the clinical practice when TCM is included as part of the treatment along side with conventional medical approaches, and it has been a common practice model in China since it may produce a better clinical effect (Lu et al. 2008). Therefore, defining TCM pattern classification becomes the underlying issue of TCM-RCTs. Before a RCT is conducted, there should be standard criteria for pattern classification of the targeted disease with the support of acceptable data and evidence.

Since pattern classification is mainly based on symptoms (including self-reported signs), tongue and pulse diagnosis, it is difficult to be understood by orthodox medical researchers. Diagnoses on symptoms, tongue and pulse are often diversified. Some of them, not closely related to the disease diagnostic parameters, are less focused upon by modern medicine, such as thirst and turbid urine and yellow tongue fur in some diseases (Lu et al. 2004; Yang et al. 2012). Although symptoms are diversified in a disease, they can be clustered into specific groups using bio-statistical analysis, even though traditionally they are classified into groups based on TCM theory and clinical experiences. A multi-center RCT study had shown that symptoms clusters in 396 patients could be classified into four factors (symptom combinations) with factor analysis. The symptom combinations are very similar to the patterns differentiated by TCM theory in RA patients, which divides RA into three basic patterns: cold, heat and deficiency patterns (He et al. 2007). The gene profile differences between the cold and heat patterns of RA patients might mainly reflect as differences in the amino acid and fat metabolism (Lu et al. 2012a; Lu et al. 2012b; van Wietmarschen et al. 2009) and the molecular mechanism of interventions in treating RA patients with corresponding TCM patterns was also analyzed based on a bioinformatics approach (Jiang et al. 2012a). In other RCTs, the TCM symptom groups in chronic gastritis was detected to be positively correlated with gastric mucosal immune reactions (Lu et al. 2005); similarly, the six typical symptoms defined in TCM in patients with asthma were identified as predictors for good response in the treatment with Xiaoqinglong granules (Zha et al. 2013). Thus TCM patterns in a disease, such as RA, can be useful as essential basis in the relation to biomedical sciences.

A report indicates that better effective treatment rate could be achieved from the RA patients some specific symptoms and the results suggest that RA patients should be treated differently based on their pattern differentiation (He et al. 2007). The application of TCM pattern classification would also be helpful to identify the innovative therapeutic methods. More importantly, pattern classification will help improvement of the clinical efficacy during practice since it further specifies the indication with TCM classification.

Above all, pattern classification based on TCM practice principles such as symptoms is important for further stratification of disease, which will help improve the treatment of disease with further specified indication of the therapy and the validity of RCTs in TCM. The idea of integrating pattern classification with disease diagnosis might be helpful in making innovations in modern clinical research, not only for TCM studies (Lu and Chen 2009).

For future progress TCM pattern classification should be incorporated into research design, producing value-added clinical evidence to identify the efficacy of TCM based on its own diagnostic & treatment principles. The innovative design of a RCT with integrating pattern information and disease diagnosis for group classification will certainly explore more valuable contribution of TCM treatment and can avoid the short-comings of some study designs in assessing TCM efficacy that utilizes orthodox medical research methods without discriminating patterns. These unique characteristics and essence of the TCM diagnosis & treatment theory should be included in future clinical studies when TCM treatments are utilized.

4.2   Randomization

It was observed from literature that the methods of allocation in studies described as randomized are poorly and infrequently reported (Jadad and Rennie 1998; Schulz et al. 1995; Vader 1998).

It is not possible to determine, in most cases, whether the investigators used proper methods to generate random sequences of allocation (Vader 1998). In reviewing an initial sample of 37,313 articles from the China National Knowledge Infrastructure electronic database, reports of RCTs were searched on 20 common diseases published from January of 1994 to June of 2005. RCTs published in some Chinese language journals lacked an adequate description of randomization, and similarly, most so-called 'randomized controlled trials' were not really randomized controlled trials due to the lack of adequate understanding on the part of the authors of the stringent clinical trial design (Wu et al. 2009).

4.3 Inclusion of Control Groups

The importance of having a control group cannot be overstated as the inclusion of a properly designed control group is one of the key factors in a RCT for TCM therapy. A review of 66 RCTs with Chinese herbal medicines for type 2 diabetes mellitus published in July 2005 indicated that a variety of control groups such as placebo, positive and waiting-list control groups (Bian et al. 2006), was included.

However, extant control strategies may not be appropriate for RCTs of TCM. In many RCTs of TCM clinical studies, positive control, which employs a conventional medicine with strong evidence of efficacy, is used widely to confirm the efficacy of TCM treatment. Most RCT outcomes from such approaches indicated that conventional drugs had better efficacy than TCM when a single disease or symptom was employed as the evaluation criterion. The effect based on TCM pattern was not publicly considered and validated, as the outcome measures lack adequately accounting for multiple statistical tests and evidence. Furthermore, conventional drugs provide more definite mechanism with a single target and treatment indication, while TCM prescriptions act in a more complicated, network-like way so that its treatment outcome often consists of a group of symptoms/pattern rather than a single disease or symptom. Thus the efficacy measurement between the two kinds of medicines is difficult to be notarized for the validity comparison.

Approved or well-used Chinese medicines are also included as control group in certain trials. In such cases, both therapeutic regimens had complex active mechanism. Nevertheless, even the indication of the two regimens proved to be the same pattern in TCM, different Chinese medicines might have diverse biological parameters/targets, which would have influenced the comparing measurement of efficacy and lead to false assessment.

It is difficult to design a perfect placebo on account of the special taste and appearance of the Chinese herbal medicines. The blindness would be revealed ahead of trial schedule by the improper placebo. Also the ethical requirements would limit the usage of placebo in many cases.

In summary, different control groups may be appropriate according to the study objectives, and several factors should be considered prior to selecting control groups in the future RCTs of Chinese herbal medicines (Bian et al. 2006): Control groups for RCTs should be selected according to study objectives; interventions as positive control groups should have the strongest evidence of efficacy with prescriptions as recommended by TCM practitioners, and act in similar ways as the test intervention; placebo should bear the physical characteristics of tested medications as closely as possible and is completely inert; no treatment control groups should be used when withholding treatment is an ethical issue, and objectives outcomes will not be subject to bias due to absent blindness. Registration through the Chinese Clinical Trial Registry (CHICTR) and getting open access to information about ongoing and completed trials will help in designing the proper control strategies.

It should be expected that interdisciplinary support from pharmacology, pathology, pharmacokinetics, pharmaceutics, and other appropriate disciplines will contribute to the innovation of control group strategies which would meet the characteristics of RCTs in TCM research.

4.4   Quality of Life (QOL), Patient Reported Outcomes (PROs) & Biomarkers

It is acceptable that Quality of Life (QOL) indicators are often used as secondary outcome indicators in many clinical studies. However, the efficacies of TCM treatment on QOL have not been particularly evident in these studies. There is a general impression among TCM practitioners that the currently available QOL instruments may not be sensitive enough to detect the health changes that are regarded as important in treatment using TCM. For examples, in TCM diagnosis and treatment regimens, appetite and digestion, routine of urination and bowel, facial and lips colour, spirit in the eyes and adaptation to climates and seasons are very important indicators of health status. However, these indicators are usually not included in common health related QOL (HRQOL) measure. Through the development of Chinese medicine based QOL (ChQOL) (Leung et al. 2005) we demonstrated this evidence-based approach using patient-reported outcomes or HRQOL measures can be utilized to evaluate treatment efficacy of Chinese medicine, thereby build a bridge for the integration of Chinese medicine into mainstream health care (Zhao and Chan 2005).

Patient-reported outcomes (PROs), generated from QOL instruments administered to patients before and after treatment intervention, refer to self-reported outcomes in the context of health care, and include any report generated directly from the person or persons involved. PROs include not only health status and quality of life but also reports on the satisfaction with the treatment and care, the adherence to prescribed regimens when directly related to end-result outcomes, and any other treatment or outcome evaluation obtained directly from the patients through interviews, self-completed questionnaires, diaries or other data collection tools, such as hand-held devices and web-based forms (Donald 2003).

PROs and HRQOL are self-reported outcomes in the context of health care. They are essential endpoints in any clinical trial in which the patient's self-report is the primary or sole indicator of the disease activity; as well as when the treatment has a small impact on survival but may have a significant impact, positive or negative, on HRQOL; the treatment may adversely affect patient's ability to function and their wellbeing; the treatment aims to offer equal clinical efficacy but differential PRO benefits; and treatment-related decisions are based on a combination of objective and patient-reported subjective parameters (Acquadro et al. 2003). In fact, PROs is not new in TCM practice. The PROs concept is actually similar to one of the four diagnostic methods in TCM: "Interrogation", which has been used since the beginning of TCM, and is a very effective diagnostic and evaluation method in TCM.

Treatment related decisions are based on a combination of objective and subjective parameters as well as PROs. The monitoring endogenous biomarkers in relation to healthy and disease conditions is an objective measurement. Biomarkers are molecular biological or physical characteristics that are used to identify risk for disease, and also to diagnose and treat a disease. Cholesterol, blood sugar, proteins and genes are some examples of biomarkers. Monitoring clinical biomarkers is an emerging strategy in future development of conventional medicine to formulate individualized or stratified medicine (Trusheim et al. 2007). The principles of adopting both objective (monitoring biomarkers and PROs) and subjective parameters (data recorded by practitioners) in assessment efficacy of TCM treatment should be encouraged for future approaches.

4.5   Quality Control on Clinical Studies

Most RCT studies of TCM have more methodological limitations than conventional medicine according to some reports (Shen and Nahas 2009), although increasing attention have been paid to quality control.

Many differences exist between clinical trials of TCM and conventional medicine (Ernst 2006). To convince the patient's compliance to TCM treatment is a critical problem especially in the west because of the absence of Chinese cultural influence in the patients' population. TCM treatment requires a long cycle in clinical trials, because herbal medicine apparently is milder in action and takes a relatively long time to manifest clinically. This means that trials must involve larger patient number and longer study period than that of conventional medicine. It is likely the drop-out rate would increase, and may affect the final statistical analysis and the credibility of the trial. It is also difficult for a western physician to fully understand and fulfill a clinical trial design in TCM. For this reason, it is challenging to organize a large-scale clinical research team for a large sampled and multi-centered RCT.

In addition to these general difficulties, clinical trials collectively encounter a range of problems that are not unique to TCM; these include size of the trial, design and other more specific obstacles to clinical research (Ernst 2006).

Many RCTs are limited by small sample sizes or inconsistencies in the TCM preparations studied (Shen and Nahas 2009). In some RCTs, the study populations differed considerably from typical primary care populations, and participants were not always screened to rule out other possible causes of their symptoms. An analysis of data on methodological quality of RCTs from 414 full length articles before 1 January 1997 in the Chinese Journal of Integrated Traditional and Western Medicine showed that only a few studies had sample sizes of 300 subjects or more (Tang et al. 1999).

Complementary medicine journals likely to publish articles on TCM are associated with a strong positive publication bias (Ernst and Pittler 1997). The concern therefore is that, due to a range of factors, bias is more of an issue in TCM than in conventional medicine.

Analysis of outcomes measures from clinical trials on TCM revealed that soft and non-validated outcome measures are often employed, e.g., percentage of patients perceiving benefit or patients' preference. Similarly, multiple outcomes are frequently used without adequately accounting for multiple statistical tests. Finally, surrogate endpoints are frequent and researchers often measure what is measurable rather than what is relevant.

Double blindness as a pre-requisite criterion can be difficult to achieve because of the taste, odour or appearance of herbal medicines that could not be distinguished from their respective placebos as exemplified by the numerous "placebo-controlled, double-blind" trials of garlic preparations for cholesterol lowering (Stevinson et al. 2000); due to the body odour caused by garlic, blinding is not a realistic option. Similarly double blind studies in clinical trial of acupuncture treatment suffer a significant difficulty. It was pointed out that blinding was used in only 15 % of the trials (Tang et al. 1999).

Quality control and safety issues of CMM preparations or composites formulae in the form of PTCM should be a pre-requisite criterion before commencement of clinical trials due to the variability of compositions and sources of origins of source materials.

Most problems related to RCTs of TCM can be solved. At present, the authority in China has increased funding source and technology inputs for clinical research on TCM, to establish an effective system of quality control and standardization for the process of RCTs, such as training communication and networking nation-wide and internationally. These measures would undoubtedly promote the quality of RCTs in TCM. More worldwide communication and collaboration with multi-fields experts will also benefit the quality of RCTs in TCM.

4.6 Safety Evaluation

Clinical trials are used not only to establish efficacy of an intervention but also to learn its most frequently occurring side-effects that can be observed from the studies. Thus report and analysis of adverse drug reactions (ADRs)/adverse events should be another focus in the outcomes. However, there seemed to be underreported adverse events in some RCTs (Shen and Nahas 2009), especially in trials of TCM, as Chinese herbal medicines were always considered as natural and thus safe products.

It is important to realize that personal experience is not a reliable basis for the exclusion of uncommon reactions to herbal remedies (Ko 1999). On the other hand, ADRs might have some correlation with the efficacy, or sometimes can be a predictive factor for the therapeutic effect in TCM clinical practice (Jiang et al. 2010; Meyer 2000; Phillips et al. 2001). Some researchers focus on the development of the predictive model of the drugs responses in complex diseases in order to find a new way of individualized treatment (Wessels et al. 2007) with the suggestions that it could be sensible for clinicians and researchers to pay more attention to ADRs both for side effect and for prediction of effectiveness.

4.7   Case Study in TCM

An often-voiced criticism of clinical trials is that such clinical experiments often inform us little about progress of individual patients after treatment intervention. In TCM, treatments are often highly individualized. Although the importance of case study has been widely recognized, the quality of the case report in TCM is still unsatisfactory.

As one of the primary methods of knowledge transmission in TCM, the case report played a critical role in the history. It is embedded in Chinese culture with its unique characteristics of focusing on key information for pattern classification without the efficacy evaluation criteria provided, which has resulted in difficulty in acceptance and comprehension by modern medical system.

It is of paramount urgency that in TCM practice the procedure for reporting of case studies should be standardized and established with a common language that can be communicated with modern conventional medicine for comparison of treatment efficacy and evidence-base discussion. To encourage the utilization of case-report as a means of evidence-based approach for assessment of TCM treatment efficacy, further analysis using modern informatics processing technology of well-kept data in TCM treatment of common diseases will contribute to the optimization of TCM treatment strategy and promote the development of individualized treatment with TCM. The quality of case-reporting in TCM can also be improved by taking the strict measure/procedure developed by the National Cancer Institute (Mesch et al. 2006) in the USA, whose current key role is committed to funding innovative treatment in cancer research by providing funding via the NCI's Office of Cancer Complementary and Alternative Medicine (OCCAM) coordinates the institute's research programs of complementary and alternative medicine (Campbell and Whitehead 1977). Such approach can be utilized to provide evidence-base validation for TCM treatment efficacy.

5   Analysis of Formulae for Female Infertility Using TCM Informatics

The efficacy of a TCM medication comes from the complex interactions of herbs or Chinese Materia Medica (CMM) in a formula. A practitioner has a repertoire of these standard formulae but they only serve as templates to be personalized for different patients. Although the records of prescription are available, to determine the true interacting herbs that contribute to the effectiveness of a treatment is still a challenging and time-consuming task. We present an approach called Interaction Rules Mining, which can find effective herbs combination with evidence. The analysis of the treatment records of female patients with infertility problem (Ainy et al. 2007) is used as illustration.

Before we get into the details of IRM, we need to introduce the *Synergy Index* (Rothman 1976) as it is important concept in our approach. In the field of epidemiology, he formalized interaction by defining the terms synergy and antagonism. This ratio was statistically approximated from the measured combined risk to the predicted combined risk. The Synergy Index compared the combined effect of two factors to that of the parts. If the combined effect of two factors is greater than that of the two factors acting independently, then this is defined as synergy, and it is antagonism when the value is sub-additive. These definitions provided the starting point for the generation of non-parametric interaction rules based on statistical significance rather than setting arbitrary thresholds as used in association rule mining.

Another important concept in our approach is complementarities which was first introduced by (Edgeworth 1881). Activities are considered complement if doing (more of) any one of them increases the returns to doing (more of) the others. The idea was later formalized (Topkis 1998) using the mathematical theory of lattices. This has become a monotone optimization problem and can be represented by the "supermodularity" of a function with respect to two or more complementary variables. Supermodularity dictates that the sum of the increases in the value of a function when the levels of the complements are changed one at a time would be less than the increase in the function's value when the levels are changed simultaneously. If complementarities among activities exist, then the gains from increasing every component are larger than the sum of the individual increases. In a more general way, a function of $f: R^k \rightarrow R$ is said to be supermodular if

$$f(x \wedge y) + f(x \vee y) \geq f(x) + f(y) \tag{1}$$

$\forall x,y \in R^k$, where $(x \vee y)$ denotes the component-wise maximum and $(x \wedge y)$ denotes the component-wise minimum of x and y (Topkis 1998). In other words, the heuristic is to measure the marginal gain over the baseline and the separate effect due to each individual variable. Suppose there are two herbs P_1 and P_2. Each herb can be used in a prescription $(P_1 = 1)$ or not $(P_1 = 0)$ and $(P_2 = 1)$ or not $(P_2 = 0)$. The function $f(P_1, P_2)$ is supermodular and P_1 and P_2 are complements only if: $f(1,1) - f(0,1) \geq f(1,0) - f(0,0)$, i.e. using an additional herb while already using the other has a higher incremental effect on outcome f than when using the herbs are used in isolation. For linear functions, this can clearly be mapped directly to the concepts of synergy and antagonism. The three concepts of epidemiological interactions, complementarities, and supermodularity are thus related, despite their different roots. Thus, the concept of complementarities can offer a useful perspective to study the complex interactions of herbs in TCM prescriptions.

5.1 Interaction Contrast (IC)

In our approach, we implement supermodularity with the measure of risk ratio based on (Poon et al. 2011). This measure has been well accepted in the domain of public health and epidemiology. We used and extended the concept of *interaction contrast* (IC) to measure two things concurrently, namely, the strength of an interaction and the reliability of that measurement by using a statistical validation. This approach simplifies the measure of interactions between probabilities of the main factors. Synergy for a 2-factor scenario is defined as positive values of IC as below

$$IC = (R_{11} - R_{01}) - (R_{10} - R_{00}) \qquad (2)$$

where R_{ij} is denotes the ratio of risk (or effect) among those in combined exposure category i, j to the risk (or effect) among those unexposed to both exposures. Synergism is defined as the increase in probability between the expected outcome and the measured outcome for a given combination of herbs. Discovered interaction rules are thus limited by statistical criteria to ensure the reliability of the generated rules. In this paper, we rely on an extension to this basic model. Interactions are represented by an increase or decrease in the probability of the 'good' outcome and the full effects of individual components are included in the model. This approach allows for a more detailed analysis of higher order interactions.

The efficacy of each combination of herbs is measured by contrasting the probability of a desirable outcome with the expected outcome due to the parts. To do this we first measure the effect of each sub-combination of the components. From this, we can construct the expected combined outcome if no interaction is present. Any interaction effect will thus be the difference between our estimated effect and the actual.

5.2   IRM Algorithm

The goal of this IRM algorithm is to systematically generate all possible herbal combinations from the clinical records; all these combinations are statistically synergistic in accordance to the previously described interaction measurement. It is computationally prohibitive to analyze every possible combination for interaction effects. Our algorithm was designed to test for the potentially significant combinations only. It was made possible using the statistical properties to be described in the next two paragraphs.

The first one is the "necessary" condition. This condition requires sufficient evidence (i.e. sufficient sample size N) to be presented in the dataset for calculating the IC described earlier. If there is insufficient data in one or more cells, k-herb interaction and its related higher-order interactions can be pruned due to insufficient evidence. The lower the N is, the lesser is the power, therefore, it is harder to get statistical significance. Extremely low sample size in any cell reduces the power of the analysis so much that the value of R cannot be determined. A valid R is required to test its value. Hence, we make use of this property to prune combinations from the model where we expect there to be too few values for R to be determined. If we do not have enough cases in a cell (strata), we cannot calculate the IC, hence there is no point to continue to calculate the subsequent IC in the sub-strata. As a result, we can discard combinations where statistical significance cannot be determined (e.g. with any N value being less than a statistical acceptable threshold).

The second one is the "sufficient" condition. This condition requires that the sets have sufficient evidence to be statistically tested based on the IC described.

Table 2 Basic statistics
of the infertility dataset

Information	Count
Number of encounters	851
Number of patients	108
Number of herbs	250
Number of good outcome	404
Min number of encounter per patient	1
Max number of encounter per patient	18

We calculate the level of synergism of each identifiable pattern of complex (high-dimensional) herb interaction from the given TCM datasets (i.e. herb combinations that have satisfied the necessary condition) then measure the statistical significance of each.

The rules generated are then analyzed for clinical significance by TCM practitioners. Clinical records of treatment were classified by the *use* or *not use* of each possible herb in a prescription. The outcome of each clinical encounter was then classified as good (1) or bad (0). From this, the probability of a good outcome was determined for each combination of herbs that could potentially have statistical significance.

5.3 Experiments and Results

A dataset of clinical treatment on female with infertility problems was obtained from a TCM hospital in Beijing. The basic statistics of this dataset can be found in Table 2. It contained the 851 encounters of 108 female patients. Two hundred and fifty different herbs were used in this dataset. Three of these herbs were frequently used; they can be found in more than 50 % of the prescriptions. The most frequently used herb was *tusizi* (菟丝子) with a frequency of 645 times, the second one was *danggui* (当归), 586 times and *baishao* (白芍) had 488 times. The highest number of encounter with a patient was 18. The outcome of each encounter was annotated by TCM clinical experts as either effective or ineffective. It was a relatively balanced dataset with 47.5 % of these encountered labeled as effective. This dataset was analyzed using the IRM algorithm. After all the statistically significant interaction rules were discovered, the rules generated were analyzed for clinical significance by TCM practitioners.

Tables 3 and 4 listed the top 10 ranking 2-way and 3-way interactions according to the *synergy-value*, with the interpretation of each of the combination in the rightmost column of the tables. Table 3(a) listed the top 2-way interactions. For the 2-way interactions, there were three pairs not having corresponding clinical interpretation. The others all had clinical values. Pair-1,3,5 were mainly related to *nourishing yin*, while the rest catered for the treatment of problems with spleen and stomach, *regulating qi*, *clearing heat* and *dredging channels*. Although the dataset was about infertility, however, the patients' symptoms were not considered in this analysis, hence, these herb-pairs might be effective to deal with the symptoms reported by the patients; they might not be related to the infertility problem. There were three combinations in Table 4 that were obviously prescribed to address

Table 3 Top 10 2-way interactions

	药1	药2	Synergy-value	Interpretation
1	石斛	生地黄	0.88623	It has practical clinical value: both herbs are useful for nourishing yin
2	石斛	菟丝子	0.88246	No such known combination
3	百合	知母	0.87846	It has practical clinical value: both herbs are useful for nourishing yin for moistening dryness
4	炒白术	紫苏梗	0.85778	They can be useful in treating the spleen and stomach, but it is not common to be used together
5	百合	龟板	0.84792	It has practical clinical value: both herbs are useful for nourishing yin. The former is for nourishing yin but not moist, while the latter herb is for nourishing kidney yin
6	党参	益智仁	0.84091	*Dangshen* is useful for regulating qi. The second herb warms the spleen and kidney, relieving diarrhoea
7	龟板	红藤	0.83893	No such known combination
8	黄芩	竹茹	0.83197	Both herbs are useful for clearing heat
9	徐长卿	金银花藤	0.83060	Both herbs are useful for dredging channels
10	夜交藤	生甘草	0.81836	No special clinical value

Table 4 Top 10 3-way interactions

	药1	药2	药3	Synergy-value	Interpretation
1	砂仁	当归	续断	0.97686	No good explanation
2	黄芩	当归	紫苏梗	0.96920	No good explanation
3	茯苓	砂仁	生甘草	0.95593	Useful for regulating stomach and spleen
★4	砂仁	当归	白芍	0.95355	The first herb is for regulating the qi to prevent miscarriage. The role of the remaining two herbs is to nourish blood. And they are two of the important herbs in the *Sijunzi* decoction
★5	莪术	延胡索	菟丝子	0.94115	The first two herbs are useful for regulating qi and promoting blood circulation. The third herb is useful for tonifying the kidney and liver, preventing miscarriage, improving eyesight and relieving diarrhea
6	麦冬	佛手	女贞子	0.93603	The first two herbs are useful for nourishing yin, while the third one is for regulating stomach
7	太子参	当归	莲子肉	0.93528	
★8	黄芩	砂仁	当归	0.93510	It is common to put these three herbs to help prevent miscarriage
9	太子参	当归	紫苏梗	0.93378	The first herb is to benefit qi. *Danggui* is to nourish blood while *Zisugeng* is to regulate qi and stomach
10	砂仁	炒枳壳	柴胡	0.93147	The combination of these three herbs has clinical value: dispersing and relieving stagnated liver qi, and regulating stomach

issues in a pregnancy, which was to prevent miscarriage. Pair-1 was useful to regulate spleen and stomach. Pair-6 aimed for *nourishing yin*. Pair 9 was useful to *benefit qi* and to regulate stomach. Pair-10 helped *disperse stagnated qi*. There were two combinations that were not easy to explain.

We had mixed response to this preliminary experiment. Firstly, the algorithm was able to find useful herb-combinations that addressed fertility problems but, secondly, other combinations that seemingly unrelated were also highlighted. We should be all aware that TCM treatment is a holistic approach. In many occasions, treatments do not necessary aim to solve the specific disease but other phenomena worth the attention. Hence, we believed this observation was largely due to the fact that many herbs were prescribed to address the symptoms reported by the patients, i.e. the spleen and stomach problem, or the stagnation of qi. We reckoned the results can be improved by first clustering the symptoms and their related herbs, then these herbs are sent to the IRM algorithm for analysis to find the effectiveness of different herbs combination.

6   Concluding Remarks

Over the past decades, increasing numbers of clinical trials on TCM treatment efficacy have emerged and we predict that there will be more RCTs with higher quality in the future to meet the needs of modern research and development, and that the quality of RCTs will be improved with the generalized RCT registration, standardization of clinical research, and the promotion of evidence-based medicine (EBM). The world-wide focus on clinical trials in TCM will continue to increase. However we are in need of modified modalities that can focus on the assessment of TCM diagnosis and treatment outcomes of holistic and individual approach.

Based on accepted and recognised models such as Interaction Rules Mining, informatics analysis of data from TCM diagnosis and treatment principles can contribute to the understanding of how complex mixture of CMM are related to the principles of TCM formulary in treatment of diseases. The success of applying information technology in deciphering TCM principles depends on the synergistic combination of knowledge from the fields of information technology, statistics, and TCM. Combining the strengths of each is essential to improving the quantitative analysis of TCM and broadening our knowledge of the principles that underlie its effectiveness. Continued feedback between the practitioners in each field will help us to refine the analytical techniques used for evaluation.

The way forward to identify evidence-base in TCM practice requires multidisciplinary collaborations among different professionals of both conventional medical and TCM practices with expertise from biomedical, bioinformatics, pharmaceutical and TCM disciplines.

References

C. Acquadro, R. Berzon, D. Dubois, N.K. Leidy, P. Marquis, D. Revicki, M. Rothman, Incorporating the patient's perspective into drug development and communication: an ad hoc task force report of the Patient-Reported Outcomes (PRO) Harmonization Group meeting at the Food and Drug Administration, February 16, 2001. Value Health 6, 522–531 (2003)

E. Ainy, P. Mirmiran, S. Zahedi Asl, F. Azizi, Prevalence of metabolic syndrome during menopausal transition Tehranian women: Tehran Lipid and Glucose Study (TLGS). Maturitas 58, 150–155 (2007)

Z.X. Bian, D. Moher, S. Dagenais, Y.P. Li, L. Liu, T.X. Wu, J.X. Miao, Improving the quality of randomized controlled trials in Chinese herbal medicine, part II: control group design. Zhong xi yi jie he xue bao (J. Chin. Integr. Med.) 4, 130–136 (2006)

S. Campbell, M. Whitehead, Oestrogen therapy and the menopausal syndrome. Clin. Obstet. Gynaecol. 4, 31–47 (1977)

K. Chan, Chinese medicinal materials and their interface with Western medical concepts. J. Ethnopharmacol. 96, 1–18 (2005)

K. Chan, L. Cheung, *Interactions between Chinese Herbal Medicinal Products and Orthodox Drugs*, Taylor & Francis Group, September 11, 2000 by CRC Press ISBN 9789057024139 Ca#TF3184

M. Deng, X.Q. Sui, S.B. Zhu, W. Ma, Y. Xu, Z.M. Chen, Clinical observation on the treatment of atrial fibrillation with amiodarone combined with Shenmai injection (). Chin. J. Integr. Med. 16, 453–456 (2010)

L. Donald, Patient-Reported Outcomes (PROs): an organizing tool for concepts, measures, and applications. Qol Newslett. 31, 1–5 (2003)

F.Y. Edgeworth, *Mathematical Psychics: An Essay on the Application of Mathematics to the Moral Sciences* (C.K. Paul & co., London, 1881)

E. Ernst, Methodological aspects of Traditional Chinese Medicine (TCM). Ann. Acad. Med. Singapore 35, 773–774 (2006)

E. Ernst, M.H. Pittler, Alternative therapy bias. Nature 385, 480 (1997)

A.Y. Fan, L. Lao, R.X. Zhang, A.N. Zhou, B.M. Berman, Preclinical safety evaluation of the aqueous acetone extract of Chinese herbal formula modified Huo Luo Xiao Ling Dan. Zhong Xi Yi Jie He Xue Bao 8, 438–447 (2010)

B. Flaws, *The Treatment of Modern Western Diseases with Chinese Medicine* (Blue Poppy Press, Boulder, 2005)

Q. Geng, B.D. Lu, X.J. Huang, Effect of modified tianxiong powder in treating oligospermia and asthenospermia. Zhongguo Zhong Xi Yi Jie He Za Zhi 30, 496–498 (2010)

Y. Gong, Q. Zha, L. Li, Y. Liu, B. Yang, L. Liu, A. Lu, Y. Lin, M. Jiang, Efficacy and safety of Fufangkushen colon-coated capsule in the treatment of ulcerative colitis compared with mesalazine: a double-blinded and randomized study. J. Ethnopharmacol. 141, 592–598 (2012)

F.L. Guo, C. Han, Q.P. Liu, L.J. Liu, Clinical observation on the effect of Tongbi Heji plus syndrome differentiation treatment for 90 rheumatoid arthritis patients. J. Tradit. Chin. Med. 10, 34–37 (2008)

Y. He, A. Lu, Y. Zha, X. Yan, Y. Song, S. Zeng, W. Liu, W. Zhu, L. Su, X. Feng, X. Qian, C. Lu, Correlations between symptoms as assessed in traditional Chinese medicine (TCM) and ACR20 efficacy response: a comparison study in 396 patients with rheumatoid arthritis treated with TCM or Western medicine. J. Clin. Rheumatol. 13, 317–321 (2007)

S.C. Hsieh, J.N. Lai, P.C. Chen, C.C. Chen, H.J. Chen, J.D. Wang, Is Duhuo Jisheng Tang containing Xixin safe? A four-week safety study. Chin. Med. 5, 6 (2010)

A.R. Jadad, D. Rennie, The randomized controlled trial gets a middle-aged checkup. JAMA 279, 319–320 (1998)

G. Jia, M.B. Meng, Z.W. Huang, X. Qing, W. Lei, X.N. Yang, S.S. Liu, J.C. Diao, S.Y. Hu, B.H. Lin, R.M. Zhang, Treatment of functional constipation with the Yun-chang capsule: a double-blind, randomized, placebo-controlled, dose-escalation trial. J. Gastroenterol. Hepatol. 25, 487–493 (2010)

M. Jiang, J. Zhao, A. Lu, Q. Zha, Y. He, Does gastrointestinal adverse drug reaction influence therapeutic effect in the treatment of rheumatoid arthritis? J. Altern. Complement. Med. **16**, 143–144 (2010)

M. Jiang, C. Lu, G. Chen, C. Xiao, Q. Zha, X. Niu, S. Chen, A. Lu, Understanding the molecular mechanism of interventions in treating rheumatoid arthritis patients with corresponding traditional Chinese medicine patterns based on bioinformatics approach. Evid. Based Complement. Alternat. Med.: eCAM **2012**, 129452 (2012a)

M. Jiang, C. Lu, C. Zhang, J. Yang, Y. Tan, A. Lu, K. Chan, Syndrome differentiation in modern research of traditional Chinese medicine. J. Ethnopharmacol. **140**, 634–642 (2012b)

M. Jiang, C. Zhang, G. Zheng, H. Guo, L. Li, J. Yang, C. Lu, W. Jia, A. Lu, Traditional Chinese medicine Zheng in the era of evidence-based medicine: a literature analysis. Evid. Based Complement. Alternat. Med.: eCAM **2012**, 409568 (2012c)

M. Jun, C. Foote, J. Lv, B. Neal, A. Patel, S.J. Nicholls, D.E. Grobbee, A. Cass, J. Chalmers, V. Perkovic, Effects of fibrates on cardiovascular outcomes: a systematic review and meta-analysis. Lancet **375**, 1875–1884 (2010)

R. Ko, Adverse reactions to watch for in patients using herbal remedies. West. J. Med. **171**, 181–186 (1999)

K.F. Leung, F.B. Liu, L. Zhao, J.Q. Fang, K. Chan, L.Z. Lin, Development and validation of the Chinese quality of life instrument. Health Qual. Life Outcomes **3**, 26 (2005)

X. Li, C. Zhang, Q. Shi, T. Yang, Q. Zhu, Y. Tian, C. Lu, Z. Zhang, Z. Jiang, H. Zhou, X. Wen, H. Yang, X. Ding, L. Liang, Y. Liu, Y. Wang, A. Lu, Improving the efficacy of conventional therapy by adding andrographolide sulfonate in the treatment of severe hand, foot, and mouth disease: a randomized controlled trial. Evid. Based Complement. Alternat. Med.: eCAM **2013**, 316250 (2013)

J.P. Liu, M. Zhang, W.Y. Wang, S. Grimsgaard, Chinese herbal medicines for type 2 diabetes mellitus. Cochrane Database Syst. Rev. **3**, CD003642 (2004)

T. Liu, C. Liu, P.X. Gao, C.P. Yu, Clinical study on method of "tonifying the lung to check the liver" for treatment of chronic cholecystitis. Chin. Acupunct. Moxib. **12**, 29–30 (2005)

D. Liu, H. Lin, X. Wang, W. Zhou, G. Chen, W. Guo, J. Ye, Z. Xu, H. Chen, X.M. Chen, Z. Lai, C. Xiang, Influence of removing blood stasis and tonifying liver and kidney method on quality of life in patients with essential hypertension: randomized controlled observation. Chin. J. Clin. Rehabil. **23**, 9–12 (2006a)

J.P. Liu, M. Yang, Y.X. Liu, M.L. Wei, S. Grimsgaard, Herbal medicines for treatment of irritable bowel syndrome. Cochrane Database Syst. Rev. **25**(1), CD004116 (2006b)

A.P. Lu, K.J. Chen, Integrative medicine in clinical practice: from pattern differentiation in traditional Chinese medicine to disease treatment. Chin. J. Integr. Med. **15**, 152 (2009)

A.P. Lu, H.W. Jia, C. Xiao, Q.P. Lu, Theory of traditional Chinese medicine and therapeutic method of diseases. World J. Gastroenterol. **10**, 1854–1856 (2004)

A.P. Lu, S.S. Zhang, Q.L. Zha, D.H. Ju, H. Wu, H.W. Jia, C. Xiao, S. Li, H. Jian, Correlation between CD4, CD8 cell infiltration in gastric mucosa, Helicobacter pylori infection and symptoms in patients with chronic gastritis. World J. Gastroenterol. **11**, 2486–2490 (2005)

A.P. Lu, X.R. Ding, K.J. Chen, Current situation and progress in integrative medicine in China. Chin. J. Integr. Med. **14**, 234–240 (2008)

C. Lu, X. Niu, C. Xiao, G. Chen, Q. Zha, H. Guo, M. Jiang, A. Lu, Network-based gene expression biomarkers for cold and heat patterns of rheumatoid arthritis in traditional Chinese medicine. Evid. Based Complement. Alternat. Med.: eCAM **2012**, 203043 (2012a)

C. Lu, C. Xiao, G. Chen, M. Jiang, Q. Zha, X. Yan, W. Kong, A. Lu, Cold and heat pattern of rheumatoid arthritis in traditional Chinese medicine: distinct molecular signatures indentified by microarray expression profiles in CD4-positive T cell. Rheumatol. Int. **32**, 61–68 (2012b)

K.S. Poon, J. Poon, M. McGrane, X. Zhou, P. Kwan, R. Zhang, B. Liu, J. Gao, C. Loy, K. Chan, D. and Sze, A Novel Approach in Discovering Significant Interactions from TCM Patient Prescription Data, International Journal of Data Mining and Bioinformatics, **5**(4), 353–367 (2011)

V.R. Mesch, L.E. Boero, N.O. Siseles, M. Royer, M. Prada, F. Sayegh, L. Schreier, H.J. Benencia, G.A. Berg, Metabolic syndrome throughout the menopausal transition: influence of age and menopausal status. Climacteric **9**, 40–48 (2006)

U.A. Meyer, Pharmacogenetics and adverse drug reactions. Lancet **356**, 1667–1671 (2000)

G. Nestler, Traditional Chinese medicine. Med. Clin. North Am. **86**, 63–73 (2002)

K.A. Phillips, D.L. Veenstra, E. Oren, J.K. Lee, W. Sadee, Potential role of pharmacogenomics in reducing adverse drug reactions: a systematic review. JAMA **286**, 2270–2279 (2001)

X.Y. Qin, X.X. Li, S. Suteanu, Comparative study on Chinese medicine and western medicine for treatment of prolapse of lumbar intervertebral disc. Chin. Acupunct. Moxib. **5**, 53–56 (2007)

H. Qing, S.F. Wang, J.M. Fan, I.L.H. Zha, J.Y. Mao, L.J. Sun, R.L. Zhang, Multi-center clinical study of Rhadiola extract injection on the treatment of stable angina pectoris of coronary heart disease with cardiac blood stasis syndrome. Chin. Tradit. Pat. Med. **3**, 20–33 (2009)

K. Rothman, The estimation of synergy or antagonism. Am. J. Epidemiol. **103**, 506–511 (1976)

K.F. Schulz, I. Chalmers, R.J. Hayes, D.G. Altman, Empirical evidence of bias. Dimensions of methodological quality associated with estimates of treatment effects in controlled trials. JAMA **273**, 408–412 (1995)

Y.H. Shen, R. Nahas, Complementary and alternative medicine for treatment of irritable bowel syndrome. Can. Fam. Physician Medecin de famille canadien **55**, 143–148 (2009)

C. Stevinson, M.H. Pittler, E. Ernst, Garlic for treating hypercholesterolemia. A meta-analysis of randomized clinical trials. Ann. Intern. Med. **133**, 420–429 (2000)

S.C. Sze, K.L. Wong, W.K. Liu, T.B. Ng, J.H. Wong, H.P. Cheung, C.M. Yow, E.S. Chu, Q. Liu, Y.M. Hu, K.W. Tsang, W.S. Lee, Y. Tong, Regulation of p21, MMP-1, and MDR-1 expression in human colon carcinoma HT29 by Tian Xian Liquid, a Chinese medicine formula. In vitro and in vivo. Integr. Cancer Ther. **10**, 58–69 (2011)

J.L. Tang, S.Y. Zhan, E. Ernst, Review of randomised controlled trials of traditional Chinese medicine. BMJ (Clinical research ed) **319**, 160–161 (1999)

X.L. Tong, Q. Ni, F.M. Lian, J.Q. Hu, F.H. Yu, Y. Ou, Q. Xue, Z. Jiang, S.T. Wu, H. Jiang, T.S. Gao, (2009)

D. Topkis, *Supermodularity and Complementarity* (Princeton University Press, Princeton, 1998)

M.R. Trusheim, E.R. Berndt, F.L. Douglas, Stratified medicine: strategic and economic implications of combining drugs and clinical biomarkers. Nat. Rev. Drug Discov. **6**, 287–293 (2007)

J.P. Vader, Randomised controlled trials: a user's guide. BMJ (Clinical research ed) **317**, 1258 (1998)

H. van Wietmarschen, K. Yuan, C. Lu, P. Gao, J. Wang, C. Xiao, X. Yan, M. Wang, J. Schroen, A. Lu, G. Xu, J. van der Greef, Systems biology guided by Chinese medicine reveals new markers for sub-typing rheumatoid arthritis patients. J. Clin. Rheumatol. **15**, 330–337 (2009)

N. Vipond, Intervertebral disc replacement (2007), http://www.acc.co.nz/PRD_EXT_CSMP/groups/external_communications/documents/reports_results/prd_ctrb091239.pdf. Accessed 28 Sep 2010

J.A. Walters, E.H. Walters, R. Wood-Baker, Oral corticosteroids for stable chronic obstructive pulmonary disease. Cochrane Database Syst. Rev., CD005374 (2005)

H. Wang, H.C. Shang, J.H. Zhang, J. Chen, B.Z. Sun, D.D. Shang, Y.Z. Xiang, H.B. Cao, M. Ren, L.P. Cuo, B.L. Zhang, Niuhuang Jiangya preparation for treatment of essential hypertension: a systematic review. Liaoning J. Tradit. Chin. Med. **35**, 649–652 (2008) [in Chinese]

S.Z. Wang, H.L. Lin, H.M. Song, W.H. Zhong, T.X. Wu, G.J. Liu, S.Q. Chen, Conservative in the treatment of protrusion of cervical vertebra intervertebral disc: a systematic review. Chin. J. Evid. Based Med. **9**, 331–336 (2009) [in Chinese]

L. Wang, R.M. Zhang, G.Y. Liu, B.L. Wei, Y. Wang, H.Y. Cai, F.S. Li, Y.L. Xu, S.P. Zheng, G. Wang, Chinese herbs in treatment of influenza: a randomized, double-blind, placebo-controlled trial. Respir. Med. **104**, 1362–1369 (2010)

C. Wang, B. Cao, Q.Q. Liu, Z.Q. Zou, Z.A. Liang, L. Gu, J.P. Dong, L.R. Liang, X.W. Li, K. Hu, X.S. He, Y.H. Sun, Y. An, T. Yang, Z.X. Cao, Y.M. Guo, X.M. Wen, Y.G. Wang, Y.L. Liu, L.D. Jiang, Oseltamivir compared with the Chinese traditional therapy maxingshigan-yinqiaosan in the treatment of H1N1 influenza: a randomized trial. Ann. Intern. Med. **155**, 217–225 (2011)

Y.G. Wang, M. Jiang, R.B. Wang, Q.L. Zha, S.J. Zhang, G.Q. Zhou, X.W. Li, Y.Y. Wang, A.P. Lv, Duration of viral shedding of influenza A (H1N1) virus infection treated with oseltamivir and/ or traditional Chinese medicine in China: a retrospective analysis. J. Tradit. Chin. Med. (Chung i tsa chih ying wen pan)//sponsored by All-China Association of Traditional Chinese Medicine, Academy of Traditional Chinese Medicine **32**, 148–155 (2012)

L.S. Wei Jinqi, H. Weining, Compared with Tagamet in treating chronic gastric ulcer. Chin. J. Integr. Tradit. West. Med. **S1**, 29–30 (1994)

J.A. Wessels, S.M. van der Kooij, S. le Cessie, W. Kievit, P. Barerra, C.F. Allaart, T.W. Huizinga, H.J. Guchelaar, A clinical pharmacogenetic model to predict the efficacy of methotrexate monotherapy in recent-onset rheumatoid arthritis. Arthritis Rheum. **56**, 1765–1775 (2007)

B. Wu, M. Liu, S. Zhang, Dan Shen agents for acute ischaemic stroke. Cochrane Database Syst. Rev. **18**(2), CD004295 (2007)

T. Wu, Y. Li, Z. Bian, G. Liu, D. Moher, Randomized trials published in some Chinese journals: how many are randomized? Trials **10**, 46 (2009)

J.X. Xie, H.T. Hu, D.N. Xiao, H.Z. Xie, C.B. Zhu, W.T. Yang, X.X. Huang, X.J. He, G.R. Liang, Z.G. Wang, Safety and efficacy of Qianlian Suppository for chronic prostatitis of damp-heat and blood-stasis syndrome: a randomized, single-blind, parallel controlled, multi-centered phase III clinical trial. Zhonghua Nan Ke Xue **15**, 1049–1052 (2009)

D.Y. Xu, J. Shu, Q.Y. Huang, L. Liu, S.P. Zhao, A comparative study of the efficacy and safety Zhibitai and atorvastatin. Zhonghua Nei Ke Za Zhi **49**, 392–395 (2010a)

D.Y. Xu, J. Shu, Q.Y. Huang, B. Wasti, C. Chen, L. Liu, S.P. Zhao, Evaluation of the lipid lowering ability, anti-inflammatory effects and clinical safety of intensive therapy with Zhibitai, a Chinese traditional medicine. Atherosclerosis **211**, 237–241 (2010b)

Y.H. Xu, J.H. Wang, F.X. Yang, X.Z. He, 8. The effects of respiratory rehabilitation training on pulmonary function and quality of life of patients with COPD. Chin. J. Rehabil. **2**, 42–44 (2010c)

H. Yang, J. Yang, Z. Wen, Q. Zha, G. Nie, X. Huang, C. Zhang, A. Lu, M. Jiang, X. Wang, Effect of combining therapy with traditional Chinese medicine-based psychotherapy and herbal medi-cines in women with menopausal syndrome: a randomized controlled clinical trial. Evid. Based Complement. Alternat. Med.: eCAM **2012**, 354145 (2012)

H.G. Yi, G.Z. Huang, G.J. Liu, Efficacy and safety of Levoamlodipine Besylate for essential hypertension: a systematic review. Chin. J. Evid. Based Med. **8**, 543–550 (2008) [in Chinese]

Z. Yu, G. Wang, G.Y. Chen, J. Chang, Y. Zhang, R.M. Zhang, Muo-luo-dan. Concentrated pill in treatment of chronic atrophic gastritis (the stomach-yin of deficiency and stagnated blood of stom-ach meridian): a prospective, randomized, controlled trial. West China Med. J. **2**, 287–289 (2007)

Q. Zha, S. Lin, C. Zhang, C. Chang, H. Xue, C. Lu, M. Jiang, Y. Liu, Z. Xiao, W. Lin, Y. Shang, J. Chen, M. Wen, A. Lu, Xiaoqinglong granules as add-on therapy for asthma: latent class analysis of symp-tom predictors of response. Evid. Based Complement. Alternat. Med.: eCAM **2013**, 759476 (2013)

L. Zhao, K. Chan, Building a bridge for integrating Chinese medicine into conventional health-care: observations drawn from the development of the Chinese quality of life instrument. Am. J. Chin. Med. **33**, 897–902 (2005)

L. Zhao, A.Y. Li, H. Lv, F.Y. Liu, F.H. Qi, Traditional Chinese medicine Ningdong granule: the beneficial effects in Tourette's disorder. J. Int. Med. Res. **38**, 169–175 (2010)

W. Zhou, Y.Q. Zhong, H.M. Yang, H.L. Jiang, J.J. Fu, W.B. Zhang, B. Mao, Traditional Chinese medicine in the treatment of chronic obstructive pulmonary disease in stable stage: a systematic review of randomized controlled trials. Chin. J. Evid. Based Med. **9**, 311–318 (2009) [in Chinese]

C.X. Zhou, X. Cui, X.Q. Li, H.L. Zeng, H.H. Ni, C.S. Huang, J. Wu, J.C. Shi, M.L. Feng, Y.G. Wu, Clinical research on combined herbal medicine and acupuncture in treating poststroke depres-sion. Shanghai J. Tradit. Chin. Med. **5**, 52–54 (2010a)

C.Y. Zhou, J.Y. Tang, D.Y. Fang, Clinical study on active rheumatoid arthritis treated with simiao xiaobi decoction. Zhongguo Zhong xi yi jie he za zhi Zhongguo Zhongxiyi jiehe zazhi (Chinese journal of integrated traditional and Western medicine//Zhongguo Zhong xi yi jie he xue hui, Zhongguo Zhong yi yan jiu yuan zhu ban) 30, 275–279 (2010b)

J. Zhu, X. Wan, Y. Zhu, X. Ma, Y. Zheng, T. Zhang, Evaluation of salidroside in vitro and in vivo genotoxicity. Drug Chem. Toxicol. **33**, 220–226 (2010)

Printed in the United States
By Bookmasters